Recent Advances and Future Challenges in Gastroenterology and Hepatology

Recent Advances and Future Challenges in Gastroenterology and Hepatology

Editors

Ludovico Abenavoli
Marcello Candelli

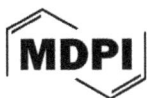

Basel • Beijing • Wuhan • Barcelona • Belgrade • Novi Sad • Cluj • Manchester

Editors

Ludovico Abenavoli
Department of Health
Sciences, Magna Graecia
University
Catanzaro, Italy

Marcello Candelli
Emergency, Anesthesiological
and Reanimation Sciences,
Fondazione Policlinico
Universitario A. Gemelli
IRCCS
Rome Italy

Editorial Office
MDPI
St. Alban-Anlage 66
4052 Basel, Switzerland

This is a reprint of articles from the Special Issue published online in the open access journal *Medicina* (ISSN 1648-9144) (available at: https://www.mdpi.com/journal/medicina/special_issues/13ZWZM293Q).

For citation purposes, cite each article independently as indicated on the article page online and as indicated below:

Lastname, A.A.; Lastname, B.B. Article Title. *Journal Name* **Year**, *Volume Number*, Page Range.

ISBN 978-3-0365-8940-4 (Hbk)
ISBN 978-3-0365-8941-1 (PDF)
doi.org/10.3390/books978-3-0365-8941-1

Cover image courtesy of Ludovico Abenavoli

© 2023 by the authors. Articles in this book are Open Access and distributed under the Creative Commons Attribution (CC BY) license. The book as a whole is distributed by MDPI under the terms and conditions of the Creative Commons Attribution-NonCommercial-NoDerivs (CC BY-NC-ND) license.

Contents

About the Editors ix

Ludovico Abenavoli and Marcello Candelli
Recent Advances and Future Challenges in the Field of Digestive Diseases
Reprinted from: *Medicina* **2023**, *59*, 208, doi:10.3390/medicina59020208 1

Cristina Maria Sabo, Daniel-Corneliu Leucuta, Constantin Simiraș, Ioana Ștefania Deac, Abdulrahman Ismaiel and Dan L. Dumitrascu
Hemogram-Derived Ratios in the Prognosis of Acute Diverticulitis
Reprinted from: *Medicina* **2023**, *59*, 1523, doi:10.3390/medicina59091523 5

Vladimir Milivojević, Jelena Bogdanović, Ivana Babić, Nevena Todorović and Ivan Ranković
Metabolic Associated Fatty Liver Disease (MAFLD) and COVID-19 Infection: An Independent Predictor of Poor Disease Outcome?
Reprinted from: *Medicina* **2023**, *59*, 1438, doi:10.3390/medicina59081438 19

Marcello Candelli, Maria Lumare, Maria Elena Riccioni, Antonio Mestice, Veronica Ojetti, Giulia Pignataro and et al.
Are Short-Stay Units Safe and Effective in the Treatment of Non-Variceal Upper Gastrointestinal Bleeding?
Reprinted from: *Medicina* **2023**, *59*, 1021, doi:10.3390/medicina59061021 35

Bogdan Miuțescu, Deiana Vuletici, Călin Burciu, Adina Turcu-Stiolica, Felix Bende, Iulia Rațiu and et al.
Identification of Microbial Species and Analysis of Antimicrobial Resistance Patterns in Acute Cholangitis Patients with Malignant and Benign Biliary Obstructions: A Comparative Study
Reprinted from: *Medicina* **2023**, *59*, 721, doi:10.3390/medicina59040721 45

Yun Suk Choi, Kyeong Deok Kim, Moon Suk Choi, Yoon Seok Heo, Jin Wook Yi and Yun-Mee Choe
Initial Experience of Robot-Assisted Transabdominal Preperitoneal (TAPP) Inguinal Hernia Repair by a Single Surgeon in South Korea
Reprinted from: *Medicina* **2023**, *59*, 582, doi:10.3390/medicina59030582 59

Sofija I. Lugonja, Ivana L. Pantic, Tamara M. Milovanovic, Vesna M. Grbovic, Bojana M. Djokovic, Željko D. Todorovic and et al.
Atherosclerotic Cardiovascular Disease in Inflammatory Bowel Disease: The Role of Chronic Inflammation and Platelet Aggregation
Reprinted from: *Medicina* **2023**, *59*, 554, doi:10.3390/medicina59030554 73

Zita Zsombor, Aladár D. Rónaszéki, Barbara Csongrády, Róbert Stollmayer, Bettina K. Budai, Anikó Folhoffer and et al.
Evaluation of Artificial Intelligence-Calculated Hepatorenal Index for Diagnosing Mild and Moderate Hepatic Steatosis in Non-Alcoholic Fatty Liver Disease
Reprinted from: *Medicina* **2023**, *59*, 469, doi:10.3390/medicina59030469 87

Yeongsoo Jo, Jai Young Cho, Ho-Seong Han, Yoo-Seok Yoon, Hae Won Lee, Jun Suh Lee and et al.
Development and Validation of a Difficulty Scoring System for Laparoscopic Liver Resection to Treat Hepatolithiasis
Reprinted from: *Medicina* **2022**, *58*, 1847, doi:10.3390/medicina58121847 101

Siti Aisyah Suhaini, Abdullah Harith Azidin, Chooi San Cheah, Wendy Lee Wei Li,
Mohammad Shukri Khoo, Noor Akmal Shareela Ismail and et al.
Kawasaki Disease with Hepatobiliary Manifestations
Reprinted from: *Medicina* 2022, 58, 1833, doi:10.3390/medicina58121833 111

Yun Suk Choi, Boram Cha, Sung Hoon Kim, Jin Wook Yi, Kyeong Deok Kim,
Moon Suk Choi and Yoon Seok Heo
Clinical Characteristics of Symptomatic Cholecystitis in Post-Gastrectomy Patients: 11 Years of
Experience in a Single Center
Reprinted from: *Medicina* 2022, 58, 1451, doi:10.3390/medicina58101451 119

Sorin Tiberiu Alexandrescu, Ioana Mihaela Dinu, Andrei Sebastian Diaconescu,
Alexandru Micu, Evelina Pasare, Cristiana Durdu and et al.
Embryologic Origin of the Primary Tumor and RAS Status Predict Survival after Resection of
Colorectal Liver Metastases
Reprinted from: *Medicina* 2022, 58, 1100, doi:10.3390/medicina58081100 131

Bianca Bartocci, Arianna Dal Buono, Roberto Gabbiadini, Anita Busacca,
Alessandro Quadarella, Alessandro Repici and et al.
Mental Illnesses in Inflammatory Bowel Diseases: *mens sana in corpore sano*
Reprinted from: *Medicina* 2023, 59, 682, doi:10.3390/medicina59040682 149

Ludovico Abenavoli, Giuseppe Guido Maria Scarlata, Emidio Scarpellini, Luigi Boccuto,
Rocco Spagnuolo, Bruno Tilocca and et al.
Metabolic-Dysfunction-Associated Fatty Liver Disease and Gut Microbiota: From Fatty Liver
to Dysmetabolic Syndrome
Reprinted from: *Medicina* 2023, 59, 594, doi:10.3390/medicina59030594 163

Mihai Adrian Eftimie, Gheorghe Potlog and Sorin Tiberiu Alexandrescu
Surgical Options for Peritoneal Surface Metastases from Digestive Malignancies—A
Comprehensive Review
Reprinted from: *Medicina* 2023, 59, 255, doi:10.3390/medicina59020255 177

Bénédicte Caron, Vipul Jairath, Ferdinando D'Amico, Sameer Al Awadhi, Axel Dignass,
Ailsa L. Hart and et al.
International Consensus on Definition of Mild-to-Moderate Ulcerative Colitis Disease Activity
in Adult Patients
Reprinted from: *Medicina* 2023, 59, 183, doi:10.3390/medicina59010183 199

Henry Sutanto and Amie Vidyani
Complex Refractory Esophageal Stricture Due to Chronic Gasoline Ingestion: A Case Report
Reprinted from: *Medicina* 2023, 59, 1020, doi:10.3390/medicina59061020 207

Stefan Lucian Popa, Abdulrahman Ismaiel, Ludovico Abenavoli,
Alexandru Marius Padureanu, Miruna Oana Dita, Roxana Bolchis and et al.
Diagnosis of Liver Fibrosis Using Artificial Intelligence: A Systematic Review
Reprinted from: *Medicina* 2023, 59, 992, doi:10.3390/medicina59050992 221

Gabriela Droc, Cristina Martac, Cristina Georgiana Buzatu, Miruna Jipa, Maria Daniela
Punga and Sebastian Isac
Orthotopic Liver Transplantation of a SARS-CoV-2 Negative Recipient from a Positive Donor:
The Border between Uncertainty and Necessity in a Pandemic Era- Case Report and Overview
of the Literature
Reprinted from: *Medicina* 2023, 59, 836, doi:10.3390/medicina59050836 237

Kei Nomura, Tomoyoshi Shibuya, Masashi Omori, Rina Odakura, Kentaro Ito, Takafumi Maruyama and et al.
Enterolith Treated with a Combination of Double-Balloon Endoscopy and Cola Dissolution Therapy
Reprinted from: *Medicina* **2023**, *59*, 573, doi:10.3390/medicina59030573 . . . . **245**

Jessica Piroddu, Maria Pina Dore, Giovanni Mario Pes, Pier Paolo Meloni and Giuseppe Manzoni
Persistence of Abdominal Pain: Did You Check for Mesenteric Vessels?
Reprinted from: *Medicina* **2023**, *59*, 442, doi:10.3390/medicina59030442 . . . . **251**

About the Editors

Ludovico Abenavoli

Ludovico Abenavoli is an Associate Professor in gastroenterology at the Department of Health Sciences, University "Magna Graecia", Catanzaro (Italy). From 2005 to 2006, he was a Fellow at the Liver Unit, Hôpital Saint Antoine, University Paris VI (France). In 2011, he was appointed as a Visiting Researcher at the Liver Unit, Hôpital "Jean Verdier" University Paris XIII (France). From 2012 to 2014, he was appointed Visiting Professor at the University of Batna (Algeria). In 2015, he was appointed Visiting Professor at the University of Novi Sad (Serbia). In 2016, he was appointed Visiting Professor at the "Iuliu Hațieganu" University of Cluj-Napoca (Romania). In 2017, he was included in the Top Italian Scientist list. In 2018, he was appointed Visiting Professor at the "Taras Shevchenko" National University of Kiev (Ukraine). From 2019, he has been included in the World's Top 2% Scientists ranking by Stanford University (USA). Since 2022, he has been an Erasmus coordinator for the Medical School at the Magna Graecia University of Catanzaro.

His main contributions in the field include: 1) chronic liver disease, 2) liver transplantation, 3) Mediterranean diet, 4) gut microbiota, 5) COVID-19, and 6) inflammatory bowel diseases.

Marcello Candelli

Marcello Candelli is an Adjunct Professor of Emergency Medicine at the Graduate School of Emergency Medicine at the Catholic University of the Sacred Heart of Rome, Faculty of Medicine and Surgery, since 2016, for years of courses I, II, III, IV, V.

He is a Medical Coordinator and is responsible for the UOS management of patients awaiting admission to the Emergency Department of the Fondazione Policlinico Universitario A. Gemelli IRCCS in Rome. He leads several research projects on emergencies and gastrointestinal diseases, in particular, mild head trauma, pulmonary embolism and PS infections.

His main research areas in gastroenterology concern the intestinal microbiota H. pylori., gastrointestinal bleeding, pancreatic diseases, and liver breath tests. He has co-authored more than 170 peer-reviewed articles published in international journals.

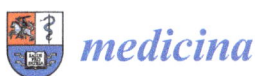

Editorial

Recent Advances and Future Challenges in the Field of Digestive Diseases

Ludovico Abenavoli [1,*] and Marcello Candelli [2]

1. Department of Health Sciences, University "Magna Graecia", Viale Europa—Germaneto, 88100 Catanzaro, Italy
2. Department of Emergency Medicine, Fondazione Policlinico Universitario "A. Gemelli" IRCCS, L. go A. Gemelli 8, 00168 Roma, Italy
* Correspondence: l.abenavoli@unicz.it; Tel.: +39-0961-3694-387

Digestive diseases are a rapidly evolving area of clinical and research. New technologies, novel therapies, and better knowledge of pathogenetic mechanisms are the main drivers of this growth [1]. However, some aspects of gastroenterology and hepatology remain insufficiently investigated and can be considered unmet medical needs that require solutions in the near future [2]. Digestive diseases comprise a multidisciplinary and interdisciplinary area of research, with many clinical aspects focused on specific organs, all of which are investigated multiple unique functional and morphological diagnostic investigations and several auxiliary disciplines, such as biochemistry, pathological anatomy, physiology, cell biology, neuroendocrinology, neuro-gastroenterology, immunology, molecular biology and genetics [3]. Moreover, there has recently been rapid development in the field of endoscopy. Complex invasive procedures are gaining visibility, and the number of potential applications is expanding. The challenge in the near future will be to balance the appropriateness of gastrointestinal endoscopy with clinical indications and the evolution of techniques [4].

The field of digestive diseases has developed considerably in recent decades due to the fruitful research of eminent scholars and researchers, which originally allowed for improvements in our knowledge of physiological and anatomical changes in various aspects of the gastrointestinal tract, some of which remain the subjects of study and development today [5]. For example, it is worth highlighting the progress made in the study of gastric acid secretion and the mechanisms that control it at the cellular level. As a result of this research, new, effective drugs with anti-secretive activity were studied and subsequently commercialized, with a consequent drastic reduction in the use of surgery to treat acid-related diseases of the upper digestive tract [6]. In addition, improved knowledge of digestive tract motility has motivated several studies that have elucidated the central role of the gastrointestinal autonomic nervous system and visceral sensitivity in various functional disorders, from the esophagus to the colon [7].

The role of infectious agents as causes of major gastrointestinal diseases has also been documented, particularly the role of Helicobacter pylori infection as the most important pathogenic factor associated with the occurrence and development of peptic ulcers. In 2005, the Nobel Prize in Physiology or Medicine was awarded to Barry Marshall and Robin Warren, which is one of the rare examples of this prestigious prize being given to clinical scholars in the field of medicine [8]. These extraordinary discoveries have led to the development of innovative and effective new therapies, such as the initial development of H2 antagonists and the later development of proton pump inhibitors and their combination with antibiotics, which have made it possible to successfully—and often definitively—treat many patients with gastrointestinal diseases [9].

The disease spectrum of non-alcoholic fatty liver disease encompasses a wide range of patients and represents a public health burden of epidemic proportions [10]. Findings from

Citation: Abenavoli, L.; Candelli, M. Recent Advances and Future Challenges in the Field of Digestive Diseases. *Medicina* **2023**, *59*, 208. https://doi.org/10.3390/medicina59020208

Received: 7 January 2023
Revised: 18 January 2023
Accepted: 19 January 2023
Published: 20 January 2023

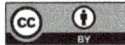

Copyright: © 2023 by the authors. Licensee MDPI, Basel, Switzerland. This article is an open access article distributed under the terms and conditions of the Creative Commons Attribution (CC BY) license (https:// creativecommons.org/licenses/by/ 4.0/).

nutrigenetics and nutrigenomics suggest the capability of nutrition to influence the clinical outcome of these patients [11]. Emerging pharmacologic strategies for the treatment of hepatic steatosis will be multi-pronged and target metabolic pathways including insulin sensitivity, oxidative stress, and fatty acid synthesis [12]. This is a burgeoning and hopeful field of study. The perspectives are bright for clinicians and researchers engaged in the study and treatment of non-alcoholic fatty liver disease.

In recent decades, the diagnosis of digestive diseases has also benefited from endoscopy and its technological advancements, which have allowed gastroenterologists to make a significant leap in the quality of diagnosis. These new technologies have strengthened the role of the clinical gastroenterologist and helped to characterize gastroenterology in every aspect as a medical specialty in its own right [13].

In addition, the recent integration of artificial intelligence into gastroenterology and hepatology will transform the field of digestive diseases in the coming years [14]. The aim is to reduce the time spent on documentation and maximize the time spent with the patient, which remains the ultimate goal of any medical practice. Present and future gastroenterologists will face new challenges in the way that health care is delivered, driven by economic and demographic changes, social trends, technological innovations, and scientific advancements.

At the end of this analysis, we can say that digestive diseases comprise a living discipline capable of impressive future developments. We strongly believe that further innovations will help specialists to apply more personalized treatments tailored to specific diagnostic procedures and therapies. We believe that, in line with recent technological advancements, including artificial intelligence and new endoscopic technologies, gastroenterologists will provide patients with new tools to improve the appropriateness and quality of treatments. In this context, we strongly believe that as gastroenterologists, we will enhance and strengthen partnerships with many other specialties, such as nutrition, diabetology, surgery, and internal medicine, to provide integrated, multidisciplinary care. Finally, myriad areas of basic and applied research can bring great satisfaction to young physicians approaching this specialty, which remains one of the most coveted in the Western world.

Author Contributions: L.A. and M.C. wrote and revised the manuscript. All authors have read and agreed to the published version of the manuscript.

Conflicts of Interest: The authors declare no conflict of interest.

References

1. Losurdo, G.; Gravina, A.G.; Maronim, L.; Gabrieletto, E.M.; Ianiro, G.; Ferrarese, A.; Young Investigator Group of SIGE the Italian Society of Gastroenterology. Future challenges in gastroenterology and hepatology, between innovations and unmet needs: A SIGE Young Editorial Board's perspective. *Dig. Liver Dis.* **2022**, *54*, 583–597. [CrossRef] [PubMed]
2. Li, J.; Li, C.; Wang, X.; Wang, Y.; Zhou, Y. Considerations and perspectives on digestive diseases during the COVID-19 pandemic: A narrative review. *Ann. Palliat. Med.* **2021**, *10*, 4858–4867. [CrossRef] [PubMed]
3. Bray, N.A.; Koloski, N.A.; Jones, M.P.; Do, A.; Pang, S.; Coombes, J.S.; McAllister, S.; Campos, J.; Arthur, L.; Stanley, P.; et al. Evaluation of a Multidisciplinary Integrated Treatment Approach Versus Standard Model of Care for Functional Gastrointestinal Disorders (FGIDS): A Matched Cohort Study. *Dig. Dis. Sci.* **2022**, *67*, 5593–5601. [CrossRef] [PubMed]
4. Karstensen, J.G.; Vilmann, P. Historical perspective on needle development: From the past to the future. *Best Pract. Res. Clin. Gastroenterol.* **2022**, *60–61*, 101814. [CrossRef] [PubMed]
5. Yamamoto, Y.; Kanayama, N.; Nakayama, Y.; Matsushima, N. Current Status, Issues and Future Prospects of Personalized Medicine for Each Disease. *J. Pers. Med.* **2022**, *12*, 444. [CrossRef] [PubMed]
6. Liang, B.; Yuan, Y.; Peng, X.J.; Liu, X.L.; Hu, X.K.; Xing, D.M. Current and future perspectives for Helicobacter pylori treatment and management: From antibiotics to probiotics. *Front. Cell Infect. Microbiol.* **2022**, *12*, 1042070. [CrossRef] [PubMed]
7. Bassotti, G.; Antonelli, E.; Villanacci, V.; Nascimbeni, R.; Dore, M.P.; Pes, G.M.; Maconi, G. Abnormal gut motility in inflammatory bowel disease: An update. *Tech. Coloproctol.* **2020**, *24*, 275–282. [CrossRef] [PubMed]
8. Goodwin, C.S.; Marshall, B.J.; Blackbourn, S.J.; Warren, J.R.; Phillips, M. Colloidal bismuth subcitrate (DE-NOL) and tinidazole healed duodenal ulceration with a low relapse rate due to elimination of Campylobacter pylori. *J. Chemother.* **1989**, *1*, 838–839. [PubMed]
9. Bell, N.J.; Hunt, R.H. Progress with proton pump inhibition. *Yale J. Biol. Med.* **1992**, *65*, 649–657. [PubMed]

10. Riazi, K.; Azhari, H.; Charette, J.H.; Underwood, F.E.; King, J.A.; Afshar, E.E.; Swain, M.G.; Congly, S.E.; Kaplan, G.G.; Shaheen, A.A. The prevalence and incidence of NAFLD worldwide: A systematic review and meta-analysis. *Lancet Gastroenterol. Hepatol.* **2022**, *7*, 851–861. [CrossRef] [PubMed]
11. Dallio, M.; Romeo, M.; Gravina, A.G.; Masarone, M.; Larussa, T.; Abenavoli, L.; Persico, M.; Loguercio, C.; Federico, A. Nutrigenomics and Nutrigenetics in Metabolic-(Dysfunction) Associated Fatty Liver Disease: Novel Insights and Future Perspectives. *Nutrients* **2021**, *13*, 1679. [CrossRef] [PubMed]
12. Filipovic, B.; Lukic, S.; Mijac, D.; Marjanovic-Haljilji, M.; Vojnovic, M.; Bogdanovic, J.; Glisic, T.; Filipovic, N.; Al Kiswani, J.; Djokovic, A.; et al. The New Therapeutic Approaches in the Treatment of Non-Alcoholic Fatty Liver Disease. *Int. J. Mol. Sci.* **2021**, *22*, 13219. [CrossRef] [PubMed]
13. Gulati, S.; Patel, M.; Emmanuel, A.; Haji, A.; Hayee, B.; Neumann, H. The future of endoscopy: Advances in endoscopic image innovations. *Dig. Endosc.* **2020**, *32*, 512–552. [CrossRef] [PubMed]
14. Cao, J.S.; Lu, Z.Y.; Chen, M.Y.; Zhang, B.; Juengpanich, S.; Hu, J.H.; Li, S.J.; Topatana, W.; Zhou, X.Y.; Feng, X.; et al. Artificial intelligence in gastroenterology and hepatology: Status and challenges. *World J. Gastroenterol.* **2021**, *27*, 1664–1690. [CrossRef] [PubMed]

Disclaimer/Publisher's Note: The statements, opinions and data contained in all publications are solely those of the individual author(s) and contributor(s) and not of MDPI and/or the editor(s). MDPI and/or the editor(s) disclaim responsibility for any injury to people or property resulting from any ideas, methods, instructions or products referred to in the content.

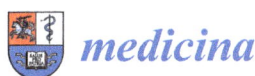

Article

Hemogram-Derived Ratios in the Prognosis of Acute Diverticulitis

Cristina Maria Sabo [1], Daniel-Corneliu Leucuta [2,*], Constantin Simiraș [3], Ioana Ștefania Deac [3], Abdulrahman Ismaiel [1] and Dan L. Dumitrascu [1]

[1] 2nd Department of Internal Medicine, "Iuliu Hatieganu" University of Medicine and Pharmacy, 400006 Cluj-Napoca, Romania; cristina.marica90@yahoo.com (C.M.S.); abdulrahman.ismaiel@yahoo.com (A.I.); ddumitrascu@umfcluj.ro (D.L.D.)

[2] Department of Medical Informatics and Biostatistics, "Iuliu Hatieganu" University of Medicine and Pharmacy, 400349 Cluj-Napoca, Romania

[3] Regional Institute of Gastroenterology and Hepatology, 400162 Cluj-Napoca, Romania; c_simiras@yahoo.com (C.S.); stefaniadeac24@gmail.com (I.Ș.D.)

* Correspondence: dleucuta@umfcluj.ro

Abstract: *Background and Objectives*: It is crucial to quickly identify those patients who need immediate treatment in order to avoid the various complications related to acute diverticulitis (AD). Although several studies evaluated the neutrophil-to-lymphocyte ratio (NLR) suggesting its predictive value in assessing the severity of AD, results have been inconclusive. Therefore, we aimed to assess the relationship between the neutrophil-to-lymphocyte ratio (NLR), the platelet-to-lymphocyte ratio (PLR), the monocyte-to-lymphocyte ratio (MLR), and systemic immune inflammation (SII) with the severity of AD, the ability to predict the presence or absence of complications, and the recurrence rate, based on the values of inflammatory markers. *Materials and Methods*: We retrospectively reviewed 147 patients diagnosed with AD between January 2012 to February 2023. Patients were divided into 2 groups, uncomplicated and complicated AD. The characteristics and full blood count between both groups were compared. *Results:* A total of 65 (44.22%) patients were classified as having complicated AD. The area under the ROC curve (AUROC) defining a Hinchey score $\geq$ 1b was as follows: SII, 0.812 (95% confidence interval (CI), 0.73 –0.888); NLR, 0.773 (95% CI, 0.676–0.857); PLR, 0.725 (95% CI, 0.63–0.813); MLR: 0.665 (95% CI, 0.542 –0.777). An SII cutoff value of > 1200 marked the highest yield for diagnosing complicated AD, with a sensitivity of 82% and a specificity of 76%. The cumulative recurrence rate was not significantly different in the groups of SII $\geq$ median vs. SII < median (p = 0.35), NLR $\geq$ median vs. NLR < median (p = 0.347), PLR $\geq$ median vs. PLR < median (p = 0.597), and MLR $\geq$ median vs. MLR < median (p = 0.651). *Conclusions*: Our study indicates that SII, NLR, and PLR are statistically significant and clinically useful classifying ratios to predict higher Hinchey scores. However, they cannot predict recurrences.

Keywords: acute diverticulitis; Hinchey score; inflammatory markers; hemogram-derived ratios

1. Introduction

Acute diverticulitis (AD) is defined as an inflammation of the diverticula and can be either uncomplicated or complicated. Around 5% of patients with diverticulosis will experience at least one episode of diverticulitis during their lifetime [1]. Most cases of AD (75%) are uncomplicated and are characterized by the presence of limited inflammation to the wall of the colon, with or without an inflammatory phlegmon confined to the colonic wall [2]. It is a relatively mild disease and one that can be safely treated in primary care [3]. Only 12% of patients with acute diverticulitis will present with complications. Among the complications, the most frequent is the presence of an abscess, followed by peritonitis, obstruction, and fistula [4]. Higher mortality rates were found among patients with complicated AD [4].

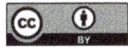

Numerous factors have been linked to a higher probability for developing AD. These factors include age [4], sex [4], genetics [5–8], adherence to a Western dietary pattern (characterized by the high consumption of red meat, high-fat dairy, and refined grains) [9], smoking [10], obesity [11–13], and the use of certain medications (such as nonsteroidal anti-inflammatory drugs [NSAIDs], opiate analgesics, and corticosteroids) [14].

The triad of symptoms consisting of left-sided lower abdomen discomfort, lack of vomiting, and a C-reactive protein (CRP) levels greater than 5 mg/dl, shows a high sensitivity for detecting AD (acute diverticulitis). However, this triad does not allow differentiating between uncomplicated and complicated diverticulitis [5]. The World Society of Emergency Surgery (WSES) recommends a comprehensive evaluation of patients, including clinical history, physical signs, laboratory inflammation markers, and radiological findings. The first choice of imaging technique is a contrast-enhanced computed tomography (CT) scan of the abdomen, or a step-up approach with CT being performed after an inconclusive or negative ultrasound (US) in patients suspected of having AD [6]. Unfortunately, this approach may lead to a significant number of patients with uncomplicated diverticulitis being referred to the emergency department, resulting in unnecessary CT scans.

Circulating cells, such as lymphocytes, monocytes, neutrophils, and platelets are essential components of the inflammatory process. Their ratios, comprising the neutrophil-to-lymphocyte ratio (NLR), platelet-to-lymphocyte ratio (PLR), monocyte-to-lymphocyte ratio (MLR), and systemic immune inflammation (SII), are simple and easily accessible inflammatory markers that have been studied as potential prognostic indicators in various medical conditions. Previous studies have found that high NLR and PLR values have been linked with complicated diverticulitis [7,8], surgical intervention [9], the failure of conservative treatment for acute first-attack colonic diverticulitis [10], shorter intervals between recurrent episodes, and longer cumulative hospitalization days [11]. The monocyte-to-lymphocyte ratio (MLR) and systemic immune inflammation (SII) have been studied as potential prognostic markers in coronavirus disease, cardiovascular diseases, sepsis, and cancer. Moreover, one study assessed their correlation with the failure of conservative management [12].

The development of a diagnostic and prognostic tool to identify complicated AD and assess the risk of complications in patients with uncomplicated AD can indeed be beneficial in reducing healthcare costs, unnecessary referrals, and the excessive use of CT scans.

Therefore, the objective of this study was to evaluate the predictive value of NLR, PLR, MLR, and SII regarding to the severity of AD, their ability to predict the presence or absence of complications, and the recurrence rate based on inflammatory marker values.

2. Materials and Methods

2.1. Study Desing, Setting, and Participants

We conducted a retrospective observational study involving subjects ≥18 years old. All patients who were admitted with acute diverticulitis (AD) at the Clinical Emergency County Hospital of Cluj-Napoca, Romania between January 2012 to February 2023 were identified, and their data were collected retrospectively using electronic medical records. The patients were searched for in the hospital database, using the ICD (International Classification of Disease) code K57 (diverticular disease of the intestine). All included patients in our study were diagnosed with AD using either a CT scan, colonoscopy, or medical/surgical report. Patients were excluded from the study based on the following criteria: (1) any malignancy, (2) a lack of confirmation of AD, and (3) a lack of laboratory parameters (leukocyte, neutrophils, lymphocytes, platelets, or monocytes) at admission.

The study was conducted according to the principles of the Declaration of Helsinki and was approved by the Ethical Committee of "Iuliu Hațieganu" University of Medicine and Pharmacy Cluj-Napoca (approval no. 139/27.06.2023).

The research has been conducted following the Strengthening the Reporting of Observational Studies in Epidemiology (STROBE) guidelines [15]. The comprehensive STROBE checklist can be found in Table S1.

2.2. Variables of Interest

The primary outcomes were to evaluate the NLR, PLR, MLR, and SII levels in patients with complicated AD and to investigate the diagnostic and prognostic accuracy of these markers.

2.3. Data Sources and Measurements

We collected the following information from patient medical records: age, sex, body mass index (BMI), clinical symptoms at admission (abdominal pain, nausea, vomiting, constipation, diarrhea, and fever), laboratory parameters, diagnosis method (CT, colonoscopy, or surgical/medical reports), length of hospital stay, recurrence rate, the time interval from the first to a recurrent episode, cumulative length of stay due to AD, and initial treatment strategy (such as careful observation, antibiotic treatment, abscess drainage or surgery, and type of intervention). Reviewing of the records was performed by three investigators (C.M.S., I.D., and S.C.).

The diagnosis of AD was based on the presence of inflammation in one or more diverticula based on CT scans, surgical reports, or colonoscopy. AD can be either uncomplicated or complicated. The classification used to define AD severity was the modified Hinchey classification based on CT findings [1]. The modified Hinchey score was as follows: stage 0—mild clinical diverticulitis; stage 1A—confined pericolic inflammation or phlegmon; stage 1B—confined pericolic abscess; stage 2—pelvic, intraabdominal, or retroperitoneal abscess; stage 3—generalized purulent peritonitis; and stage 4—fecal peritonitis [1].

Laboratory parameters included leukocytes, neutrophils (N), lymphocytes (Ly), monocytes (M), platelets (P), red cell distribution width (RDW), platelet distribution width (PDW), urea, and creatinine. NLR (the neutrophil-to-lymphocyte ratio) and PLR (the platelet-to-lymphocyte ratio) were defined as neutrophil or platelet counts divided by the total number of lymphocytes. MLR (the monocyte to lymphocyte ratio) was defined as the absolute monocyte count, divided by the absolute lymphocyte count. The systemic immune-inflammatory index (SII) was calculated using the formula $SII = (P \times N)/L$.

The number of cases with AD diagnosis in our hospital during the study period determined the sample size. We grouped the patients into two categories of uncomplicated (0, IA) vs. complicated diverticulitis (1B–4). Moreover, for a more detailed analysis, the patients were further divided into three groups according to the modified Hinchey grade. Patients with a modified Hinchey score of 0 or IA were considered the uncomplicated AD group, while patients with a modified Hinchey score of IB or II were diagnosed as having complicated AD with an abscess, and patients with modified Hinchey score of III were diagnosed as belonging to the complicated AD with perforation group.

2.4. Statistical Analysis

Data were presented as counts and percentages when the variables were categorical, as means and standard deviations when the variables were quantitative and with a normal distribution, or as medians and interquartile ranges when the variables were quantitative and did not follow a normal distribution. The comparisons between two independent groups concerning categorical data were conducted using a chi-squared test or Fisher's exact test. For quantitative data that did not follow a normal distribution, we used the Mann-Whitney U test. For quantitative data that followed a normal distribution, the analysis was performed using an independent t-test. Comparisons between three independent groups concerning quantitative data that did not follow a normal distribution were made using the Kruskal–Wallis method. The discriminating qualities of inflammatory markers were assessed using receiver operating characteristic (ROC) curves, using their area under the curve (with a 95% bootstrapped computed confidence interval [CI]), as well as by identifying the best cutoff point by maximizing the Youden index and computing its sensitivity and specificity. Comparisons between ROC curves were performed with the De Long test. The intervals between episodes were compared using Kaplan–Meier survival curves, and the Cox proportional hazards regression model was used to analyze associations of several factors such as NLR, PLR, MLR, and SII with cumulative recurrence rate. For all statistical tests, a two-tailed p-value was computed, and a value of ≤ 0.05 was considered to be statistically significant. All analyses were computed in the R environment for statistical computing and graphics, version 4.1.2 (R Foundation for Statistical Computing, Vienna, Austria).

3. Results

3.1. General Characteristics

The cohort included 147 patients, of which, 71 (49.98%) patients were females. The mean age was 60.8 years, ranging from 25–89 years. Only 23% of the patients (n = 34) were younger than 50 years of age. According to the modified Hinchey classification [13,14], 70 (47.61%) patients were diagnosed with uncomplicated acute diverticulitis, and 57 (38.77%) were diagnosed with complicated disease. Of the complicated diverticulitis group, 44 (29.93%) patients showed CT findings that were compatible with Hinchey stage III disease, and none with Hinchey stage IV disease. The demographic and clinical characteristics of the subjects are presented in Table 1.

Table 1. Demographic characteristics of patients with acute diverticulitis.

Characteristic	Number (%) (n = 147)	Uncomplicated AD (n = 82)	Complicated AD (n = 65)	p-Value
Age (years), mean (SD)	60.8 (14.05)	62.05 (14)	59.22 (14.06)	0.226
Sex				
female	72 (48,97)	40 (57.14)	32 (56.14)	0.957
Location of diverticula				
rectum	1 (0.79)	1 (1.43)	0 (0)	1
sigmoid colon	85 (66.93)	38 (54.29)	47 (82.46)	<0.001
descending colon	13 (10.24)	6 (8.57)	7 (12.28)	0.493
transverse colon	4 (3.15)	4 (5.71)	0 (0)	0.127
ascending colon	3 (2.36)	2 (2.86)	1 (1.75)	1
cecum	0 (0)			
Symptoms				
abdominal pain	133 (91.72)	72 (87.8)	61 (96.83)	0.051
right iliac region	10 (6.9)	5 (6.1)	5 (7.94)	0.747
right lumbar region	4 (2.76)	3 (3.66)	1 (1.59)	0.633
right hypochondriac region	3 (2.07)	3 (3.66)	0 (0)	0.258
epigastric region	3 (2.07)	3 (3.66)	0 (0)	0.258
left hypochondriac region	5 (3.45)	5 (6.1)	0 (0)	0.069
left lumbar region	30 (20.69)	20 (24.39)	10 (15.87)	0.209
left iliac region	63 (43.45)	38 (46.34)	25 (39.68)	0.423
hypogastric region	19 (13.1)	9 (10.98)	10 (15.87)	0.386
umbilical region	1 (0.69)	1 (1.22)	0 (0)	1
diffuse	37 (25.52)	13 (15.85)	24 (38.1)	0.002
diarrhea at admission	43 (29.66)	29 (35.37)	14 (22.22)	0.086
constipation at admission	17 (11.72)	14 (17.07)	3 (4.76)	0.022
nausea	19 (13.1)	12 (14.63)	7 (11.11)	0.533
vomiting	17 (11.72)	8 (9.76)	9 (14.29)	0.401
fever	27 (18.62)	11 (13.41)	16 (25.4)	0.066
Hinchey classification				
stage 0	43 (29.25)			
stage IA	39 (26.53)			
stage IB	10 (6.8)			
stage II	11 (7.48)			
stage III	44 (29.93)			
stage IV	0 (0)			
Treatment				
conservative	106 (72.11)	80 (97.56)	26 (40)	<0.001
drainage	22 (14.97)	1 (1.22)	21 (32.31)	<0.001

Table 1. Cont.

Characteristic	Number (%) (n = 147)	Uncomplicated AD (n = 82)	Complicated AD (n = 65)	p-Value
surgery				
without	103 (70.07)	80 (97.56)	23 (35.38)	
emergency	37 (25.17)	1 (1.22)	36 (55.38)	<0.001
elective	7 (4.76)	1 (1.22)	6 (9.23)	
Recurrence				
one episode	12			
two episodes	2			
≥ three episodes	1			
unknown	1			

SD, standard deviation; AD, acute diverticulitis.

3.2. Patients' Characteristics According to the Severity of Diverticulitis

The patients were categorized into two groups based on the presence or absence of complications. The characteristics of patients between uncomplicated AD and complicated AD are compared in Table 1. A total of 65 subjects were diagnosed with complicated acute diverticulitis and 82 subjects with uncomplicated acute diverticulitis. Compared to uncomplicated AD, complicated AD patients presented statistically significant differences in terms of the location of the diverticula in the sigmoid colon ($n = 47$ (82.46%) vs. $n = 38$ (54.29%), $p < 0.001$), the presence of diffuse abdominal pain ($n = 24$ (38.1%) vs. $n = 13$ (15.85%), $p = 0.002$) and constipation ($n = 3$ (4.76%) vs. $n = 14$ (17.07%), $p = 0.022$), as well as the treatment. There was no significant difference between uncomplicated and complicated AD groups in other factors, such as age, sex, abdominal pain, diarrhea, nausea, vomiting, and fever.

3.3. Inflammatory Markers in Patients with AD

The patients were classified into three groups, based on the Hinchey classification, namely the 0/IA group (uncomplicated AD) ($n = 82$), the IB/II group (complicated AD with abscess) ($n = 21$), and the III group (complicated AD with perforation) ($n = 44$). We compared total and differential white blood cell (WBC) counts, along with six novel inflammatory ratios in uncomplicated AD patients, complicated AD patients with an abscess, and complicated AD with perforation, as demonstrated in Tables 2 and 3. These inflammatory ratios included MLR, NLR, PDW, PLR, RDW, and SII.

Table 2. Total and differential leukocyte counts in the uncomplicated and complicated AD groups.

Hinchey Classification	0/Ia (n = 82)	Ib/II (n = 21)	III (n = 44)	p-Value
WBC ($\times 10^9$/mL), median (IQR)	7.95 (6.45–9.84)	11.11 (9.67–16.34)	11.18 (7.29–13.26)	<0.001 (0.003/0.01/0.742) [n1 = 79, n2 = 20, n3 = 43]
WBC, n (%)				< 0.001
Below NR	0 (0)	0 (0)	2 (4.65)	
NR	64 (81.01)	10 (50)	19 (44.19)	
Above NR	15 (18.99)	10 (50)	22 (51.16)	
Ly ($\times 10^9$/mL), median (IQR)	1.6 (1.24–2)	1.35 (1.05–1.72)	1.44 (0.9–1.76)	0.096 (0.336/0.233/1) [n1 = 75, n2 = 14, n3 = 36]
Ly, n (%)				0.012
Below NR	9 (12)	3 (21.43)	13 (36.11)	
NR	66 (88)	11 (78.57)	23 (63.89)	

Table 2. Cont.

Hinchey Classification	0/Ia (n = 82)	Ib/II (n = 21)	III (n = 44)	p-Value
M (×10^9/mL), median (IQR)	0.47 (0.37–0.71)	0.76 (0.52–0.92)	0.55 (0.4–0.74)	0.169 (0.163/0.85/0.523) [n1 = 69, n2 = 10, n3 = 25]
M, n (%)				0.017
Below NR	0 (0)	0 (0)	2 (8)	
NR	58 (84.06)	5 (50)	18 (72)	
Above NR	11 (15.94)	5 (50)	5 (20)	
N (×10^9/mL), median (IQR)	5.38 (4.16–7.36)	8.69 (6.96–12.3)	9.48 (5.38–11.96)	<0.001 (0.004/0.009/0.983) [n1 = 75, n2 = 14, n3 = 36]
N, n (%)				<0.001
Below NR	1 (1.33)	0 (0)	1 (2.78)	
NR	54 (72)	4 (28.57)	13 (36.11)	
Above NR	20 (26.67)	10 (71.43)	22 (61.11)	
P (×10^3/mL), median (IQR)	239 (195.5–273.5)	300 (272.5–447.5)	257 (227–354)	<0.001 (<0.001/0.175/0.051) [n1 = 79, n2 = 20, n3 = 42]
P, n (%)				0.01
Below NR	4 (5.06)	0 (0)	4 (9.52)	
NR	72 (91.14)	15 (75)	31 (73.81)	
Above NR	3 (3.8)	5 (25)	7 (16.67)	

IQR, interquartile range; NR, normal range; WBC, white blood cell (NR = 4–11); Ly, lymphocyte (NR = 1–4.8); M, monocytes (NR = 0.2–0.8); N, neutrophil (NR = 2.5–7); P, platelet (NR = 150–450); values between the square brackets represent the number of observations per group.

Table 3. Inflammatory ratio values in the uncomplicated and complicated AD groups.

Hinchey Classification	0/Ia (n = 82)	Ib/II (n = 21)	III (n = 44)	p-Value
MLR, median (IQR)	0.35 (0.21–0.42)	0.43 (0.4–0.6)	0.42 (0.28–0.62)	0.013 (0.101/0.133/0.738) [n1 = 69, n2 = 10, n3 = 25]
NLR, median (IQR)	3.53 (2.51–4.81)	5.86 (4.14–13.18)	6.96 (5.1–10.52)	<0.001 (0.006/<0.001/0.976) [n1 = 75, n2 = 14, n3 = 36]
PDW, median (IQR)	13.75 (11.83–16)	12.9 (10.75–15.75)	13.95 (11.12–15.9)	0.318 (0.383/0.614/0.767) [n1 = 70, n2 = 16, n3 = 40]
PLR, median (IQR)	140.15 (108.1–214.34)	278.32 (204.28–426.21)	228.7 (149.68–400.46)	<0.001 (0.002/0.006/0.541) [n1 = 75, n2 = 14, n3 = 36]
RDW, median (IQR)	42.3 (40.1–46.6)	44.65 (41.18–50.9)	43.3 (41.5–46.2)	0.443 (0.584/0.755/0.782) [n1 = 65, n2 = 12, n3 = 29]
SII, median (IQR)	773.24 (539.28–1173.68)	2856.29 (1434.65–3631.29)	1689.24 (1310.22–3532.76)	<0.001 (<0.001/<0.001/0.775) [n1 = 75, n2 = 14, n3 = 36]

IQR, interquartile range; NLR, neutrophil-to-lymphocyte ratio; PLR, platelet-to-lymphocyte ratio; MLR, monocyte-to-lymphocyte ratio; SII, systemic immune inflammation; PDW, platelet distribution width; RDW, red blood cell distribution width; values between square brackets represent the number of observations per group.

Firstly, the WBC (p-value < 0.001), neutrophil (N) (p-value < 0.001), and platelet (P) (p-value < 0.001) values were significantly different between the three groups. Secondly, three inflammatory ratios demonstrated a statistically significant difference between the three groups, including NLR (p-value < 0.001), PLR (p-value < 0.001), and SII (p-value <0.001). Comparing every two groups, WBC, N, P, NLR, PLR, and SII were significantly different between the uncomplicated AD group and the complicated AD with abscess group, and no statistically significant difference between complicated AD with abscess group and the complicated AD with perforation group. These values, except in the case of platelets, were significantly higher in patients with complicated AD with perforation, compared to those with uncomplicated AD group.

The above results showed that SII, NLR, and PLR levels were significantly higher in the complicated AD group (modified Hinchey grade of > IA). We studied the cutoff point, the area under the curve (AUC), Se, and Sp for these inflammatory ratios (Table 4). The ROC predicting curve analysis (Figure 1) showed an AUC and 95% CI of SII, NLR, PLR, and MLR in predicting complicated AD of 0.812 (95% CI [0.73–0.888]), 0.773 (95% CI [0.676 –0.857]), 0.725 (95% CI [0.63–0.813]), 0.665 (95% CI [0.542–0.777]), respectively. The diagnostic value of SII was the highest. When the cutoff value of SII was 1200, the sensitivity and specificity were 82% and 76%, respectively. There was no significant difference in AUC compared with each other ($p > 0.05$) (Table 4).

Table 4. The area under the receiver operating characteristic (ROC) curve (AUC) and cutoff values for MLR, NLR, PLR, and SII in the complicated AD (modified Hinchey grade > IA), as well as comparisons between the ROC curves.

Characteristic	AUROC (95% CI)	Cutoff	Se	Sp
MLR	0.665 (0.542–0.777)	0.38	65.7	65.2
NLR	0.773 (0.676–0.857)	4.06	80	69.3
PLR	0.725 (0.63–0.813)	144.38	80	56
SII	0.812 (0.73–0.888)	1200	82	76
SII vs. NLR	$p = 0.111$			
SII vs. MLR	$p = 0.027$			
SII vs. PLR	$p = 0.019$			
NLR vs. PLR	$p = 0.323$			

AUROC, the area under the receiver operating characteristic curve; CI, confidence interval; NLR, neutrophil-to-lymphocyte ratio; PLR, platelet-to-lymphocyte ratio; MLR, monocyte-to-lymphocyte ratio; SII, systemic immune inflammation; Se, sensitivity; Sp, specificity.

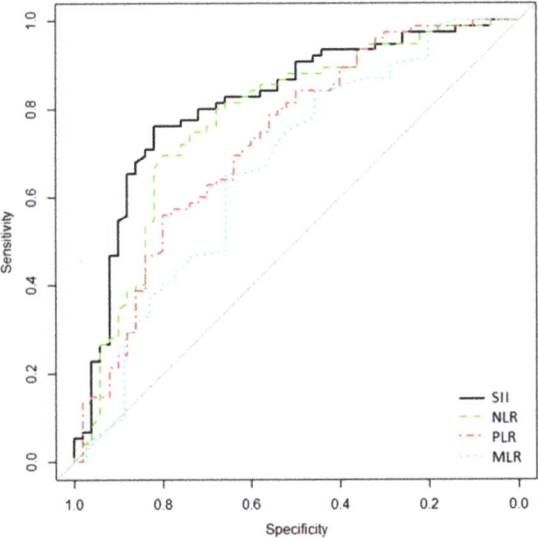

Figure 1. Receiver operating characteristics (ROC) curves for SII, NLR, PLR, and MLR to discriminate the complicated AD group (modified Hinchey grade > IA). The x-axis shows false-positive/1-specificity, and on the y-axis, true positive/sensitivity is expressed.

The ROC curve (Figure 2) showed that the AUC of SII, NLR, PLR, and MLR in the diagnosis of complicated AD with perforation (modified Hinchey grade III) were 0.738 (95% CI [0.632–0.831]), 0.737 (95% CI [0.629–0.834]), 0.65 (95% CI [0.53–0.754]), and 0.614 (95% CI [0.474–0.738]), respectively. The diagnostic value of SII was the highest. When the cutoff value of SII was 1200, the sensitivity and specificity were 83.3% and 67.4%, respectively (Table 5).

Table 5. The area under the ROC curve (AUROC) for MLR, NLR, PLR, and SII in the complicated AD with perforation group (modified Hinchey grade III).

Characteristic	AUROC (95% CI)	Cutoff	Se	Sp
MLR	0.614 (0.474–0.738)	0.51	48	81
NLR	0.737 (0.629–0.834)	5.61	72.2	76.4
PLR	0.65 (0.53–0.754)	144.38	77.8	49.4
SII	0.738 (0.632–0.831)	1200	83.3	67.4

NLR, neutrophil-to-lymphocyte ratio; PLR, platelet-to-lymphocyte ratio; MLR, monocyte-to-lymphocyte ratio; SII, systemic immune inflammation; Se, sensitivity; Sp, specificity.

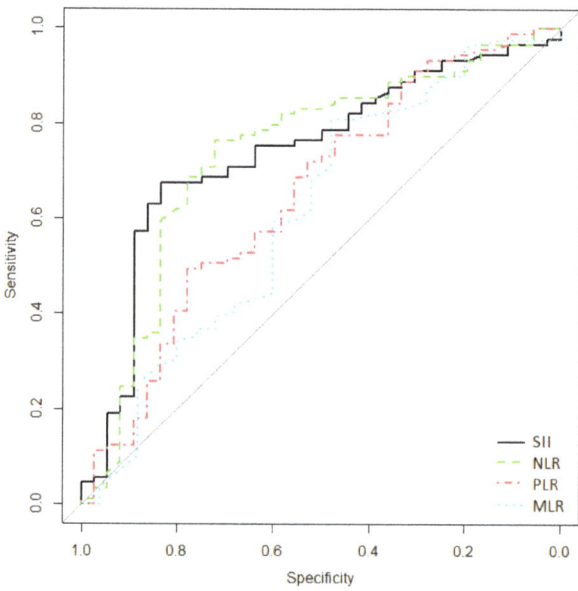

Figure 2. Receiver operating characteristics (ROC) curves for SII, NLR, PLR, and MLR, used to discriminate cases of complicated AD with perforation (modified Hinchey grade III). On the x-axis, false-positive/1-specificity is shown, and on the y-axis, true positive/sensitivity is expressed.

Additional episodes of acute diverticulitis occurred in 15 (10.20%) patients; of these, 4 (26.66%) patients presented more than one episode of acute diverticulitis. Survival analysis was used to assess the predictive value of SII, NLR, PLR, and MLR regarding the intervals between episodes. The intervals between episodes were compared using Kaplan–Meier survival curves (Figure 3). Using the log-rank test, there were no statistically significant differences in the cumulative recurrence rate between SII $\geq$ median (=1101.57) vs. SII < median group ($p = 0.35$), NLR $\geq$ median (=4.06) vs. NLR < median ($p = 0.347$), PLR $\geq$ median (=168.64) vs. PLR < median ($p = 0.597$), and MLR $\geq$ median (=0.36) vs. MLR < median ($p = 0.651$) in patients with acute diverticulitis. Using the Cox proportional hazards regression model, we observed that the interval between episodes was higher in the PLR < median group and MLR < median group compared with PLR $\geq$ median group and MLR $\geq$ median group. However, it was lower in the NLR < median group and SII < median group compared with the NLR $\geq$ median group and SII $\geq$ median group, albeit not being statistically significant (Table 6).

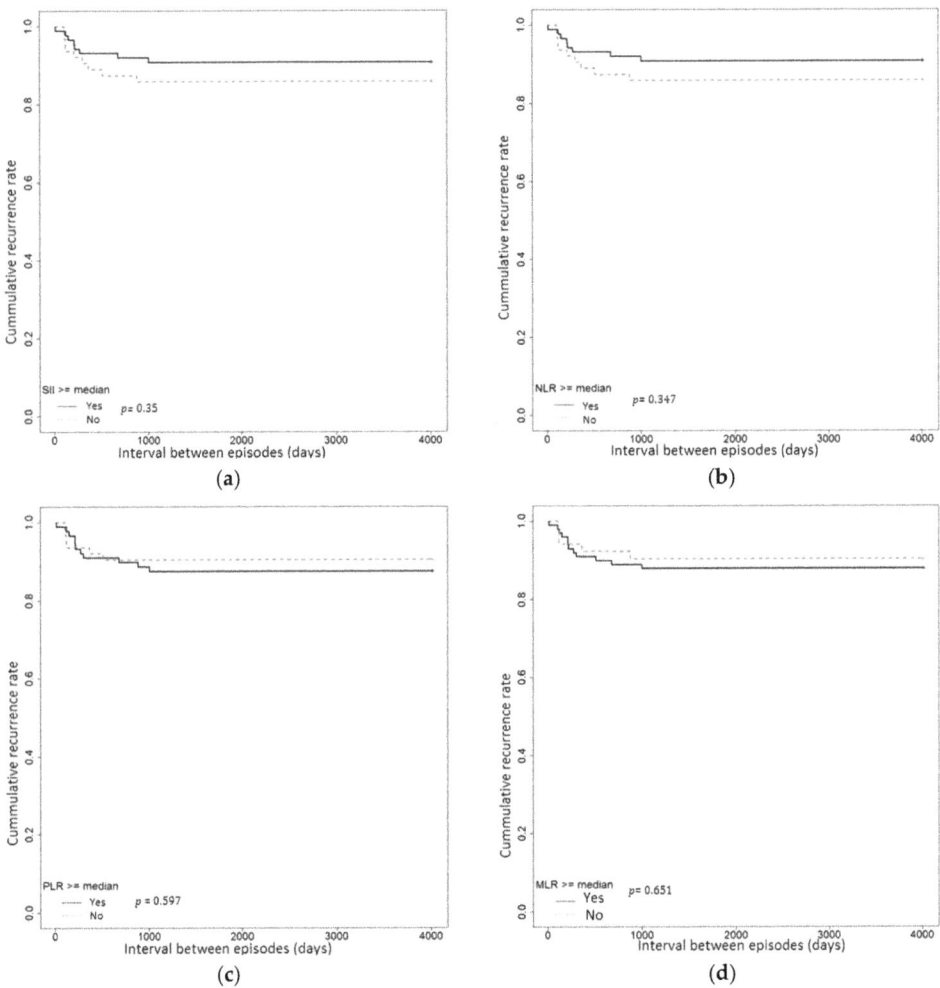

Figure 3. Kaplan–Meier analysis of the intervals between episodes of AD: (**a**) among patients with SII ≥ median (**b**) among patients with an NLR ≥ median; (**c**) among patients with a PLR ≥ median; (**d**) among patients with an MLR ≥ median.

Table 6. The hazard ratio (HR) for MLR, NLR, PLR, and SII using the Cox proportional hazards regression model.

Characteristic	HR	p-Value
MLR ≥ median	1.27 (95% CI 0.45–3.6)	0.651
NLR ≥ median	1.57 (95% CI 0.61–4.08)	0.347
PLR ≥ median	1.31 (95% CI 0.48–3.53)	0.597
SII ≥ median	1.57 (95% CI 0.61–4.08)	0.347

NLR, neutrophil-to-lymphocyte ratio; PLR, platelet-to-lymphocyte ratio; MLR, monocyte-to-lymphocyte ratio; SII, systemic immune inflammation; HR, hazard ratio.

4. Discussion

It is crucial to recognize complicated AD at an early admission stage for prognosis, risk assessment, the allocation of resources, appropriate disease management, and informed clinical decision-making. This allows for tailored interventions based on the severity of the disease and helps optimize patient outcomes. A CT scan is the gold standard of diagnostic tools for acute diverticulitis since it is, effective in evaluating its severity, and excluding alternative diagnoses. To optimize the use of CT scans, it is recommended to consider the clinical and laboratory findings when dealing with suspected complicated diverticulitis. This approach helps minimize the treatment expenses and potential radiation risks.

This retrospective study assessed the associations between NLR, PLR, MLR, and SII regarding the severity of acute diverticulitis. The values for these hemogram-derived ratios were easily and quickly obtained. Moreover, we also evaluated the ability of these ratios to predict the presence of complications and the disease recurrence rate, based on these inflammatory ratio values. We included a total population of 147 patients who were admitted with acute diverticulitis, out of whom 44.2% (n = 65) of patients presented with complicated AD. Firstly, we observed that the SII, NLR, and PLR levels were significantly higher in the complicated AD group (modified Hinchey grade >IA), but no statistically significant difference was reported between the complicated AD with abscess group and the complicated AD with perforation group. Secondly, the SII, NLR, and PLR were the most accurate inflammatory ratios associated with complicated AD. Lastly, we did not observe a correlation between the SII, NLR, and PLR levels and the interval between episodes of acute diverticulitis. To the best of our knowledge, this is the first study to evaluate the utility of the SII and MLR levels for diagnosing AD.

The mean age in our study was 60.8 years, with patients ranging from 25 to 89 years. Only 23% were younger than 50 years of age. According to the World Society of Emergency Surgery (WSES) guidelines [16], caution is advised against solely relying on the patient's clinical signs, symptoms, and laboratory tests for diagnosing left colonic AD in the elderly population. To confirm the diagnosis and distinguish between complicated and uncomplicated AD in elderly patients, the guidelines recommend using a CT scan with IV-contrast dye. Alternatively, when intravenous contrast enhanced CT scan is not feasible, ultrasound (US), magnetic resonance imaging (MRI), or a CT scan without IV contrast dye may be considered based on resource availability.

The prevalence of complicated AD in our study was similar to that reported by Zager et al. [11] (44.2% (n= 65) vs. 32.7% (n = 149]), but was different from that reported by Palacios Huatuco et al. [17] and Bharucha et al. [4] (44.2% (n = 65) vs. 9 % (n = 30) vs. (12% (n = 386)). In the complicated diverticulitis group, 29.93% (n = 44) of patients had CT findings compatible with a diagnosis of Hinchey stage III. Recurrent episodes of acute diverticulitis occurred in 10.20% (n = 15) of patients, of whom 26.66% (n = 4) presented more than one episode of acute diverticulitis. We also found that patients with complicated AD were of a similar age to those with uncomplicated AD (median age, 59.22 vs. 62.05 years, p = 0.226). These findings are similar to those reported by Palacios Huatuco et al. [17] and are different from those reported by Chang et al. [18].

In our study, WBC, neutrophil, platelet, and monocyte counts were higher in the complicated AD group (Hinchey IB/II and Hinchey III), while lymphocytes were lower in this group, suggesting an inflammatory response and immune system activation. Only WBC, neutrophil, and platelet counts have a statistically significant association with complicated AD. However, we did not find any statistically significant differences related to these values in the group with perforation compared to those with abscesses, as we would have expected. This unexpected finding may indicate that other factors beyond these specific markers play a significant role in differentiating between these two types of complications in AD.

Circulating cells, such as lymphocytes, monocytes, neutrophils, and platelets are essential components of the inflammatory process. In contrast to measuring each WBC component separately, measuring the divergence among them has been thought to be more accurate for predicting poor clinical outcomes [19]. Previous studies that have used two hemogram-derived ratios, namely, the NLR and PLR, have found that high NLR or PLR have been linked with complicated diverticulitis [7,8], surgical intervention [9], the failure of conservative treatment for acute first-attack colonic diverticulitis [10], a shorter interval between recurrent episodes, and longer cumulative hospitalization days [11]. Several studies have studied MLR and SII as potential prognostic markers in coronavirus disease, cardiovascular diseases, sepsis, and cancer; however, one study has assessed their correlation with the failure of conservative disease management [12]. In our cohort, we found that SII, NLR, and PLR levels were significantly higher in the complicated AD group (modified Hinchey grade >IA), but the MLR level was not significantly different between the uncomplicated AD and complicated AD groups.

In our study, the SII cutoff of 1200 had a sensitivity of 82% and a specificity of 76%; the NLR cutoff of 4.06 had a sensitivity of 80% and a specificity of 69.3%; and the PLR cutoff of 144.38 had a sensitivity of 80% and a specificity of 56%. The diagnostic accuracy of the SII, NLR, and PLR for complicated AD is good and is also comparable, but MLR could only predict those patients who had complicated AD with low accuracy (AUC = 0.665, Se = 65.7%, Sp = 65.2%). The SII showed the highest AUROC value of 0.812, indicating its ability to discriminate effectively between patients with and without complicated AD. This finding is particularly interesting since the SII showed a diagnostic potential similar to that of procalcitonin, a well-known biomarker for infection and inflammation [20]. Regarding the cutoff values for the NLR and PLR, we found that the reported values in the literature align with our observations. The cutoff values for the NLR and PLR vary according to the specific clinical context. In cases of malignancy, the cutoff value of NLR typically hovers around 3, while sepsis situations tend to require a higher cutoff value of approximately 5 [21]. In our study, we found a NLR cutoff value of 4.06, which is within the range reported for sepsis situations. This suggests that NLR may be a relevant marker for distinguishing sepsis-related conditions, such as complicated acute diverticulitis. This finding aligns with a study by Palacios Huatuco et al. [17] who found a value of NLR 4.2 (Se: 80%, Sp: 64.1%), with the best diagnostic yield to define severity. The cut-off value of above 150 for PLR is widely reported and published by various authors both in oncology [22] and sepsis conditions [23]. In our study, we calculated a PLR cutoff value of 144.38, which is remarkably close to the reported value. This correspondence with the internationally reported cutoff value strengthens the validity of our study and endorses the reliability of PLR as a potential diagnostic marker for complicated AD. Mari et al. found that the PLR demonstrated lower diagnostic accuracy than the NLR (AUC values of 0.73, and 0.77, respectively) [7]. Zager et al. did not find an independent association between a high PLR (>120) and complicated disease [11]. The PLR cutoff value of 120 used by Zager et al. might have been lower than the optimal threshold that is required to detect an independent association with complicated disease. Park et al. [12] showed that NLR, lymphocyte-to-monocyte ratio (LMR), PLR, and SII levels were not predictive factors in ascertaining the success or failure of conservative management in patients with right colonic diverticulitis.

In a previous study conducted by Zager et al. [11], it was reported that elevated levels of NLR (>5.4) were associated with shorter intervals between episodes of acute diverticulitis, an increased number of readmissions, and a longer hospital stay. In our study, we did not find statistically significant differences in the cumulative reoccurrence rates between the groups based on SII, NLR, PLR, and MLR. This suggests that these inflammatory ratios may not be strongly associated with the interval between episodes of acute diverticulitis.

Our research has several limitations. First, the data were collected retrospectively; hence, a selection bias may exist, and also, some medical records did not contain all variables. Second, this was a single-center study conducted in Eastern Europe with a relatively small sample size, which may affect the statistical power of our findings and limit their generalizability to other populations or settings. Third, smoking status, medication use, and BMI could not be included in the analysis due to lack of data. Most patients with diverticulosis are obese and are diagnosed concurrently with metabolic dysfunction-associated steatotic liver disease (MASLD) [24]. It has been observed that overweight and obesity are associated with an increased risk of moderate/severe diverticular disease, complicated diverticular disease with abscesses or perforation, the need for emergency surgical intervention, and diverticular bleeding in both sexes. A recent meta-analysis, which included six studies, calculated a relative risk (RR) of 1.31 (95% CI 1.09–1.56) and 1.20 (95% CI 1.04–1.40) for diverticular disease and complicated diverticular disease, respectively [25]. The presence of obesity and metabolic syndrome was not determined in our study cohort due to the lack of data in each patient's medical records. Obesity influences NLR; therefore, the absence of this data represents another limitation of the current study.

However, despite these limitations, our study also has several important strengths. It provides a valuable and comprehensive evaluation of multiple inflammatory markers and hemogram-derived ratios in complicated AD. It is the first study to evaluate the utility of SII and MLR for diagnosing complicated AD and establish their prognostic utility. Additionally, the associated complications were accurately evaluated using CT scan or surgical report.

We believe that the clinical significance of this study lies in its potential to improve diagnostic accuracy, guide treatment decisions, optimize healthcare resource utilization, and contribute to the existing knowledge in the field of complicated acute diverticulitis. By evaluating multiple inflammatory markers, including SII and MLR, this study expands the range of diagnostic tools available for complicated acute diverticulitis, enhancing the accuracy and efficiency of diagnosing the severity of the disease. The early recognition of complicated AD allows for timely and targeted interventions, such as performing additional imaging studies or initiating more intensive monitoring, guiding decisions about the need for surgical consultation or aggressive medical management. Furthermore, by ruling out complicated AD in a considerable proportion of cases with good specificity, the inflammatory parameters can help avoid unnecessary CT scans and hospitalizations, thus optimizing healthcare resource utilization. Finally, it fills a gap in the literature by being the first to evaluate the utility of SII and MLR in diagnosing complicated acute diverticulitis, expanding the understanding of inflammatory markers in this specific context and opening avenues for further research and validation.

Therefore, future studies with larger sample sizes, multi-center designs, and prospective data collection methods are needed to confirm our results on the predictive role of hemogram-derived ratios in complicated AD and to refine the optimized cutoff values for the assessed parameters.

5. Conclusions

SII, NLR, and PLR can predict complicated AD, with an SII of >1200 having the highest yield for diagnosing complicated AD. Incorporating these hemogram-derived ratios into a comprehensive predictive model may improve accuracy and aid in clinical decision-making for patients with AD.

Supplementary Materials: The following supporting information can be downloaded at: https://www.mdpi.com/article/10.3390/medicina59091523/s1, Table S1: STROBE Statement—checklist of items that should be included in reports of observational studies.

Author Contributions: C.M.S.: conceptualization, methodology, data curation, result interpretation, writing—original draft preparation and editing; C.S. and I.Ș.D.: data collection, data curation; D.-C.L.: conceptualization, methodology, formal analysis, result interpretation and revised the manuscript; A.I.: performed result interpretation and revised the manuscript; D.L.D.: conceptualization, methodology, revision of the manuscript, and approved the final text. All authors have read and agreed to the published version of the manuscript.

Funding: This research received no external funding.

Institutional Review Board Statement: The study was conducted according to the principles of the Declaration of Helsinki and was approved by the Ethical Committee of "Iuliu Hațieganu" University of Medicine and Pharmacy Cluj-Napoca (approval no. 139/27.06.2023).

Informed Consent Statement: Patient consent was waived due to the retrospective design of this study, which does not affect patient care.

Data Availability Statement: The data used to support the findings of this study are available from the corresponding author upon request.

Conflicts of Interest: The authors declare no conflict of interest.

References

1. Swanson, S.M.; Strate, L.L. Acute Colonic Diverticulitis. *Ann. Intern. Med.* **2018**, *168*, ITC65–ITC80. [CrossRef]
2. Tursi, A.; Scarpignato, C.; Strate, L.L.; Lanas, A.; Kruis, W.; Lahat, A.; Danese, S. Colonic diverticular disease. *Nat. Rev. Dis. Prim.* **2020**, *6*, 20. [CrossRef]
3. Trifan, A.; Gheorghe, C.; Marica Sabo, C.; Diculescu, M.; Nedelcu, L.; Singeap, A.M.; Sfarti, C.; Gheorghe, L.; Sporea, I.; Tanțău, M.; et al. Diagnosis and Treatment of Colonic Diverticular Disease: Position Paper of the Romanian Society of Gastroenterology and Hepatology. *J. Gastrointest. Liver Dis. JGLD* **2018**, *27*, 449–457. [CrossRef] [PubMed]
4. Bharucha, A.E.; Parthasarathy, G.; Ditah, I.; Fletcher, J.G.; Ewelukwa, O.; Pendlimari, R.; Yawn, B.P.; Melton, L.J.; Schleck, C.; Zinsmeister, A.R. Temporal Trends in the Incidence and Natural History of Diverticulitis: A Population-Based Study. *Am. J. Gastroenterol.* **2015**, *110*, 1589–1596. [CrossRef] [PubMed]
5. Laméris, W.; van Randen, A.; van Gulik, T.M.; Busch, O.R.; Winkelhagen, J.; Bossuyt, P.M.; Stoker, J.; Boermeester, M.A. A Clinical decision rule to establish the diagnosis of acute diverticulitis at the emergency department. *Dis. Colon Rectum* **2010**, *53*, 896–904. [CrossRef] [PubMed]
6. Sartelli, M.; Weber, D.G.; Kluger, Y.; Ansaloni, L.; Coccolini, F.; Abu-Zidan, F.; Augustin, G.; Ben-Ishay, O.; Biffl, W.L.; Bouliaris, K.; et al. 2020 update of the WSES guidelines for the management of acute colonic diverticulitis in the emergency setting. *World J. Emerg. Surg. WJES* **2020**, *15*, 32. [CrossRef]
7. Mari, A.; Khoury, T.; Lubany, A.; Safadi, M.; Farraj, M.; Farah, A.; Kadah, A.; Sbeit, W.; Mahamid, M. Neutrophil-to-Lymphocyte and Platelet-to-Lymphocyte Ratios Are Correlated with Complicated Diverticulitis and Hinchey Classification: A Simple Tool to Assess Disease Severity in the Emergency Department. *Emerg. Med. Int.* **2019**, *2019*, 6321060. [CrossRef]
8. Hogan, J.; Sehgal, R.; Murphy, D.; O'Leary, P.; Coffey, J.C. Do Inflammatory Indices Play a Role in Distinguishing between Uncomplicated and Complicated Diverticulitis? *Dig. Surg.* **2017**, *34*, 7–11. [CrossRef]
9. Reynolds, I.S.; Heaney, R.M.; Khan, W.; Khan, I.Z.; Waldron, R.; Barry, K. The Utility of Neutrophil to Lymphocyte Ratio as a Predictor of Intervention in Acute Diverticulitis. *Dig. Surg.* **2017**, *34*, 227–232. [CrossRef]
10. Kim, J.H.; Han, S.H.; Lee, J.-W.; Kim, H.; Han, J. Platelet to lymphocyte ratio is a risk factor for failure of non-operative treatment of colonic diverticulitis. *Sci. Rep.* **2023**, *13*, 4377. [CrossRef]
11. Zager, Y.; Horesh, N.; Dan, A.; Aharoni, M.; Khalilieh, S.; Cordoba, M.; Nevler, A.; Gutman, M.; Rosin, D. Associations of novel inflammatory markers with long-term outcomes and recurrence of diverticulitis. *ANZ J. Surg.* **2020**, *90*, 2041–2045. [CrossRef] [PubMed]
12. Park, Y.Y.; Nam, S.; Han, J.H.; Lee, J.; Cheong, C. Predictive factors for conservative treatment failure of right colonic diverticulitis. *Ann. Surg. Treat. Res.* **2021**, *100*, 347–355. [CrossRef] [PubMed]
13. Wasvary, H.; Turfah, F.; Kadro, O.; Beauregard, W. Same hospitalization resection for acute diverticulitis. *Am. Surg.* **1999**, *65*, 632–635; discussion 636. [CrossRef] [PubMed]
14. Kaiser, A.M.; Jiang, J.-K.; Lake, J.P.; Ault, G.; Artinyan, A.; Gonzalez-Ruiz, C.; Essani, R.; Beart, R.W., Jr. The management of complicated diverticulitis and the role of computed tomography. *Am. J. Gastroenterol.* **2005**, *100*, 910–917. [CrossRef]
15. Vandenbroucke, J.P.; von Elm, E.; Altman, D.G.; Gøtzsche, P.C.; Mulrow, C.D.; Pocock, S.J.; Poole, C.; Schlesselman, J.J.; Egger, M. Strengthening the Reporting of Observational Studies in Epidemiology (STROBE): Explanation and elaboration. *PLoS Med.* **2007**, *4*, e297. [CrossRef]
16. Fugazzola, P.; Ceresoli, M.; Coccolini, F.; Gabrielli, F.; Puzziello, A.; Monzani, F.; Amato, B.; Sganga, G.; Sartelli, M.; Menichetti, F.; et al. The WSES/SICG/ACOI/SICUT/AcEMC/SIFIPAC guidelines for diagnosis and treatment of acute left colonic diverticulitis in the elderly. *World J. Emerg. Surg. WJES* **2022**, *17*, 5. [CrossRef]
17. Palacios Huatuco, R.M.; Pantoja Pachajoa, D.A.; Bruera, N.; Pinsak, A.E.; Llahi, F.; Doniquian, A.M.; Alvarez, F.A.; Parodi, M. Neutrophil-to-lymphocyte ratio as a predictor of complicated acute diverticulitis: A retrospective cohort study. *Ann. Med. Surg.* **2021**, *63*, 102128. [CrossRef]
18. Chang, C.-Y.; Hsu, T.-Y.; He, G.-Y.; Shih, H.-M.; Wu, S.-H.; Huang, F.-W.; Chen, P.-C.; Tsai, W.-C. Utility of monocyte distribution width in the differential diagnosis between simple and complicated diverticulitis: A retrospective cohort study. *BMC Gastroenterol.* **2023**, *23*, 96. [CrossRef]
19. Suppiah, A.; Malde, D.; Arab, T.; Hamed, M.; Allgar, V.; Smith, A.M.; Morris-Stiff, G. The prognostic value of the neutrophil–lymphocyte ratio (NLR) in acute pancreatitis: Identification of an optimal NLR. *J. Gastrointest. Surg.* **2013**, *17*, 675–681. [CrossRef]
20. Jeger, V.; Pop, R.; Forudastan, F.; Barras, J.P.; Zuber, M.; Piso, R.J. Is there a role for procalcitonin in differentiating uncomplicated and complicated diverticulitis in order to reduce antibiotic therapy? A prospective diagnostic cohort study. *Swiss Med. Wkly.* **2017**, *147*, w14555. [CrossRef]

21. Shelat, V.G. Role of inflammatory indices in management of hepatocellular carcinoma—Neutrophil to lymphocyte ratio. *Ann. Transl. Med.* **2020**, *8*, 912. [CrossRef]
22. Li, D.-Z.; Guo, J.; Song, Q.-K.; Hu, X.-J.; Bao, X.-L.; Lu, J. Prognostic prediction of the platelet-to-lymphocyte ratio in hepatocellular carcinoma: A systematic review and meta-analysis. *Transl. Cancer Res.* **2022**, *11*, 4037–4050. [CrossRef] [PubMed]
23. Botoș, I.D.; Pantiș, C.; Bodolea, C.; Nemes, A.; Crișan, D.; Avram, L.; Negrău, M.O.; Hirișcău, I.E.; Crăciun, R.; Puia, C.I. The Dynamics of the Neutrophil-to-Lymphocyte and Platelet-to-Lymphocyte Ratios Predict Progression to Septic Shock and Death in Patients with Prolonged Intensive Care Unit Stay. *Medicina* **2023**, *59*, 32. [CrossRef] [PubMed]
24. Pantic, I.; Lugonja, S.; Rajovic, N.; Dumic, I.; Milovanovic, T. Colonic Diverticulosis and Non-Alcoholic Fatty Liver Disease: Is There a Connection? *Medicina* **2021**, *58*, 38. [CrossRef] [PubMed]
25. Aune, D.; Sen, A.; Leitzmann, M.F.; Norat, T.; Tonstad, S.; Vatten, L.J. Body mass index and physical activity and the risk of diverticular disease: A systematic review and meta-analysis of prospective studies. *Eur. J. Nutr.* **2017**, *56*, 2423–2438. [CrossRef]

Disclaimer/Publisher's Note: The statements, opinions and data contained in all publications are solely those of the individual author(s) and contributor(s) and not of MDPI and/or the editor(s). MDPI and/or the editor(s) disclaim responsibility for any injury to people or property resulting from any ideas, methods, instructions or products referred to in the content.

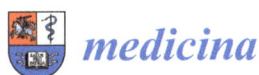

Article

Metabolic Associated Fatty Liver Disease (MAFLD) and COVID-19 Infection: An Independent Predictor of Poor Disease Outcome?

Vladimir Milivojević [1,2,*], Jelena Bogdanović [2,3], Ivana Babić [3], Nevena Todorović [4] and Ivan Ranković [5]

1. Clinic for Gastroenterology and Hepatology University Clinical Centre of Serbia, Dr Koste Todorovica 2, 11000 Belgrade, Serbia
2. Faculty of Medicine, University of Belgrade, Dr Subotica 8, 11000 Belgrade, Serbia
3. Clinic for Endocrinology, Diabetes and Metabolic Diseases University Clinical Centre of Serbia, Dr Subotica 13, 11000 Belgrade, Serbia
4. Clinic for Infectious and Tropical Diseases University Clinical Centre of Serbia, Bulevar Oslobođenja 16, 11000 Belgrade, Serbia
5. Department of Gastroenterology, Royal Cornwall Hospitals NHS Trust, Truro TR1 3LJ, UK; doctorranke@gmail.com
* Correspondence: dotorevlada@gmail.com; Tel.: +381-66-8302-675

Citation: Milivojević, V.; Bogdanović, J.; Babić, I.; Todorović, N.; Ranković, I. Metabolic Associated Fatty Liver Disease (MAFLD) and COVID-19 Infection: An Independent Predictor of Poor Disease Outcome?. *Medicina* **2023**, *59*, 1438. https://doi.org/10.3390/medicina59081438

Academic Editors: Ludovico Abenavoli and Marcello Candelli

Received: 9 July 2023
Revised: 3 August 2023
Accepted: 4 August 2023
Published: 8 August 2023

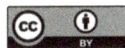

Copyright: © 2023 by the authors. Licensee MDPI, Basel, Switzerland. This article is an open access article distributed under the terms and conditions of the Creative Commons Attribution (CC BY) license (https://creativecommons.org/licenses/by/4.0/).

Abstract: *Background and Objectives*: Early reports on COVID-19 infection suggested that the SARS-CoV-2 virus solely attacks respiratory tract cells. As the pandemic spread, it became clear that the infection is multiorganic. Metabolic associated fatty liver disease (MAFLD) is a chronic liver disease strongly associated with insulin resistance and diabetes. The aim of this study was to assess a possible interplay between MAFLD and COVID-19 infection and its implication in COVID-19 outcome. *Materials and Methods*: A retrospective observational study, including 130 COVID-19 positive patients was conducted. MAFLD diagnosis was made based on the International Consensus criteria. Patients were divided into two groups, group A (MAFLD) and group B (nonMAFLD). Anthropometric and laboratory analysis were obtained. COVID-19 severity was assessed using the NEWS2 score. Disease outcome was threefold and regarded as discharged, patients who required mechanical ventilation (MV), and deceased patients. *Results*: MAFLD prevalence was 42%, 67% of patients were discharged, and 19% needed MV. Mortality rate was 14%. MAFLD patients were significantly younger ($p < 0.001$), and had higher body mass index ($p < 0.05$), respiratory rate ($p < 0.05$) and systolic blood pressure ($p < 0.05$) than nonMAFLD patients. Regarding metabolic syndrome and inflammatory markers: group A had significantly higher glycemia at admission ($p = 0.008$), lower HDL-c ($p < 0.01$), higher triglycerides ($p < 0.01$), CRP ($p < 0.001$), IL-6 ($p < 0.05$) and ferritin ($p < 0.05$) than group B. MAFLD was associated with more prevalent type 2 diabetes ($p = 0.035$) and hypertension ($p < 0.05$). MAFLD patients had a more severe disease course (NEWS2 score, 6.5 ± 0.5 vs. 3 ± 1.0, $p < 0.05$). MAFLD presence was associated with lower patient discharge ($p < 0.01$) and increased need for MV ($p = 0.024$). Multiple regression analysis showed that BMI ($p = 0.045$), IL-6 ($p = 0.03$), and MAFLD ($p < 0.05$) are significant independent risk factors for a poor COVID-19 outcome. *Conclusions*: The prevalence of MAFLD is relatively high. MAFLD patients had a more severe COVID-19 clinical course and worse disease outcome. Our results imply that early patient stratification and risk assessment are mandatory in order to avoid poor outcomes.

Keywords: COVID-19; MAFLD; disease outcome; severity

1. Introduction

Coronavirus disease 19 (COVID-19) is a disease that originated in China in December of 2019 and has, by now, reached a pandemic level [1]. It is caused by a pathogen, a novel coronavirus called the severe acute respiratory syndrome coronavirus (SARS-CoV-2). Similar infections from the same family of viruses have been noted before (SARS and MERS in 2003 and 2012, respectively), both reaching epidemic levels [2]. SARS-CoV-2 infection begins with the viral spike protein's attachment to an adequate host cell receptor. It has been shown that angiotensin-converting enzyme 2 (ACE2) is the prime surface protein that enables virus cell entrance [3]. However, the SARS-CoV-2 spike protein harbors a single mutation that significantly increases its affinity towards the ACE2 receptor, thus suggesting that this novel virus has evolved with an increased ability to spread among humans [4].

Early reports focused solely on respiratory tract involvement, but as the pandemic spread and further investigation was conducted, it became clear that COVID-19 affects other organs as well [5]. Accumulating evidence suggests that while the virus primarily affects the lungs, it can also affect other organs, causing systemic consequences, coagulopathy and multiple organ injuries. The etiology of the systemic effects of COVID-19 is multifold.

It has been suggested that there are several other receptors and coreceptors that facilitate virus entry, thus enabling one of the possible systemic effect mechanisms of SARS-CoV-2. Liver tropism of SARS-CoV-2 has been postulated before, considering ACE2 receptors have been found in the liver during biopsy [6,7]. However, mechanisms of liver injury in COVID-19 infection are multifold, including direct cytopathic effect, drug-induced injury, hypoxic injury, and cytokine-storm-enhanced inflammation in patients with chronic liver disease (CLD) [7]. The relationship between CLD and COVID-19 seems to be bidirectional, with COVID-19 worsening CLD through its systemic complications while at the same time, compromised liver function in patients with CLD may lead to adverse events in patients with concomitant COVID-19 infection [7].

Fatty liver disease (SLD) as a CLD was first described in 1886 and later further divided into alcoholic liver disease (ALD) and non-alcoholic fatty liver disease (NAFLD) [8]. By global consensus, a novel term of metabolic associated fatty liver disease (MAFLD) was proposed as a way of lifting the stigma off of patients with ALD, considering MAFLD is an inclusive diagnosis made based on the presence of several metabolic syndrome parameters, including obesity and/or diabetes [9]. Some scientists regard MAFLD as a hepatic complication of diabetes, considering the role of insulin resistance, low-grade inflammation, and oxidative stress in its pathogenesis [10]. MAFLD covers a broad spectrum of different disease phenotypes, from simple liver steatosis to fibrosis and ultimately liver failure [8].

Considering that previous studies have identified diabetes and obesity as risk factors for COVID-19 infection and having in mind that both diabetes and obesity, by definition, can accompany MAFLD, it places these patients in a vulnerable, COVID-19-susceptible group, potentially prone to adverse clinical outcomes. However, it is still controversial whether MAFLD is a causal factor in promoting the progression of COVID-19 infection or the said infection exacerbates the existing chronic disease, which in turn leads to poor disease outcome.

In that sense, the aim of our study was to assess a possible interplay between MAFLD and COVID-19 infection and its implication in COVID-19 outcomes.

2. Materials and Methods

2.1. Study Design

A retrospective observational study was conducted. A total of 130 patients treated at a tertiary health care center from June 2021 until November 2021 were included.

A COVID-19 infection diagnosis was made following a positive RT-PCR nasopharyngeal swab test. Patients were divided into two groups according to the presence of MAFLD. MAFLD diagnosis was made based on the international consensus criteria [9]. Hepatic steatosis was detected by imaging techniques (ultrasound of the abdomen) and blood biomarkers (fatty liver index, FLI). Patients were measured for waist circumeference and body mass index (BMI, kg/m^2), and classified as normal weight (<25 kg/m^2), overweight (25–29.9 kg/m^2), or obese (>30 kg/m^2). FLI was calculated by using the BMI, waist circumference, serum triglycerides, and gamma-glutamyl transferase (g-GT) levels. Type 2 diabetes (T2D) was diagnosed based on the patient's medical history or defined as: 1. fasting plasma glucose $\geq$ 7 mmol/L (126 mg/dL), 2. random plasma glucose $\geq$ 11.1 mmol/L (200 mg/dL), 3. HbA1c $\geq$ 7%, according to the American Diabetes Association (ADA) criteria [11]. Atherosclerotic cardiovascular disease (ASCVD) was regarded as the presence of coronary heart disease (CHD) such as myocardial infarction, angina or coronary artery disease, cerebrovascular disease, or peripheral artery disease [12]. Chronic kidney disease (CKD) was defined as decreased glomerular filtration (GFR) of less than 60 mL/min/1.73m^2 for at least three months [13]. Upon admission, vital parameters, including heart rate (HR), respiratory rate (RR), oxygen saturation (sO2), systolic (SBP) and diastolic blood pressure (DBP), body temperature (t), and state of consciousness, were assessed.

COVID-19 severity was determined using the National Early Warning Score 2 (NEWS2). The initial score, NEWS, was developed in 2012 by the Royal College of Physicians (RCP) in order to detect all-cause deterioration and predict disease outcome [14]. It comprises RR, oxygen saturation, SBP, body temperature, and state of consciousness. An upgraded version, NEWS2, differs from the previous in terms of the addition of new-onset confusion and a new oxygen saturation scale for hypercapnic respiratory failure (scale 2) [15]. Each category is scored 0–3 and combined to give an overall score with two and three additional points for the use of supplemental oxygen and altered state of consciousness (alert, verbal, pain, unresponsive (respectively). A total score ranges from 0 to 20, with patients being divided into three categories based on the clinical risk assessed: low (aggregate score 0–4), medium (aggregate score 5–6), and high (aggregate score 7 or more). If the patient scores 3 in any individual category, they are immediately classified as high-risk. It has been demonstrated that a higher NEWS2 score is a good predictor of short-term mortality in COVID-19 patients [16].

Disease outcome was regarded as: 1. discharged patients (survivors, not treated in the Intensive Care Unit (ICU)), 2. patients needing mechanical ventilation (MV), thus being transferred to the ICU, and 3. deceased patients (non-survivors).

2.2. Inclusion and Exclusion Criteria

Inclusion criteria consisted of COVID-19-positive consecutive patients aged > 18 years old. Exclusion criteria were pregnancy, previous viral hepatitis, cirrhosis, liver tumors (benign or malignant), or ALD.

2.3. Measurements

Data on comorbidities and vital, anthropometric, and biochemical parameters were obtained.

Assessed vital parameters were: RR (n/min), HR (n/min), SBP (mmHg), DBP (mmHg), body temperature (C), oxygen saturation (%), and state of consciousness (AVPU).

BMI was measured according to the equation weight (kg)/height (m^2). Biochemical data consisted of metabolic syndrome parameters taken after an 8 h fasting (glycemia (mmol/L and mg/dL), triglyceride levels (mmol/L and mg/dL) and HDL-cholesterol (mmol/L and mg/dL)) and synthetic liver function markers (AST (U/L), ALT (U/L), g-GT (U/L), ALP (U/L), albumins (g/L), and platelets (g/L)). The De Ritis coefficient was measured as the AST/ALT ratio and inflammatory markers (C-reactive protein (CRP) (mg/L), fibrinogen (g/L), ferritin (ug/L), and interleukin-6 (IL-6) (pg/mL)).

2.4. Ethical Compliance

Considering this is a retrospective study, all discharged participants were informed of the details of the study and signed an informed consent form for participation (regarding their medical data) in accordance with the Declaration of Helsinki. Regarding the medical dataset of the deceased patients, their representative family members were informed of the study details and signed an informed consent form. All procedures were conducted in accordance with standard clinical settings. The study was approved by the Ethics Committee of the University Clinical Centre of Serbia.

2.5. Statistical Analysis

Descriptive statistical analyses were performed. The normality test was performed for numerical variables and based on the test results, numerical variables were presented as means and standard deviation (SD). Categorial variables were presented as percentages (%). Comparisons of anthropometric and clinical variables between two groups were conducted using the Student *t*-test (for continuous variables) and the Chi square test (for categorical variables). The correlation was assessed using the Pearson correlation coefficient (r) for continuous variables. Univariate and multivariate logistic regression analyses were used to determine factors for disease outcome. The odds ratio (OR) and relative risk (RR) were measured with death and need for mechanical ventilation being used as a composite poor disease outcome. Results were expressed as OR and RR (respectively), with a corresponding 95% confidence interval (CI). The level of significance was set at 0.05. All statistical analyses were performed using SPSS 21.0.

3. Results

Among 130 COVID-19-positive patients, based on the international consensus criteria, 42% (n = 55) were placed in the MAFLD group (group A), while 58% (n = 75) of patients were placed in the nonMAFLD group (group B). The selection process is presented in Figure 1.

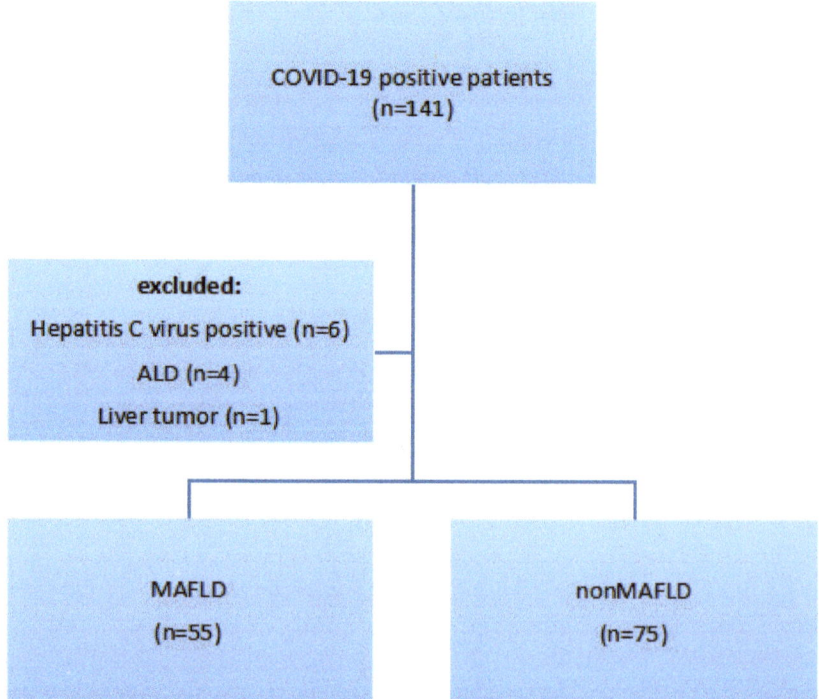

Figure 1. Inclusion process.

Concerning anthropometric parameters, age, gender, and BMI were evaluated. There was no statistically significant difference between groups concerning gender (male/female, 29/26 vs. 40/35, $p = 0.94$). MAFLD patients were significantly younger (53.5 ± 4.5 vs. 62.3 ± 4.2, $p < 0.001$) and had a higher BMI (28.5 ± 2.8 vs. 24.8 ± 3.1, $p < 0.001$), as seen in the Table 1.

Table 1. Anthropometric and vital parameters comparison at admission.

Anthropometric and Vital Parameters	MAFLD	nonMAFLD	p Value
Gender (male vs. female)	29/26	40/35	0.94
Age (years)	53.5 ± 4.5	62.3 ± 4.2	<0.001
Body mass index (BMI, kg/m^2)	28.5 ± 2.8	24.8 ± 3.1	<0.001
Respiratory rate (RR, n/min)	19.5 ± 3.1	16.2 ± 4.1	<0.001
Heart rate (HR, n/min)	89.1 ± 14.2	82.1 ± 11.9	0.6
Systolic blood pressure * (>140 mmHg, yes)	14	21	<0.05
Diastolic blood pressure * (<90 mmHg, yes)	7	11	0.43
Body temperature	37.4 ± 1.1	37.1 ± 0.9	0.09
Oxygen saturation * (supplemental oxygen, yes)	14	12	0.52

* number of patients.

Having assessed vital parameters, we noticed that MAFLD patients had a higher SBP (142.5 ± 10.1 vs. 130.4 ± 7.9, $p < 0.001$) while there was no difference considering DBP, RR, or HR (Table 1).

In order to evaluate the comorbidities-related differences between groups, we evaluated the prevalence and potential differences regarding T2D, ASCVD, heart failure (HF), arterial hypertension, CKD, and chronic obstructive pulmonary disease or asthma (COPD). It was noted that T2D was significantly more prevalent in the MAFLD group (63% vs. 37%, $p = 0.005$). Regarding other comorbidities, no significant difference between groups was observed (Figure 2).

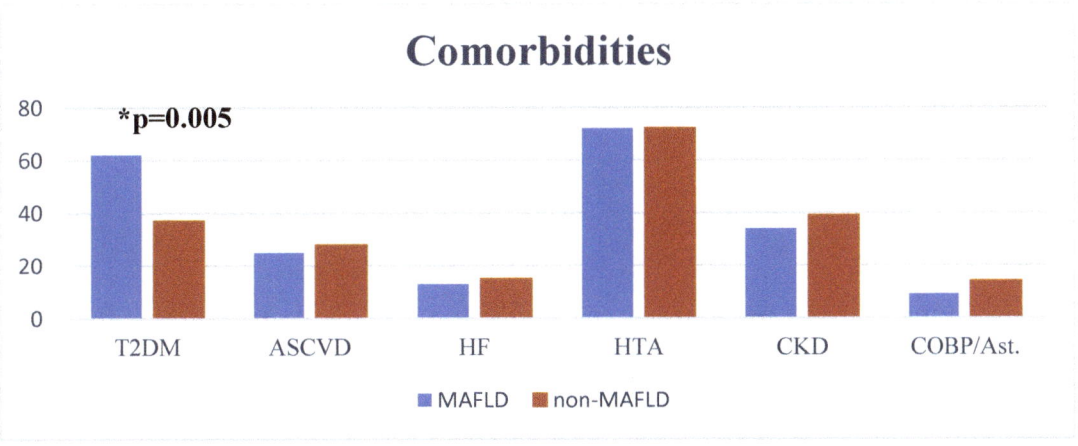

Figure 2. Comorbidites prevalence comparison.

Evaluation of liver function parameters showed significant in-between-group differences regarding aspartate aminotransferase (AST), alanine aminotransferase (ALT), gamma glutamyl transferase (g-GT), alkaline phosphatase (ALP), platelets, and albumin levels. Group A had significantly higher levels of AST (52.3 ± 11.2 vs. 45.5 ± 8.9, $p = 0.002$), ALT (64.4 ± 12.5 vs. 47.5 ± 10.2, $p = 0.001$), and ALP (108.3 ± 10.3 vs. 101.4 ± 13.3, $p = 0.001$) as presented in the Table 2. Simultaneously, no significant difference was noted regarding g-GT. On the other hand, the MAFLD group had significantly lower platelets (145 ± 14.2 vs. 179.5 ± 11.6, $p < 0.001$) and albumin levels (31 ± 4.5 vs. 38.5 ± 5.1, $p < 0.001$). A between-group difference was also observed for the AST to ALT (AST/ALT) ratio (De Ritis ratio), with a lower level in the MAFLD group (0.84 ± 0.04) as opposed to the nonMAFLD group (0.91 ± 0.03) ($p < 0.001$) (Table 2).

Table 2. Liver function markers: comparison.

Liver Function Parameters	MAFLD	nonMAFLD	p Value
AST (U/L)	52.3 ± 11.2	45.5 ± 8.9	0.002
ALT (U/L)	64.4 ± 12.5	47.5 ± 10.2	<0.001
ALP (U/L)	108.3 ± 10.3	101.4 ± 13.3	0.0017
g-GT (U/L)	40.4 ± 11.0	41.5 ± 9.9	0.55
De Ritis coefficient	0.84 ± 0.04	0.91 ± 0.03	<0.001
Albumins (g/L)	31 ± 4.5	38.5 ± 5.1	<0.001
Platelets (g/L)	145 ± 14.2	179.5 ± 11.6	<0.001

Notes: upper normal limits: AST 37 U/L, ALT 41 U/L, g-GT 38 U/L, ALP 120 U/L, albumins 53 g/L, platelets 424×10^9/L.

Having assessed inflammatory markers, we observed a significant difference regarding C-reactive protein (CRP), interleukin-6 (IL-6), and ferritin, with the MAFLD group having higher levels of the aforementioned markers compared with nonMAFLD patients (CRP: 29.5 ± 11.0 vs. 21.2 ± 7.9, $p < 0.001$, IL-6: 56.5 ± 5.1 vs. 54.2 ± 4.1, $p < 0.05$, ferritin: 331.2 ± 31.0 vs. 256.2 ± 28.5, $p < 0.05$). There was no significant in-between-group difference regarding fibrinogen levels (4.6 ± 1.2 vs. 4.5 ± 1.1, $p = 0.62$) as shown in Table 3.

Table 3. Inflammatory markers: comparison.

Inflammatory Markers	MAFLD	nonMAFLD	p Value
CRP (mg/L)	29.5 ± 11.0	21.2 ± 7.9	<0.001
IL-6 (pg/mL)	56.5 ± 5.1	54.2 ± 4.1	<0.05
Ferritin (µg/L)	331.2 ± 31.0	256.2 ± 28.5	<0.05
Fibrinogen (g/L)	4.6 ± 1.2	4.5 ± 1.1	0.62

Notes: upper normal limits: CRP 5.0 g/L, IL-6 7.0 pg/mL, ferritin 150.0 ug/L, fibrinogen 4.0 g/L.

Concerning metabolic syndrome parameters, MAFLD patients had higher triglycerides (Tg) (59.4 ± 16.2) and fasting glycemia levels (151.2 ± 21.6) as compared with the nonMAFLD group: Tg 50.4 ± 18.0 ($p < 0.001$), glycemia 127.8 ± 46.8 ($p = 0.008$). At the same time, HDL-cholesterol (HDL-c) levels were lower in group A than in group B (12.6 ± 1.8 vs. 18.0 ± 7.2, $p < 0.01$) (Table 4).

Table 4. Metabolic syndrome parameters: comparison.

Metabolic Syndrome Parameters	MAFLD	nonMAFLD	p Value
HDL-cholesterol (mg/dL)	12.6 ± 1.8	18.0 ± 7.2	<0.01
Triglycerides (mg/dL)	59.4 ± 16.2	50.4 ± 18.0	<0.001
Fasting glycemia (mg/dL)	151.2 ± 21.6	127.8 ± 46.8	0.008
SBP (mmHg)	142.5 ± 10.1	130.4 ± 7.9	<0.001
DBP (mmHg)	82.2 ± 5.6	83.0 ± 5.8	0.43

Analysis of disease severity was made using the validated NEWS2 score, with higher values indicating higher risk of COVID-19 severity and expressed as mean ± SD.

Results showed that MAFLD patients had a higher NEWS2 score (5.5 ± 1.1) than nonMAFLD patients (3.6 ± 0.9) ($p < 0.001$), as presented in Figure 3.

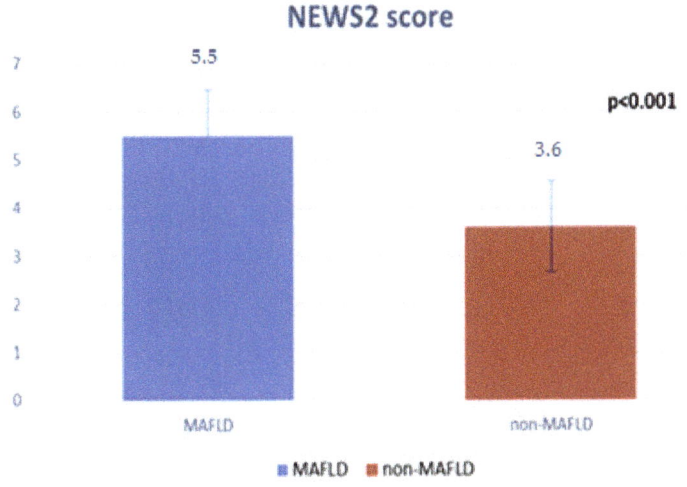

Figure 3. Disease severity: comparison.

Further subanalysis of disease severity by dividing patients into low, medium, and high risk groups revealed a gradual increase in the number of MAFLD patients in the medium and high risk groups as compared to the low risk patient group. Results presented in Figure 4 indicate only MAFLD patients were stratified into medium and high risk groups.

Disease outcome was threefold and was regarded as discharged patients, patients needing MV, and deceased patients. Group A had a lower number of discharged patients than Group B (60% vs. 81%, $p = 0.007$). Further, MAFLD patients had a higher need for MV than nonMAFLD patients (22% vs. 8%, $p = 0.024$), while no significant difference was noted concerning the death rate (18% vs. 11%, $p = 0.24$) between groups (Figure 5). In further analysis, a composite outcome of need for MV and death was used as a marker for poor disease outcome.

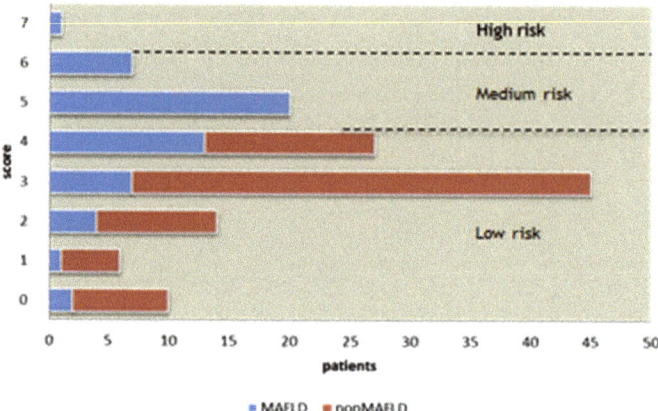

Figure 4. Patient stratification in risk-groups according to NEWS2 score: comparison.

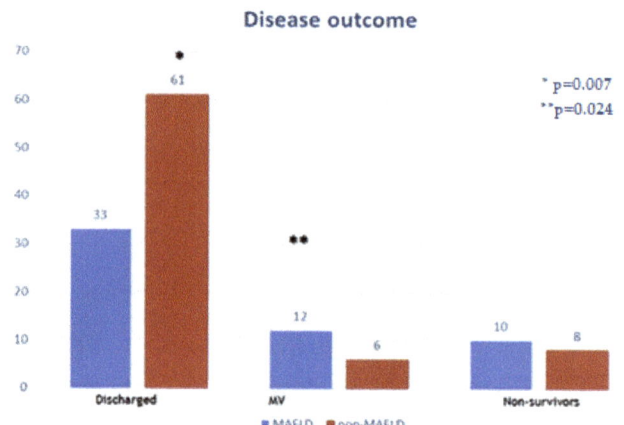

Figure 5. Individual disease outcome parameters: comparison.

Using univariate logistic regression analysis, MAFLD presence, BMI, HDL-c, Tg, SBP, and IL-6 were found to be significantly associated with poor disease outcome. In the final multivariate regression analysis, three predictors of poor COVID-19 outcome, namely MAFLD (odds ratio (OR) 3.4, 95% confidence interval (CI) 3.0–6.3; $p < 0.001$), BMI (OR 2.3, 95% CI 1.7–3.1; $p = 0.045$), and IL-6 (OR 2.1, 95% CI (1.2–2.3); $p = 0.03$), remained significant (Figure 6, Table 5). In order to avoid overestimating the effect of MAFLD presence on poor COVID-19 outcomes, a risk ratio was further calculated. A relative risk of MAFLD patients having a poor disease outcome was 2.1 (95% CI 1.2–3.8, $p < 0.001$).

Table 5. Multivariate regression analysis: predictors of COVID-19 outcome.

Variables	B	SE	OR (95% CI)	p Value
MAFLD (yes vs. no)	2.1	0.30	3.5 (3.1–6.5)	<0.001
BMI	1.9	0.05	2.5 (1.5–3.4)	0.045
IL-6	2.0	0.60	2.2 (1.8–2.7)	0.03

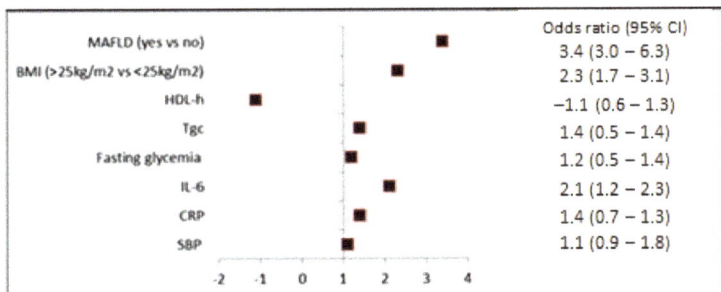

Figure 6. Regression analysis: odds ratio for predictors of COVID-19 outcome.

4. Discussion

In the present study, we provide vital insight into the prevalence of MAFLD and its possible association with COVID-19 severity and outcome.

Metabolic syndrome represents a cluster of diseases such as type 2 diabetes, obesity, hypertension, and dyslipidemia [17]. All of these conditions have been proven to pose a risk for poor outcome of COVID-19 infection [17,18]. MAFLD is often regarded as a hepatic complication of diabetes and, in that sense, may contribute to the development of a more severe form of COVID-19 [19].

In our retrospective observational study, MAFLD was diagnosed in 42% of COVID-19-positive patients. The prevalence of MAFLD has been steadily growing in the past two decades, from 25.5% before 2005 to 38.9% in 2020, with the highest prevalence reported in the Middle East (31.79%) and South America (30.45%) and the lowest in Africa (13.48%) [20].

It is thought that the increasing burden of other metabolic diseases such as type 2 diabetes (T2D), dyslipidemia, and obesity is the main driving force behind the increase in MAFLD prevalence. Notably, in the last two years, concurrent with the global COVID-19 pandemic, a much greater increase (2.16 annual rate of change) in the prevalence of MAFLD has been reported [21]. It is estimated that by 2040, the prevalence of MAFLD will be 55.7%, which is a three-fold increase since 1990 and a 43.2% increase from the 2020 prevalence of 38.9% [21]. As of now, MAFLD is the most common chronic liver disease (CLD) and a leading cause of liver-related morbidity and mortality [22].

The diagnosis of MAFLD in the setting of COVID-19 infection is challenging, considering numerous studies have shown an increase in liver enzyme levels during COVID-19 infection [6,7,23]. It is still not fully understood what the driving mechanism behind this process is. Noticeably, in our study MAFLD patients had significantly elevated hepatocellular dysfunction markers. This is interesting considering our findings dominantly point to liver injury on a hepatocellular level. However, previous studies on extrapulmonary manifestations of COVID-19 and conducted liver biopsies proved ACE2 receptors were dominantly present on cholangiocytes [7]. Nevertheless, this could be explained by the multifold nature of COVID-19-mediated liver injury [23]. Additionally, this can be attributed to the condition itself, considering elevated liver enzymes are part of the MAFLD diagnostic criteria. Patients with preexisting liver disease (LD) are more susceptible to disease deterioration during an infection, with COVID-19 being one of the most challenging ones [24]. However, this phenomenon was also noted in patients without previous liver dysfunction [25]. It has been postulated that an uncontrolled immune response with a high release of cytokines causing hyperinflammation and consequently multi-organ damage may be one of the possible causators [23]. On the other hand, metabolic diseases, such as MAFLD, T2D, and obesity, cause low-grade inflammation through certain proinflammatory cytokines such as TNFalpha and IL-6, which can act as a steppingstone in a vicious cycle of hyperinflammation and cytokine storm, resulting in target organ damage [7]. In highly specific circumstances, such as COVID-19 infection, in order to exclude confounding factors in diagnosing MAFLD, imaging techniques such as ultrasound and CT scan are of great help and should be used as diagnostic tools alongside other criteria as proposed by the International Consensus Report Guidelines [9].

The presence of MAFLD was evaluated upon patient admission and regarded as a newly diagnosed condition for the majority of our patients, highlighting the fact that most of our patients were unaware of LD presence even when harboring multiple risk factors. Studies have shown a lack of awareness regarding the prevalence and diagnosis of MAFLD, which suggests the need for large-scale implementations of educational programs [26].

In our study, MAFLD patients were significantly younger and expectedly had a higher BMI. However, mean BMI did not reach the obesity grade level. Nevertheless, it has been reported that not only obese patients but also overweight patients are at a higher risk of developing a severe form of COVID-19 and needing respiratory support as well as invasive ventilation [27]. The patophysiological mechanisms underlying the association between BMI and COVID-19 severity are multifold and probably a result of the bidirectional relationship between virus and host impairment [28]. The immunomodulatory effect of chronic low-grade inflammation present in overweight people simultaneously with suboptimal T-cell and B-cell responses and possible dysfunctional respiratory capacity in overweight people suggests the possibility of invasive ventilation susceptibility [29]. Studies have shown that overweight and obesity are independent risk factors for a critical clinical course of COVID-19 infection even in the young population, which is in line with our findings, considering our MAFLD patients were significantly younger than the nonMAFLD patient group [30].

Our patients had a higher respiratory rate (RR) and a higher systolic blood pressure (SBP). Both of these parameters have been shown to indicate a poor prognosis in sepsis-related critical conditions [31]. It has been shown that RR is an indicator of lower respiratory tract infection and is deemed an important tool for assessing disease severity in clinical settings [32]. Additionally, it has been shown that not only arterial hypertension as a chronic disease but also acutely elevated SBP values were associated with poor disease outcome [33]. High SBP was identified as a covariate in both mortality and survival prediction models and was present in deceased COVID-19 patients as compared to discharged individuals [33]. Even though there was no statistical difference noted in the presence of hypertension in our patient groups, it is worth noting that elevated SBP could be a marker of pre-existing hypertension-mediated subclinical organ damage (HMOD, i.e., vascular stiffness), thus representing an important comorbidity factor [34]. Higher SBP could also be the consequence of reduced enzymatic activity of ACE2 caused by the binding of a higher SARS-CoV-2 load [35].

Secondary to hypertension, type 2 diabetes (T2D) was proven to be the most common comorbidity in patients with COVID-19 infection as well as the most common concomitant disease in patients with MAFLD [18,36]. In keeping with that, in our study, T2D was significantly more prevalent in MAFLD than in the nonMAFLD group. The impact of T2D on COVID-19 severity and outcome still remains a controversial topic. Early reports have proposed diabetes as a major risk factor for COVID-19 development. A Chinese meta-analysis showed a 9.8% prevalence of diabetes among COVID-19 hospitalized patients, which is the equivalence of overall diabetes prevalence in China [37]. In a similarly structured large study conducted in the UK, 32% of participants had T2D [38]. However, it was later established that diabetes per se does not contribute to COVID-19 susceptibility, but poorly controlled diabetes and acute hyperglycemia are risk factors for hospital admission, disease severity, and its poor outcome [39]. Recent meta-analyses showed that diabetes increases the risk of severity by three times, and two-and-a-half times the risk of COVID-19-associated death [40]. Studies have shown that even short-term hyperglycemia can cause an impaired immune system response and compromise both innate and adaptive mechanisms of action [41]. Moreover, diabetes causes decreased expression of ACE2, which in turn has antioxidative capacity and lowers inflammation, thus making COVID-19 diabetics more susceptible to hyper-inflammation and cytokine storm [42].

It is established that insulin resistance can be regarded as a cornerstone for fatty liver development [36]. Perturbations in insulin action lead to increased liver lipid accumulation, a process called lipotoxicity. While assessing lipid status of our patients, lipid abnormalities regarding triglycerides (Tg) and HDL-cholesterol (HDL-c) were noted. MAFLD patients had a significantly higher level of Tg and a significantly lower level of HDL-c as opposed to the nonMAFLD group. Recently, studies have emerged proposing that atherogenic dyslipidemia be used as a predictor of the critical COVID-19 course [43]. Apart from being closely linked to insulin resistance and diabetes, whose pathophysiological mechanisms of damage in COVID-19 were previously discussed, atherogenic dyslipidemia itself, regardless of diabetes status, may play a role in poor clinical outcome in COVID-19 hospitalized patients. In a retrospective Italian study, Bellia et al. found atherogenic dyslipidemia to be significantly more prevalent in critically ill patients and was associated with mortality in both the diabetes cohort and overall population of COVID-19 hospitalized patients [43]. This association was more potentiated if paired with visceral and/or overall obesity, as marked by the BMI. This is in accordance with our results, considering MAFLD patients were predominantly overweight and had a significantly higher BMI than nonMAFLD group. However, when adjusted for sex, age, and other confounding factors, Tg and HDL-c did not show significant contributions regarding disease course and outcome.

Regarding pro-inflammatory markers, MAFLD patients had significantly higher levels of CRP and ferritin. CRP is an acute-phase protein synthesized in the liver and is expectedly elevated in inflammatory states such as infection or tissue injury [44]. Considering MAFLD is closely related to greater derangements in the metabolic profile and linked to low-grade inflammation, it has been postulated that CRP can potentially be used as a valuable tool in predicting its progression. CRP is a proven independent risk factor for cardiovascular and all-cause mortality in a number of chronic diseases, LD included [45]. However, its role in predicting liver-related morbidity and mortality remains controversial [46]. Even though MAFLD patients had higher CRP levels than the nonMAFLD group, in further analysis, CRP failed to reach statistical significance regarding its independent contribution to COVID-19 outcomes. Furthermore, ferritin is another acute phase reactant that has emerged as a potential marker for MAFLD disease activity considering insulin resistance, inflammation, and steatosis (all found in MAFLD) lead to an altered iron metabolism, thus causing elevated ferritin levels [47]. Numerous studies have confirmed increased ferritin in patients with MAFLD/NAFLD [48]. Kowdley et al. showed an independent association between ferritin level and increased risk for liver fibrosis in patients with NAFLD [48]. On the contrary, two large retrospective studies concluded that even though ferritin was associated with liver steatosis, it was a poor predictor of fibrosis stage and disease progression [49]. This was in keeping with our results. Both MAFLD and nonMALD patients had ferritin levels above the reference range, with the MAFLD group having significantly higher levels. However, that could be contributed to the over-inflammation response caused by the SARS-CoV-2 virus targeting already inflamed liver tissue. Further analysis excluded ferritin as an independent predictor of COVID-19 outcome.

It is widely accepted that cytokines play a critical role in the pathogenesis of MAFLD by activating various signaling pathways that interfere with insulin signaling [50]. Pro-inflammatory cytokines secreted by adipose tissue involved in this process include, among others, interleukin-6 (IL-6). It has been postulated that IL-6 plays a critical role in virus-induced cytokine storm, hence, a recombinant humanized monoclonal antibody IL-6 receptor inhibitor, tocilizumab, has recently emerged as an alternative treatment for COVID-19 [51]. On the other hand, considering MAFLD is closely related to immunologically activated adipose tissue, studies have shown IL-6 levels to be elevated in patients with this condition [52]. Our study confirmed what was expected: all COVID-19 patients had increased IL-6, with MAFLD patients expressing significantly higher levels. This could be attributed to IL-6 being a marker of inflamed liver and/or adipose tissue. Even though the MAFLD group had a higher BMI, robustly indicating a higher source of adipose tissue as a possible explanation for the difference in IL-6, studies have shown that regardless of body fat percentage, MAFLD is associated with higher IL-6 [53]. It has been noted that in the setting of COVID-19 infection, IL-6 has additive potential for indicating disease severity [54]. In that sense, we noted that IL-6 was an independent predictor of disease outcome, with higher levels of the cytokine corresponding to higher mortality and mechanical ventilation as markers for disease outcome.

Following the first reports of certain patient groups suffering rapid health deterioration and needing invasive respiratory support, it became clear that patient stratification would be mandatory. Efforts have been made in order to produce the best tool possible for early patient triage.

The National Early Warning Score (NEWS) had been recommended by the Royal College of Physicians in 2012 as a standardized track and trigger early warning system to grade acute illness severity, detect acute clinical deterioration, and help guide clinical decision-making [14]. An updated version of NEWS, NEWS2, was developed in 2017 and, by 2020, was widely used across the UK for early disease stratification in acutely ill patients with undifferentiated illness or sepsis. In the setting of COVID-19, NEWS2 showed superiority to other similarly constructed scores, with high sensitivity and specificity in early risk assessment [16].

MAFLD patients showed an overall higher score rating upon admission as opposed to the nonMAFLD group, with higher ratings in almost every NEWS2 parameter. Noticeably, the prevalence of nonMAFLD patients was significantly higher in the low clinical risk group. However, there were zero nonMAFLD patients stratified into medium and high clinical risk.

Regarding clinical outcome, MAFLD patients more significantly showed the need for mechanical ventilation, while nonMAFLD patients were more frequently discharged. There was no significant difference regarding death as a clinical outcome. When assessing a composite outcome consisting of MV need and death, again, the nonMAFLD group showed favorable results.

Assessing individual risk factors, MAFLD presence, higher BMI, and elevated IL-6 showed statistically significant unfavorable effects of the COVID-19 outcome.

Based on our results, poor clinical course and worse disease outcome of MAFLD patients could be attributed to various factors that, unfortunately, in this vulnerable patient group seem to act simultaneously. Higher cardiometabolic risk (reflected by dyslipidemia, dysglycemia, and higher BMI), low grade inflammation (further potentiated by the COVID-19 infection) and the burden of having more than one chronic-metabolic-dysfunction associated disease, contribute to further compromisation of patients' immune defense mechanisms, ultimately leading to worse COVID-19 outcome.

Our study has certain limitations. It is an observational retrospective study; hence, a certain level of bias is hard to avoid. Direct patient comparison was made at the beginning of their hospital stay and hence may not have reflected the interrelationship between MAFLD and COVID-19 in the best way. Additionally, a moderate number of MAFLD patients were included. However, to the best of our knowledge, this is the first study reporting Serbian experience regarding MAFLD prevalence and association with COVID-19 course and outcome.

5. Conclusions

MAFLD prevalence has been on the rise in the last two decades following the increase in global prevalence of other closely related metabolic disorders. Immunomodulatory effects, hyper-inflammation, and chronic oxidative stress have made this already vulnerable population more susceptible to respiratory derangement. COVID-19-positive patients with MAFLD are at a higher risk of developing a more severe form of the disease as well as a worse disease outcome. Early patient stratification with the assessment of independent risk factors is mandatory in order to make specific recommendations, and provide guidance on therapy, all in order to ultimately achieve better treatment results.

Author Contributions: Conceptualization, V.M., I.R. and I.B.; methodology, I.B. and N.T.; investigation, V.M., J.B. and I.B.; software, I.B.; validation, V.M.; formal analysis, V.M. and I.B.; resources, V.M. and I.R.; data curation, J.B. and I.R.; writing—original draft preparation, V.M. and I.B.; writing—review and editing, I.R.; visualization, I.B. and N.T.; supervision, V.M. and I.R. All authors have read and agreed to the published version of the manuscript.

Funding: This research received no external funding.

Institutional Review Board Statement: The study was approved by the Ethics Committee of the University Clinical Centre of Serbia (No 788/21, September 2021).

Informed Consent Statement: All patients were informed regarding the aim of the study and provided written informed consent in accordance with the Declaration of Helsinki.

Data Availability Statement: Data regarding investigated patients and statistical analysis will not be made publicly available.

Conflicts of Interest: The authors declare no conflict of interest.

References

1. Kumar, A.; Singh, R.; Kaur, J.; Pandey, S.; Sharma, V.; Thakur, L.; Sati, S.; Mani, S.; Asthana, S.; Sharma, T.K.; et al. Wuhan to World: The COVID-19 Pandemic. *Front. Cell. Infect. Microbiol.* **2021**, *11*, 596201. [CrossRef]
2. Petrosillo, N.; Viceconte, G.; Ergonul, O.; Ippolito, G.; Petersen, E. COVID-19, SARS and MERS: Are they closely related? *Clin. Microbiol. Infect.* **2020**, *26*, 729–734. Available online: https://www.clinicalmicrobiologyandinfection.com/article/S1198-743X(20)30171-3/fulltext (accessed on 5 July 2023). [CrossRef] [PubMed]
3. Wu, C.; Liu, Y.; Yang, Y.; Zhang, P.; Zhong, W.; Wang, Y.; Wang, Q.; Xu, Y.; Li, M.; Li, X.; et al. Analysis of therapeutic targets for SARS-CoV-2 and discovery of potential drugs by computational methods. *Acta Pharm. Sin. B* **2020**, *10*, 766–788. [CrossRef] [PubMed]
4. Amicone, M.; Borges, V.; Alves, M.J.; Isidro, J.; Zé-Zé, L.; Duarte, S.; Vieira, L.; Guiomar, R.; Gomes, J.P.; Gordo, I. Mutation rate of SARS-CoV-2 and emergence of mutators during experimental evolution. *Evol. Med. Public Health* **2022**, *10*, 142–155. [CrossRef]
5. Puelles, V.G.; Lütgehetmann, M.; Lindenmeyer, M.T.; Sperhake, J.P.; Wong, M.N.; Allweiss, L.; Chilla, S.; Heinemann, A.; Wanner, N.; Liu, S.; et al. Multiorgan and Renal Tropism of SARS-CoV-2. *N. Engl. J. Med.* **2020**, *383*, 590–592. [CrossRef]
6. Sarkesh, A.; Sorkhabi, A.D.; Sheykhsaran, E.; Alinezhad, F.; Mohammadzadeh, N.; Hemmat, N.; Baghi, H.B. Extrapulmonary Clinical Manifestations in COVID-19 Patients. *Am. J. Trop. Med. Hyg.* **2020**, *103*, 1783–1796. [CrossRef]
7. Marjot, T.; Moon, A.; Stamataki, Z.; Wong, V.; Webb, G.; Barnes, E.; Barritt, A. COVID-19 and liver disease: Mechanistic and clinical perspectives. *Nat. Rev. Gastroenterol. Hepatol.* **2021**, *18*, 348–364. [CrossRef] [PubMed]
8. Riazi, K.; Azhari, H.; Charette, J.H.; Underwood, F.E.; King, J.A.; Afshar, E.E.; Swain, M.G.; Congly, S.E.; Kaplan, G.G.; Shaheen, A.-A. The prevalence and incidence of NAFLD worldwide: A systematic review and meta-analysis. *Lancet Gastroenterol. Hepatol.* **2022**, *7*, 851–861. [CrossRef] [PubMed]
9. Eslam, M.; Sanyal, A.J.; George, J.; International Consensus Panel. MAFLD: A Consensus-Driven Proposed Nomenclature for Metabolic Associated Fatty Liver Disease. *Gastroenterology* **2020**, *158*, 1999–2014.e1. [CrossRef]
10. Fouad, Y.; Waked, I.; Bollipo, S.; Gomaa, A.; Ajlouni, Y.; Attia, D. What's in a name? Renaming 'NAFLD' to 'MAFLD'. *Liver Int.* **2020**, *40*, 1254–1261. [CrossRef]
11. American Diabetes Association Professional Practice Committee. 2. Classification and Diagnosis of Diabetes: Standards of Medical Care in Diabetes—2022. *Diabetes Care* **2022**, *45* (Suppl. S1), S17–S38. [CrossRef]
12. Wong, N.D.; Budoff, M.J.; Ferdinand, K.; Graham, I.M.; Michos, E.D.; Reddy, T.; Shapiro, M.D.; Toth, P.P. Atherosclerotic cardiovascular disease risk assessment: An American Society for Preventive Cardiology clinical practice statement. *Am. J. Prev. Cardiol.* **2022**, *10*, 100335. [CrossRef]
13. Kidney Disease: Improving Global Outcomes (KDIGO) Diabetes Work Group. KDIGO 2022 Clinical Practice Guideline for Diabetes Management in Chronic Kidney Disease. *Kidney Int.* **2022**, *102* (Suppl. S5), S1–S127. [CrossRef] [PubMed]
14. Jones, M. NEWSDIG: The National Early Warning Score Development and Implementation Group. *Clin. Med.* **2012**, *12*, 501–503. Available online: https://www.rcpjournals.org/content/clinmedicine/12/6/501 (accessed on 5 July 2023). [CrossRef] [PubMed]
15. Williams, B. The National Early Warning Score 2 (NEWS2) in patients with hypercapnic respiratory failure. *Clin. Med.* **2019**, *19*, 94–95. [CrossRef]
16. Gidari, A.; De Socio, G.V.; Sabbatini, S.; Francisci, D. Predictive value of National Early Warning Score 2 (NEWS2) for intensive care unit admission in patients with SARS-CoV-2 infection. *Infect. Dis.* **2020**, *52*, 698–704. [CrossRef] [PubMed]
17. Mendrick, D.L.; Diehl, A.M.; Topor, L.S.; Dietert, R.R.; Will, Y.; La Merrill, M.A.; Bouret, S.; Varma, V.; Hastings, K.L.; Schug, T.T.; et al. Metabolic Syndrome and Associated Diseases: From the Bench to the Clinic. *Toxicol. Sci.* **2018**, *162*, 36–42. [CrossRef] [PubMed]
18. Russell, C.D.; Lone, N.I.; Baillie, J.K. Comorbidities, multimorbidity and COVID-19. *Nat. Med.* **2023**, *29*, 334–343. [CrossRef] [PubMed]

19. Mare, R.; Sporea, I. Gastrointestinal and Liver Complications in Patients with Diabetes Mellitus—A Review of the Literature. *J. Clin. Med.* **2022**, *11*, 5223. [CrossRef]
20. Younossi, Z.M.; Golabi, P.; Paik, J.M.; Henry, A.; Van Dongen, C.; Henry, L. The global epidemiology of nonalcoholic fatty liver disease (NAFLD) and nonalcoholic steatohepatitis (NASH): A systematic review. *Hepatology* **2023**, *77*, 1335–1347. [CrossRef]
21. Cheung, K.S.; Mok, C.H.; Mao, X.; Zhang, R.; Hung, I.F.; Seto, W.K.; Yuen, M.F. COVID-19 vaccine immunogenicity among chronic liver disease patients and liver transplant recipients: A meta-analysis. *Clin. Mol. Hepatol.* **2022**, *28*, 890–911. [CrossRef]
22. Pouwels, S.; Sakran, N.; Graham, Y.; Leal, A.; Pintar, T.; Yang, W.; Kassir, R.; Singhal, R.; Mahawar, K.; Ramnarain, D. Non-alcoholic fatty liver disease (NAFLD): A review of pathophysiology, clinical management and effects of weight loss. *BMC Endocr. Disord.* **2022**, *22*, 63. [CrossRef] [PubMed]
23. Ning, Q.; Wu, D.; Wang, X.; Xi, D.; Chen, T.; Chen, G.; Wang, H.; Lu, H.; Wang, M.; Zhu, L.; et al. The mechanism underlying extrapulmonary complications of the coronavirus disease 2019 and its therapeutic implication. *Signal Transduct. Target. Ther.* **2022**, *7*, 57. [CrossRef] [PubMed]
24. Hu, X.; Sun, L.; Guo, Z.; Wu, C.; Yu, X.; Li, J. Management of COVID-19 patients with chronic liver diseases and liver transplants: COVID-19 and liver diseases. *Ann. Hepatol.* **2022**, *27*, 100653. [CrossRef]
25. Khawaja, J.; Bawa, A.; Omer, H.; Ashraf, F.; Zulfiqar, P. COVID-19 Infection Presenting as an Isolated Severe Acute Liver Failure. *Cureus* **2022**, *14*, e24873. [CrossRef] [PubMed]
26. Vrsaljko, N.; Samadan, L.; Viskovic, K.; Mehmedović, A.; Budimir, J.; Vince, A.; Papic, N. Association of Nonalcoholic Fatty Liver Disease With COVID-19 Severity and Pulmonary Thrombosis: CovidFAT, a Prospective, Observational Cohort Study. *Open Forum Infect. Dis.* **2022**, *9*, ofac073. Available online: https://academic.oup.com/ofid/article/9/4/ofac073/6524775 (accessed on 5 July 2023). [CrossRef] [PubMed]
27. Longmore, D.K.; Miller, J.E.; Bekkering, S.; Saner, C.; Mifsud, E.; Zhu, Y.; Saffery, R.; Nichol, A.; Colditz, G.; Short, K.R.; et al. Diabetes and Overweight/Obesity Are Independent, Nonadditive Risk Factors for In-Hospital Severity of COVID-19: An International, Multicenter Retrospective Meta-analysis. *Diabetes Care* **2021**, *44*, 1281–1290. [CrossRef]
28. Tanaka, M.; Itoh, M.; Ogawa, Y.; Suganami, T. Molecular mechanism of obesity-induced 'metabolic' tissue remodeling. *J. Diabetes Investig.* **2018**, *9*, 256–261. [CrossRef]
29. Paich, H.A.; Sheridan, P.A.; Handy, J.; Karlsson, E.A.; Schultz-Cherry, S.; Hudgens, M.G.; Noah, T.L.; Weir, S.S.; Beck, M.A. Overweight and obese adult humans have a defective cellular immune response to pandemic H1N1 Influenza a virus. *Obesity* **2013**, *21*, 2377–2386. [CrossRef]
30. Deng, Y.; Qi, Y.; Deng, L.; Wang, H.; Xu, Y.; Li, Z.; Meng, Z.; Tang, J.; Dai, Z. Obesity as a Potential Predictor of Disease Severity in Young COVID-19 Patients: A Retrospective Study. *Obesity* **2020**, *28*, 1815–1825. [CrossRef]
31. Asiimwe, S.B.; Abdallah, A.; Ssekitoleko, R. A simple prognostic index based on admission vital signs data among patients with sepsis in a resource-limited setting. *Crit. Care* **2015**, *19*, 86. [CrossRef] [PubMed]
32. Strauß, R.; Ewig, S.; Richter, K.; König, T.; Heller, G.; Bauer, T.T. The prognostic significance of respiratory rate in patients with pneumonia: A retrospective analysis of data from 705 928 hospitalized patients in Germany from 2010–2012. *Dtsch. Arztebl. Int.* **2014**, *111*, 503–508. [PubMed]
33. Du, Y.; Zhou, N.; Zha, W.; Lv, Y. Hypertension is a clinically important risk factor for critical illness and mortality in COVID-19: A meta-analysis. *Nutr. Metab. Cardiovasc. Dis.* **2021**, *31*, 745–755. Available online: https://www.nmcd-journal.com/article/S0939-4753(20)30518-4/fulltext (accessed on 5 July 2023). [CrossRef] [PubMed]
34. Gallo, G.; Calvez, V.; Savoia, C. Hypertension and COVID-19: Current Evidence and Perspectives. *High Blood Press. Cardiovasc. Prev.* **2022**, *29*, 115–123. [CrossRef] [PubMed]
35. Delalić, Đ.; Jug, J.; Prkačin, I. Arterial hypertension following COVID-19: A retrospective study of patients in a Central European tertiary care center. *Acta Clin. Croat.* **2022**, *61*, 23–27.
36. Yuan, Q.; Wang, H.; Gao, P.; Chen, W.; Lv, M.; Bai, S.; Wu, J. Prevalence and Risk Factors of Metabolic-Associated Fatty Liver Disease among 73,566 Individuals in Beijing, China. *Int. J. Environ. Res. Public Health* **2022**, *19*, 2096. [CrossRef]
37. Li, H.; Tian, S.; Chen, T.; Cui, Z.; Shi, N.; Zhong, X.; Qiu, K.; Zhang, J.; Zeng, T.; Chen, L.; et al. Newly diagnosed diabetes is associated with a higher risk of mortality than known diabetes in hospitalized patients with COVID-19. *Diabetes Obes. Metab.* **2020**, *22*, 1897–1906. [CrossRef]
38. Ramanathan, K.; Antognini, D.; Combes, A.; Paden, M.; Zakhary, B.; Ogino, M.; MacLaren, G.; Brodie, D.; Shekar, K. Planning and provision of ECMO services for severe ARDS during the COVID-19 pandemic and other outbreaks of emerging infectious diseases. *Lancet Respir. Med.* **2020**, *8*, 518–526. Available online: https://www.thelancet.com/journals/lanres/article/PIIS2213-2600(20)30121-1/fulltext (accessed on 5 July 2023). [CrossRef]
39. Gerganova, A.; Assyov, Y.; Kamenov, Z. Stress Hyperglycemia, Diabetes Mellitus and COVID-19 Infection: Risk Factors, Clinical Outcomes and Post-Discharge Implications. *Front. Clin. Diabetes Healthc.* **2022**, *3*, 826006. [CrossRef]
40. Lima-Martínez, M.M.; Boada, C.C.; Madera-Silva, M.D.; Marín, W.; Contreras, M. COVID-19 and diabetes: A bidirectional relationship. *Clin. Investig. Arterioscler.* **2021**, *33*, 151–157. [CrossRef]
41. Jafar, N.; Edriss, H.; Nugent, K. The Effect of Short-Term Hyperglycemia on the Innate Immune System. *Am. J. Med. Sci.* **2016**, *351*, 201–211. [CrossRef] [PubMed]

42. Roberts, J.; Pritchard, A.L.; Treweeke, A.T.; Rossi, A.G.; Brace, N.; Cahill, P.; MacRury, S.M.; Wei, J.; Megson, I.L. Why Is COVID-19 More Severe in Patients with Diabetes? The Role of Angiotensin-Converting Enzyme 2, Endothelial Dysfunction and the Immunoinflammatory System. *Front. Cardiovasc. Med.* **2021**, *7*, 629933. [CrossRef] [PubMed]
43. Bellia, A.; Andreadi, A.; Giudice, L.; De Taddeo, S.; Maiorino, A.; D'ippolito, I.; Giorgino, F.M.; Ruotolo, V.; Romano, M.; Magrini, A.; et al. Atherogenic Dyslipidemia on Admission Is Associated with Poorer Outcome in People With and Without Diabetes Hospitalized for COVID-19. *Diabetes Care* **2021**, *44*, 2149–2157. [CrossRef] [PubMed]
44. Sproston, N.R.; Ashworth, J.J. Role of C-Reactive Protein at Sites of Inflammation and Infection. *Front. Immunol.* **2018**, *9*, 754. [CrossRef] [PubMed]
45. Tian, R.; Tian, M.; Wang, L.; Qian, H.; Zhang, S.; Pang, H.; Liu, Z.; Fang, L.; Shen, Z. C-reactive protein for predicting cardiovascular and all-cause mortality in type 2 diabetic patients: A meta-analysis. *Cytokine* **2019**, *117*, 59–64. [CrossRef]
46. Lambrecht, J.; Tacke, F. Controversies and Opportunities in the Use of Inflammatory Markers for Diagnosis or Risk Prediction in Fatty Liver Disease. *Front. Immunol.* **2021**, *11*, 634409. [CrossRef] [PubMed]
47. Mousavi, S.R.M.; Geramizadeh, B.; Anushiravani, A.; Ejtehadi, F.; Anbardar, M.H.; Moini, M. Correlation between Serum Ferritin Level and Histopathological Disease Severity in Non-alcoholic Fatty Liver Disease. *Middle East J. Dig. Dis.* **2018**, *10*, 90–95. [CrossRef]
48. Kowdley, K.V.; Belt, P.; Wilson, L.A.; Yeh, M.M.; Neuschwander-Tetri, B.A.; Chalasani, N.; Sanyal, A.J.; Nelson, J.E.; the NASH Clinical Research Network. Serum ferritin is an independent predictor of histologic severity and advanced fibrosis in patients with nonalcoholic fatty liver disease. *Hepatology* **2012**, *55*, 77–85. [CrossRef]
49. Wang, H.; Sun, R.; Yang, S.; Ma, X.; Yu, C. Association between serum ferritin level and the various stages of non-alcoholic fatty liver disease: A systematic review. *Front. Med.* **2022**, *9*, 934989. [CrossRef]
50. Das, S.K.; Balakrishnan, V. Role of Cytokines in the Pathogenesis of Non-Alcoholic Fatty Liver Disease. *Indian J. Clin. Biochem.* **2011**, *26*, 202–209. [CrossRef]
51. Shekhawat, J.; Gauba, K.; Gupta, S.; Purohit, P.; Mitra, P.; Garg, M.; Misra, S.; Sharma, P.; Banerjee, M. Interleukin-6 Perpetrator of the COVID-19 Cytokine Storm. *Indian J. Clin. Biochem.* **2021**, *36*, 440–450. [CrossRef] [PubMed]
52. Singh, P. Evaluation of Pro-Inflammatory Markers IL-6 and TNF-a and their Correlation with Non-Alcoholic Fatty Liver Disease. *J. Adv. Res. Med.* **2019**, *6*, 1–6. [CrossRef]
53. Kuchay, M.S.; Martínez-Montoro, J.I.; Choudhary, N.S.; Fernández-García, J.C.; Ramos-Molina, B. Non-Alcoholic Fatty Liver Disease in Lean and Non-Obese Individuals: Current and Future Challenges. *Biomedicines* **2021**, *9*, 1346. [CrossRef]
54. Papic, N.; Samadan, L.; Vrsaljko, N.; Radmanic, L.; Jelicic, K.; Simicic, P.; Svoboda, P.; Lepej, S.Z.; Vince, A. Distinct Cytokine Profiles in Severe COVID-19 and Non-Alcoholic Fatty Liver Disease. *Life* **2022**, *12*, 795. [CrossRef] [PubMed]

Disclaimer/Publisher's Note: The statements, opinions and data contained in all publications are solely those of the individual author(s) and contributor(s) and not of MDPI and/or the editor(s). MDPI and/or the editor(s) disclaim responsibility for any injury to people or property resulting from any ideas, methods, instructions or products referred to in the content.

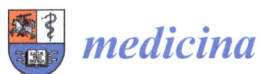

Article

Are Short-Stay Units Safe and Effective in the Treatment of Non-Variceal Upper Gastrointestinal Bleeding?

Marcello Candelli [1,*], Maria Lumare [1], Maria Elena Riccioni [2], Antonio Mestice [1], Veronica Ojetti [1], Giulia Pignataro [1], Giuseppe Merra [3], Andrea Piccioni [1], Maurizio Gabrielli [1], Antonio Gasbarrini [2] and Francesco Franceschi [1]

[1] Emergency, Anesthesiological and Reanimation Sciencese Department, Fondazione Policlinico Universitario A. Gemelli—IRCCS of Rome, 00168 Rome, Italy; maria.lumare01@icatt.it (M.L.); antonio.mestice01@icatt.it (A.M.); veronica.ojetti@policlinicogemelli.it (V.O.); giulia.pignataro@policlinicogemelli.it (G.P.); andrea.piccioni@policlinicogemelli.it (A.P.); maurizio.gabrielli@policlinicogemelli.it (M.G.)

[2] Medical and Abdominal Surgery and Endocrine-Metabolic Scienze, Fondazione Policlinico Universitario A. Gemelli—IRCCS of Rome, 00168 Rome, Italy; mariaelena.riccioni@policlinicogemelli.it (M.E.R.)

[3] Biomedicine and Prevention Department, Section of Clinical Nutrition and Nutrigenomics, Facoltà di Medicina e Chirurgia, Università degli Studi di Roma Tor Vergata, 00133 Rome, Italy; giuseppe.merra@uniroma2.it

* Correspondence: marcello.candelli@policlinicogemelli.it; Tel.: +39-0630153161

Abstract: *Introduction*: Emergency Department (ED) overcrowding is a health, political, and economic problem of concern worldwide. The causes of overcrowding are an aging population, an increase in chronic diseases, a lack of access to primary care, and a lack of resources in communities. Overcrowding has been associated with an increased risk of mortality. The establishment of a Short Stay Unit (SSU) for conditions that cannot be treated at home but require treatment and hospitalization for up to 72 h may be a solution. SSU can significantly reduce hospital length of stay (LOS) for certain conditions but does not appear to be useful for other diseases. Currently, there are no studies addressing the efficacy of SSU in the treatment of non-variceal upper gastrointestinal bleeding (NVUGIB). Our study aims to evaluate the efficacy of SSU in reducing the need for hospitalization, LOS, hospital readmission, and mortality in patients with NVUGIB compared with admission to the regular ward. *Materials and Methods*: This was a retrospective, single-center observational study. Medical records of patients presenting with NVUGIB to ED between 1 April 2021, and 30 September 2022, were analyzed. We included patients aged >18 years who presented to ED with acute upper gastrointestinal tract blood loss. The test population was divided into two groups: Patients admitted to a normal inpatient ward (control) and patients treated at SSU (intervention). Clinical and medical history data were collected for both groups. The hospital LOS was the primary outcome. Secondary outcomes were time to endoscopy, number of blood units transfused, readmission to the hospital at 30 days, and in-hospital mortality. *Results*: The analysis included 120 patients with a mean age of 70 years, 54% of whom were men. Sixty patients were admitted to SSU. Patients admitted to the medical ward had a higher mean age. The Glasgow-Blatchford score, used to assess bleeding risk, mortality, and hospital readmission were similar in the study groups. Multivariate analysis after adjustment for confounders found that the only factor independently associated with shorter LOS was admission to SSU ($p < 0.0001$). Admission to SSU was also independently and significantly associated with a shorter time to endoscopy ($p < 0.001$). The only other factor associated with a shorter time to EGDS was creatinine level ($p = 0.05$), while home treatment with PPI was associated with a longer time to endoscopy. LOS, time to endoscopy, number of patients requiring transfusion, and number of units of blood transfused were significantly lower in patients admitted to SSU than in the control group. *Conclusions*: The results of the study show that treatment of NVUGIB in SSU can significantly reduce the time required for endoscopy, the hospital LOS, and the number of transfused blood units without increasing mortality and hospital readmission. Treatment of NVUGIB at SSU may therefore help to reduce ED overcrowding but multicenter randomized controlled trials are needed to confirm these data.

Citation: Candelli, M.; Lumare, M.; Riccioni, M.E.; Mestice, A.; Ojetti, V.; Pignataro, G.; Merra, G.; Piccioni, A.; Gabrielli, M.; Gasbarrini, A.; et al. Are Short-Stay Units Safe and Effective in the Treatment of Non-Variceal Upper Gastrointestinal Bleeding?. *Medicina* **2023**, *59*, 1021. https://doi.org/10.3390/medicina59061021

Academic Editor: Adolfo Francesco Attili

Received: 28 March 2023
Revised: 5 May 2023
Accepted: 23 May 2023
Published: 25 May 2023

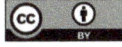

Copyright: © 2023 by the authors. Licensee MDPI, Basel, Switzerland. This article is an open access article distributed under the terms and conditions of the Creative Commons Attribution (CC BY) license (https://creativecommons.org/licenses/by/4.0/).

Keywords: gastrointestinal bleeding; short stay unit; emergency department; overcrowding; peptic ulcer; anticoagulant

1. Introduction

Emergency department (ED) overcrowding is a worldwide problem of great concern to health care systems, policy makers, and the public. ED overcrowding is defined as a situation in which demand for ED services exceeds the capacity of ED, resulting in patients waiting longer for care, longer wait times, and even boarding of patients at ED. The causes of ED overcrowding are complex and multifactorial and can include factors related to patient demand, hospital resources, and system-level issues. Key factors contributing to ED overcrowding include increased patient demand, a shortage of hospital beds, lack of resources in the community, and delays in patient flow within the hospital. ED is often the first point of contact for patients with acute illnesses or injuries, and demand for ED services has steadily increased over the years. This increase in patient demand is caused by factors such as an aging population, an increase in chronic diseases, and a lack of access to primary care. The shortage of hospital beds can lead to longer waiting times at ED as patients wait for a bed to become available. This is especially true for patients who need to be admitted to the hospital. The lack of resources in the community, such as primary care clinics and mental health services, can lead to patients seeking care at ED rather than receiving it through channels that are more appropriate. Delays in patient flow within the hospital, such as delays in test results, consultation with specialists, or admission to the hospital, can also contribute to overcrowding [1]. The consequences of ED overcrowding can be severe, leading to delays in treatment, increased patient morbidity and mortality, and lower patient satisfaction. ED overcrowding can also lead to higher health care costs, as patients may require more complex and expensive treatment when delays in care occur. To address ED overcrowding, several solutions have been proposed around the world. These include initiatives to improve patient flow, such as fast-track pathways for patients with minor injuries or illnesses, and the use of clinical decision units to care for patients who do not require hospitalization. Interventions to reduce unnecessary visits ED have also been proposed, such as improving access to primary care and promoting patient education [2]. It is important to note that while these solutions have proven effective in some cases, there is no one-size-fits-all solution for ED crowding. Implementing these solutions may require a tailored approach that considers the specific needs of each health system and population. Short-stay units (SSUs) in ED have been suggested as a potential solution to reduce overcrowding and improve patient flow. SSUs are designated areas within the ED, where patients can be treated for up to 24–72 h before either being discharged or transferred to another hospital unit. Several studies suggest that SSUs can effectively reduce ED overcrowding and improve patient flow. For example, an Italian review found that the introduction of a SSU resulted in a significant reduction in ED length of stay, risk of in–hospital acquired infections, and boarding time [3]. Other studies found that SSUs could reduce length of stay (LOS) and mortality in patients with chronic obstructive pulmonary disease (COPD) and acute heart failure (AHF), but at the cost of higher readmission rates [4,5]. Even in elderly patients, the incidence of adverse events may be lower when admitted to SSU than to a medical ward, as shown by Strom C et al. in an observational study in Denmark [6]. However, a review of 10 studies highlighted that the quality and evidence of safety and efficacy of SSU are low and that further studies are needed to compare usual care and SSU to better understand the potential benefits and limitations [7]. SSUs have been proposed for several conditions. Upper gastrointestinal bleeding (UGIB) is a common emergency that often requires urgent investigation and treatment and is one of the possible indications for hospital admission to a SSU. Studies evaluating SSUs are often performed on all patients who have access to them and include patients with UGIB [8]. At now, there are no studies that address the safety and efficacy of SSUs in the management of UGIB. The aim of our study was to evaluate the efficacy of SSU in reducing the need for hospitalization, length of hospital stay, hospital readmission, number of blood units transfused and mortality in patients with non-variceal UGIB (NVUGIB) presenting to ED.

2. Materials and Methods

This is a retrospective, monocentric observational study conducted using electronic medical records (EMR) of 120 patients presenting with NVUGIB from 1 April 2022 to 30 September 2022 at ED of Fondazione Policlinico Agostino Gemelli Hospital—IRCCS of Rome. Patients with gastrointestinal bleeding come to our ED in a variety of ways. They may present to our emergency department on their own, or they may call the public emergency service and be transported by ambulance, and finally, they may be transferred from other lower level hospitals that do not have the appropriate resources to diagnose, treat, and manage the pathology affecting the patient (spoke centres). In our study, we only included patients who came to our hospital on their own or through emergency services, and not those who were referred by our spoke centres. At our hospital, patients who come to the emergency department with a diagnosis of suspected gastrointestinal bleeding and do not require intensive care are admitted to our SSU as their first choice. If beds are not available at SSU, patients are assigned to a gastroenterology or internal medicine department. The medical staff of our SSU consists of all the doctors of ED, who take turns to take care of the patients admitted there, and a chief physician with expertise in gastroenterology.

We enrolled 60 patients who were admitted to our SSU from April 2022 to June 2022, and 60 patients who were admitted to a medical ward from July 2022 to September 2022, when the SSU was closed. The study aims is to compare patient outcomes and resource utilization between two groups: those admitted to a regular medical ward (control group) and those treated at ED in a SSU (intervention group). The study population consists of adult patients (18 years or older) who present to ED with UGIB, defined as acute blood loss from the upper gastrointestinal tract (hematemesis or melena). Patients with chronic UGIB, variceal bleeding and those requiring immediate surgical intervention or admission to intensive care unit (ICU), palliative care and patients with an initial prognosis of less than 6 months of life were excluded. Electronic medical recorder data were collected for each patient, including demographic information, medical history, vital signs, laboratory and endoscopic results, treatment, therapies, disposition (admission or discharge), hospital length of stay (LOS), time to endoscopy, healthcare utilization (e.g., number of blood units transfused) and, Rockwood clinical frailty scale. Outcome measures: The primary outcome measure was hospital LOS (from triage registration to discharge). Secondary outcomes include time to endoscopy (from triage registration to endoscopy), number of blood units consumed, hospital readmission at 30 days, and in-hospital mortality. Statistical analysis: Descriptive statistics has been used to summarize the patient characteristics and outcome measures for each group. Continuous data were described as mean and standard deviation or median and interquartile range. Categorical data were described as percentages. Bivariate analysis was used to compare the characteristics and outcomes between the control and intervention groups (Chi square test or Fisher's exact test for categorical data and Student's T-Test or Mann-Whitney U test for continuous data). Multivariate regression analysis has been used to adjust for potential confounding factors (e.g., age, comorbidities, severity of illness) and to estimate the effect of SSUs on the primary and secondary outcomes.

Ethics and approvals: This study has been conducted in accordance with ethical guidelines and regulations, and approved from the Ethical Board of Catholic University of the Sacred heart of Rome, Italy, (ID:5378)

3. Results

The current analysis includes 120 patients (mean age 69.6 ± 0.7 years), of whom 54% were men. Overall, 60 of the patients (50) were admitted to short stay unit (SSU) and

60 (50%) were admitted to an internal medicine ward. In Table 1 are showed patients demographic, clinical and laboratory and outcomes data.

Table 1. Patients' demographic, comorbidities, laboratory, and outcomes data.

	All Patients (N = 120)	SSU (N = 60)	Medical Ward (N = 60)	p
Demographic data				
Age (years, M ± SD)	69.6 ± 16	66.4 ± 16	72.6 ± 16	**0.03**
Males N (%)	65 (54)	29 (48)	36 (60)	0.2
RCFS (Median and IQR)	4 (2–5)	4 (3–5)	4 (2–4)	0.83
Clinical presentation at ED				
Melena N (%)	110 (91.6)	55 (91.6)	55 (91.6)	1
Hematemesis N (%)	8 (6.7)	4 (6.7)	4 (6.7)	1
Rectal bleeding + UGIB N (%)	2 (1.7)	1 (1.7)	1 (1.7)	1
Duration of symptoms at admission (M ± SD)	34 ± 23	32 ± 25	35 ± 22	0.09
Comorbidities N (%)				
Diabetes	25 (21)	10 (17)	15 (25)	0.26
Hypertension	48 (40)	34 (57)	22 (37)	0.46
Coronary Heart Disease	21 (17)	9 (15)	12 (20)	0.52
Congestive Heart Failure	10 (8)	5 (8)	5 (8)	1
Chronic Liver Disease	6 (5)	2 (3)	4 (7)	0.7
Atrial Fibrillation	32 (27)	12 (20)	20 (33)	0.1
COPD	15 (12)	5 (8)	10 (17)	0.17
Active cancer	22 (18)	4 (7)	18 (30)	**0.002**
History of stroke	9 (7)	1 (2)	8 (13)	**0.03**
Chronic Kidney Disease	11 (9)	4 (7)	7 (12)	0.53
Previous bariatric surgery	6 (5)	4 (7)	2 (3)	0.7
Autoimmune diseases	6 (5)	3 (5)	3 (5)	1
VTE	6 (5)	3 (5)	3 (5)	1
N. of comorbidities >1	54 (45)	21 (35)	33 (55)	**0.03**
RCFS > 4	32 (27)	14 (23)	18 (30)	0.68
At-home treatment N (%)				
Anticoagulants	33 (27)	12 (20)	21 (35)	0.07
VKA	5 (4)	0 (0)	5 (4)	0.21
DOAC	22 (18)	10 (17)	12 (20)	0.64
Dabigatran	4 (3)	3 (5)	1 (2)	0.62
Apixaban	4 (3)	1 (2)	3 (5)	0.62
Rivaroxaban	4 (3)	0 (0)	4 (7)	0.36
Edoxaban	12 (10)	6 (10)	4 (7)	0.74
LMWH	5 (7)	1 (2)	4 (7)	0.36
Fondaparinux	1 (2)	1 (3)	0 (0)	0.81
Antiplatelets	29 (24)	13 (22)	16 (27)	0.52
ASA	23 (27)	11 (18)	12 (20)	0.82
Clopidogrel	10 (8)	5 (8)	5 (8)	1
Others antiplatelets	4 (3)	0 (0)	4 (7)	0.36
Dual antiplatelets therapy	8 ((7)	3 (5)	5 (8)	0.77
Anticoagulant + Antiplatelets	3 (2)	1 (2)	2 (3)	1
NSAIDs	12 (10)	5 (8)	7 (12)	0.54
Corticosteroids	8 (7)	2 (3)	6 (10)	0.27
PPI	33 (27)	15 (25)	28 (47)	**0.01**
Laboratory and vital signs (M ± DS)				
Hemoglobin (g/dL)	8.7 ± 2	9.0 ± 2	8.3 ± 2	0.11
WBC ($\times 10^9$/L)	8794 ± 3350	8960 ± 3270	8629 ± 3447	0.62
Neutrophils ($\times 10^7$/L)	7040 ± 6564	6450 ± 2900	7633 ± 8819	0.31
Plt ($\times 10^9$/L)	260 ± 97	273 ± 104	247 ± 90	0.15
INR	1.2 ± 1	1.1 ± 1	1.3 ± 1	**0.04**
Na$^+$ (mmol/L)	139 ± 3	139 ± 3	138 ± 4	0.43
K+ (mmol/L)	4.2 ± 1	4.3 ± 1	4.1 ± 1	0.15
Creatinine (mg/dL)	1.2 ± 1	1.1 ± 1	1.4 ± 1	0.06
SBP (mm/Hg)	110 ± 18	109 ± 16	112 ± 17	0.34
Heart Rate (beats/min)	94 ± 12	95 ± 14	93 ± 10	0.62
BUN (mmol/L)	9.6 ± 7	9.6 ± 6	9.7 ± 7	0.98
Glasgow-Blatchford Score *	10 (7–12)	10 (7–13)	10 (8–12)	0.89

Table 1. Cont.

	All Patients (N = 120)	SSU (N = 60)	Medical Ward (N = 60)	p
Outcome N (%)				
Patients who need transfusion	69 (57)	28 (47)	41 (68)	**0.02**
Blood unit transfused *	1 (0–2)	0 (0–2)	2 (0–2)	**0.04**
Readmission at 30 days	3 (3)	1 (2)	2 (3)	1
In-hospital death	2 (2)	0 (0)	2 (3)	0.76
Admission to hospital	67 (56)	7 (12)	60 (100)	**<0.0001**
Outcome (M ± SD)				
Length of Hospital stay (h)	214 ± 209	126 ± 133	298 ± 212	**<0.0001**
Time to endoscopy (h)	66 ± 14	31 ± 39	104 ± 119	**<0.0001**
Time to admission (h)	45 ± 26	33 ± 21	67 ± 30	**<0.001**
Time from endoscopy to discharge	145 ± 181	99 ± 131	199 ± 207	**<0.0001**

Legend. SSU: short stay unit, M: media, SD: standard deviation, N: number, IQR: interquartile range, RCFS: Rackwood clinical frailty scale, ED: emergency department, COPD: chronic obstructive pulmunary disease, VTE: venous thromboembolism, VKA: vitamine K antagonist, DOAC: direct oral anticoagulants, LMWH: low molecular weight heparin, ASA: actylsalicyclic acid, NSAIDS: non steroidal anti-inflammatory drugs, PPI: proton pump inhibitor, WBC: white blood cells, Plt: platelets, INR: international normalized ratio, Na^+: sodium, K^+: potassium, SBP: systolic blood pressure, BUN: Blood urea nitrogen, h: hours. * (Median and Interquartile Range). Significant p values are written in bold.

The main duration of symptom before admission was 34 ± 23 h with a wide range (2–72 h). However no difference in duration of symptoms before admission was found between patients admitted in the SSU and controls (32 ± 25 vs. 35 ± 22 h, p = 0.09). The distribution of symptoms duration before addmission was similar between groups (p = 0.68). Patients admitted directly to medical ward has a higher mean age (72.6 ± 16 vs. 66.4 ± 16 years; p = 0.03), a higher probability to have 2 or more comorbidities (55 vs. 35%; p = 0.03)), a higher chance to had a history of cerebrovasculare disease (13 vs. 2%; p = 0.03) and active cancer (30 vs. 7%; p = 0.03). No difference in use of anticoagulants or antiplatelets drugs was found between groups. The at-home use of proton pump inhibitors (PPI) was statistically lower in patients admitted to SSU then in controls (25 vs. 47%: p = 0.01). Among evaluated laboratory data only the international normalized ratio (INR) was found slightly but significantly higher in patients admitted to medical ward then in patients admitted to SSU (1.3 ± 1 vs. 1.1 ± 1; p = 0.04). The number of comorbidities between groups was showed in Figure 1. To evaluate the risk of bleeding in enrolled patients we used the Glasgow Blatchford bleeding Score (GBS). Study and control groups showed similar GBS). Both the median scores and the distribution of the Rockwood Fraility Clinical Score did not differ between case and control (p = 0.83 and 0.64, respectively). Finally, the number of patients with a RCFS > 4 was similar between patients admitted in the SSU and in the medical ward (Table 1).

Thirty-two patients had an history of previous gastrointestinal beeding, 13 in the SSU group and 19 in control group (22 vs. 32%; p: 0.22) In hospital mortality and readmisson to the hospital at 30 days were very low and similar between group. LOS, time to endoscopy, number of patients who need trasfusion, number of unit of blood transfused were significantly lower in patients admitted to SSU then in controls. Finally, we found no differences in mortality and the need for hospital readmission 30 days after discharge (Table 1). In Table 2 are showed the sources of UIGB.

Other sources non described in the table were 3 gastric antral vascular ectasias (GAVE, 1 in SSU), 2 Dieulafoy's lesion (1 in SSU) and 5 neoplasms (1 gastric malignancy in SSU and 2 in control group, 1 duodenal malignancy in control group and 1 biliary neoplasm infiltrating duodenum in SSU). In Table 3 are described the Forrest's classification of peptic ulcers in our patients. No statistical difference was found between studied groups.

None of the patients participating in the study required urgent or elective surgery during their hospital stay.

No difference in the number and type of hemostatic techniques was found between the study groups. Mechanical hemostasis with endoscopic clips was the most commonly used means of controlling and treating the source of bleeding. Thermocoagulation (with argon plasma coagulation or heater bipolar probe), injection of diluted (1:10,000) epinephrine, and injection of fibrin glue were also used alone or in conjunction with mechanical hemostasis. Table 4 lists all hemostatic techniques used in the patients studied.

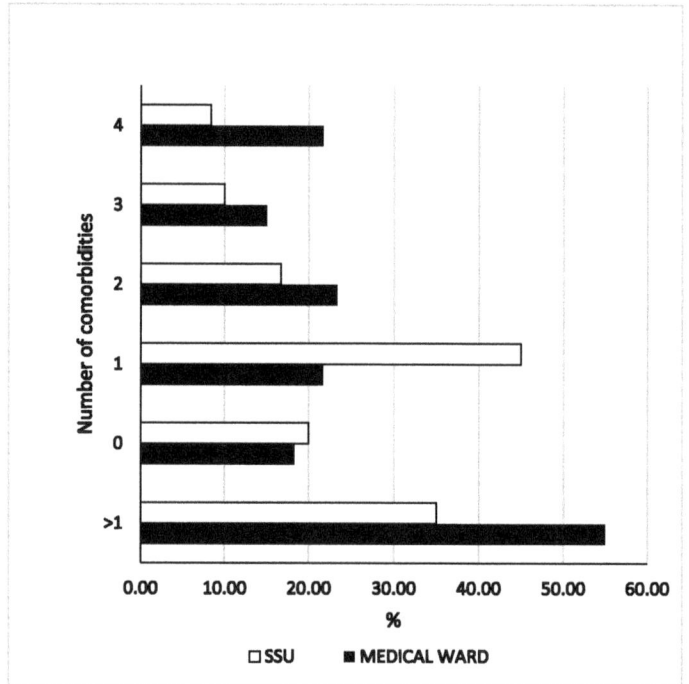

Figure 1. Number of comorbidities in patients admitted to medical ward or SSU. SSU: short stay unit. $p = 0.03$ between groups for 2 comorbidities or more.

Table 2. Sources of gastrointestinal bleeding.

Type of NVUGIB N (%)	All Patients (120)	SSU (60)	Medical Ward (60)	p
Peptic Ulcer	66 (55)	42 (70)	24 (40)	**0.001**
Gastric Ulcer	35 (29)	23 (38)	12 (20)	**0.03**
Duodenal Ulcer	31 (26)	19 (32)	12 (20)	0.14
Erosive hemorrhagic gastritis	15 (12)	4 (7)	11 (18)	0.1
Angiodysplasia	8 (7)	3 (5)	5 (8)	0.72
Obscure gastrointestinal bleeding	10 (8)	4 (7)	6 (10)	0.51
Esophagitis	11 (9)	3 (5)	8 (13)	0.20
Other sources	10 (8)	4 (7)	6 (10)	0.74

Legend. NVUGIB: non-variceal upper gastrointestinal bleeding; N: number, SSU: short stay unit. Significant p values are written in bold

Finally, we performed two multivariate linear regression for the two continue outcomes we found related with SSU admission (LOS and time to endoscopy). We corrected for age, sex and all the variables that at univariate analyses had a p level of at least 0.1. The only factor that resulted independently associated to a reduced LOS were the SSU admission ($p < 0.0001$). The atrial fibrillation was associated to an increased LOS ($p < 0.01$). The SSU admission resulted independently and significantly associated to a shorter time to endoscopy ($p < 0.001$). The others only factor associated to a reduced time to EGDS was the creatinine levels ($p = 0.05$). At the contrary, the at-home treatment with PPI was associated to a longer time to endoscopy ($p < 0.05$).

Table 3. Forrest's classification in patients with peptic ulcer disease between groups.

Forrest Classification	All Patients (66)	SSU (42)	Medical Ward (24)	p
III	40 (61)	25 (60)	15 (62)	0.90
IIc	7 (11)	5 (12)	2 (8)	1.00
IIb	3 (4.5)	1 (2)	2 (8)	0.55
IIa	11 (17)	9 (21)	2 (8)	0.30
I	5 (7)	2 (5)	3 (12)	0.34

Legend. NVUGIB: non-variceal upper gastrointestinal bleeding; SSU: short stay unit.

Table 4. Endoscopic hemostatic treatment used.

Hemostasis N (%)	All Patients (120)	SSU (60)	Medical Ward (60)	p
Any techniques	35 (29)	17 (28)	18 (30)	0.84
Endoscopic clip	23 (19)	11 (18)	12 (20)	0.81
Epinephrine injection	9 (8)	5 (8)	4 (7)	0.99
Thermocoagulation	8 (7)	5 (8)	3 (5)	0.72
Fibrin glue	7 (7)	5 (8)	2 (3)	0.44
2 or more combined tool	s15 (13)	10 (17)	5 (8)	0.27

4. Discussion

SSUs are used worldwide to reduce ED waiting times, overcrowding, and hospital admissions. However, according to a recent meta-analysis, there is still inconclusive evidence of their efficacy and safety due to heterogeneity of outcomes, pathologies considered, and admission criteria to SSU [7]. For example, a recent study of patients with heart failure showed that there were no differences in safety and efficacy between patients discharged from SSU and patients discharged directly from ED [9]. In contrast, other studies have found that SSU can reduce LOS for patients with atrial fibrillation, chest pain, and syncope [10–12]. The extreme diversity of pathologies studied in a SSU is likely the main cause of the conflicting results in the literature. Our study focused on NVUGIB, a condition not previously treated in a SSU. NVUGIBs are an important cause of ED visits and result in a high number of admissions to internal medicine and gastroenterology departments [13]. We retrospectively compared outcomes of patients with NVUGIB treated in a SSU or in a medical ward of our tertiary teaching hospital. Bleeding severity was assessed by GBS and did not differ between the 2 groups. Patient frailty assessed with the Rockwood Clinical Frailty Scale and time of onset of symptoms on arrival at the emergency department did not differ between the two groups studied and therefore do not appear to be factors that could explain the observed differences in LOS. However, some variables evaluated such as, age and the number of concomitant diseases were higher in patients treated as inpatients than in those admitted at SSU. For this reason, we adjusted the results for these potential confounders and for variables that showed significant differences between groups in univariate analysis. Even after correction, patients treated in the SSU had significantly lower LOS than patients admitted to an internal medicine ward. The shorter time from triage to admission underscores that at least part of the overall reduction in length of stay is due to the faster bed turnover in SSU compared with medical wards. Regarding the shortening of the time from endoscopy to discharge by SSU compared to the medical department, we can hypothesize that physicians in the internal medicine departments are more likely to look at the patient from all sides and spend more time resolving other, non-acute problems of the patient. The availability of diagnostic tools and care providers at any point in the day may have facilitated timely decision-making in the SSU compared to hospitalized patients. In addition, the emergency doctor treating patients at the SSU may face increased pressure from the ED to expedite discharge. Finally, the reduction in time to endoscopy we observed for patients admitted to SSU is certainly another important factor in reducing overall LOS. The time to endoscopy determined in our study was high and certainly higher than the time to endoscopy recommended in the main international guidelines. However, time to endoscopy was calculated based on triage registration rather than visit to ED. Given the overcrowding in emergency departments, the time between triage registration and physician visit can be very long. In addition, urgent endoscopy, especially for patients seen at night or on holidays, is performed in the operating room reserved for emergencies and competes with other surgical procedures. Obviously, unstable surgical patients are prioritized over stabilized patients with suspected gastrointestinal bleeding. We believe that the shorter time to endoscopy for patients admitted to SSU is related to endoscopists' perception of a requests from the ED, which includes SSU, as more urgent than requests for in-hospital admitted patients. The shorter time to endoscopy is probably related to the lower number of transfusions in patients admitted to SSU. It is likely that earlier treatment of the bleeding source contributes to a lower need for red blood cell units. However, the lower hemoglobin levels in the control group are also a factor influencing this outcome. Creatinine is the only factor besides SSU admission associated with shortened time to endoscopy. Higher creatinine levels are associated with higher patient frailty and complexity, although the correlation with creatinine level remains after adjusting for these factors in this study. However, creatinine is an important risk factor for gastrointestinal bleeding and has been associated with increased mortality in several studies [14–16]. For this reason, the emergency physicians and endoscopists could be more motivated to request and perform early EGDS in these patients. In addition, the increase in creatinine levels in patients taking anticoagulants and antiplatelet agents could increase the concentrations of these agents and contribute to greater bleeding and clinical severity explaining the shorter time to endoscopy. In contrast, taking PPIs at home, as opposed to creatinine, is a factor that "reassures" physicians and reduces the extent of bleeding, resulting in a longer time to endoscopy. Another finding of our analysis concerns the INR value, which seems to be slightly but significantly higher in patients admitted to the internal medicine ward than in patients admitted to SSU. We also found that AF is associated with a significant increase in hospital LOS. These two findings are likely related. Some patients with AF are treated with vitamin K antagonists (anticoagulant medications) that increase INR; this means that gastrointestinal bleeding may be more important in these patients, require more time to ensure patients' clinical stability, and have a higher risk of recurrence. Therefore, a longer LOS is required in patients with AF, regardless of the hospital unit to which they are admitted (SSU or medical department). Our study has limitations. It is a retrospective study, and any biases inherent in this model may be present. In particular, selection bias cannot be excluded. The study was conducted at a single center with extensive experience in the treatment of gastrointestinal pathologies, so generalization of the results is not possible. In addition, the study sample was designed to analyze differences in the primary outcome (LOS) rather than the other end-points, so the lack of a difference in mortality and rehospitalization at 30 days between groups may be due to a relatively small number of patients included.

5. Conclusions

Management of NVUGIB in SSU allowed a significant reduction in time to endoscopy, length of hospital stay, and number of blood units transfused without increasing mortality and hospital readmission. Treatment of NVUGIB in SSU could help reduce overcrowding in ED. Multicenter randomized controlled trials are needed to confirm these results.

Author Contributions: Conceptualization, G.P. and M.G.; methodology, V.O.; validation, A.G. and F.F.; formal analysis, A.P. and M.C.; investigation, M.L., M.G. and A.M.; data curation, M.C.; writing—original draft preparation, G.M. and G.P.; writing—review and editing, M.E.R.; supervision, M.C. All authors have read and agreed to the published version of the manuscript.

Funding: This research received no external funding.

Institutional Review Board Statement: The study was conducted in accordance with the Declaration of Helsinki, and approved by the Institutional Ethics Committee of Catholic University of the Sacred Heart of Rome. (Protocol code 5378, 7 December 2022).

Informed Consent Statement: Informed consent was obtained from all subjects involved in the study.

Data Availability Statement: Data are available upon reasonable requests to corresponding author.

Conflicts of Interest: The authors declare no conflict of interest.

References

1. Savioli, G.; Ceresa, I.F.; Gri, N.; Bavestrello Piccini, G.; Longhitano, Y.; Zanza, C.; Piccioni, A.; Esposito, C.; Ricevuti, G.; Bressan, M.A. Emergency Department Overcrowding: Understanding the Factors to Find Corresponding Solutions. *J. Pers. Med.* **2022**, *12*, 279. [CrossRef] [PubMed]
2. Pines, J.M.; Hilton, J.A.; Weber, E.J.; Alkemade, A.J.; Al Shabanah, H.; Anderson, P.D.; Bernhard, M.; Bertini, A.; Gries, A.; Ferrandiz, S.; et al. International perspectives on emergency department crowding. *Acad. Emerg. Med.* **2011**, *18*, 1358–1370. [CrossRef] [PubMed]
3. Damiani, G.; Pinnarelli, L.; Sommella, L.; Vena, V.; Magrini, P.; Ricciardi, W. The Short Stay Unit as a new option for hospitals: A review of the scientific literature. *Med. Sci. Monit.* **2011**, *17*, 15–19. [CrossRef] [PubMed]
4. Juan, A.; Salazar, A.; Alvarez, A.; Perez, J.R.; Garcia, L.; Corbella, X. Effectiveness and safety of an emergency department short-stay unit as an alternative to standard inpatient hospitalisation. *Emerg. Med. J.* **2006**, *23*, 833–837. [CrossRef] [PubMed]
5. Miró, Ò.; Carbajosa, V.; Peacock, W.F.; Llorens, P.; Herrero, P.; Jacob, J.; Collins, S.P.; Fernández, C.; Pastor, A.J.; Martín-Sánchez, F.J.; et al. The effect of a short-stay unit on hospital admission and length of stay in acute heart failure: REDUCE-AHF study. *Eur. J. Intern. Med.* **2017**, *40*, 30–36. [CrossRef] [PubMed]
6. Strøm, C.; Mollerup, T.K.; Kromberg, L.S.; Rasmussen, L.S.; Schmidt, T.A. Hospitalisation in an emergency department short-stay unit compared to an internal medicine department is associated with fewer complications in older patients—An observational study. *Scand. J. Trauma Resusc. Emerg. Med.* **2017**, *25*, 80. [CrossRef] [PubMed]
7. Strøm, C.; Stefansson, J.S.; Fabritius, M.L.; Rasmussen, L.S.; Schmidt, T.A.; Jakobsen, J.C. Hospitalisation in short-stay units for adults with internal medicine diseases and conditions. *Cochrane Database Syst. Rev.* **2018**, *8*, CD012370. [CrossRef] [PubMed]
8. Downing, H.; Scott, C.; Kelly, C. Evaluation of a dedicated short-stay unit for acute medical admissions. *Clin. Med.* **2008**, *8*, 18–20. [CrossRef] [PubMed]
9. Sánchez-Marcos, C.; Jacob, J.; Llorens, P.; López-Díez, M.P.; Millán, J.; Martín-Sánchez, F.J.; Tost, J.; Aguirre, A.; Juan, M.Á.; Garrido, J.M.; et al. Emergency department direct discharge compared to short-stay unit admission for selected patients with acute heart failure: Analysis of short-term outcomes. *Intern. Emerg. Med.* **2023**. Online ahead of print. [CrossRef] [PubMed]
10. Decker, W.W.; Smars, P.A.; Vaidyanathan, L.; Goyal, D.G.; Boie, E.T.; Stead, L.G.; Packer, D.L.; Meloy, T.D.; Boggust, A.J.; Haro, L.H.; et al. A prospective, randomized trial of an emergency department observation unit for acute onset atrial fibrillation. *Ann. Emerg. Med.* **2008**, *52*, 322–328. [CrossRef] [PubMed]
11. Miller, C.D.; Case, L.D.; Little, W.C.; Mahler, S.A.; Burke, G.L.; Harper, E.N.; Lefebvre, C.; Hiestand, B.; Hoekstra, J.W.; Hamilton, C.A.; et al. Stress cardiac magnetic resonance imaging reduces revascularization, hospital readmission, and recurrent cardiac testing in intermediate risk patients with acute chest pain: A randomized trial. *J. Am. Coll. Cardiol. Cardiovasc. Imaging* **2013**, *6*, 785–794. [CrossRef] [PubMed]
12. Sun, B.C.; McCreath, H.; Liang, L.J.; Bohan, S.; Baugh, C.; Ragsdale, L.; Henderson, S.O.; Clark, C.; Bastani, A.; Keeler, E.; et al. Randomised clinical trial of an emergency department observation syncope protocol vs. routine inpatient admission. *Ann. Emerg. Med.* **2014**, *64*, 167–175. [CrossRef] [PubMed]
13. Lanas, A.; Dumonceau, J.M.; Hunt, R.H.; Fujishiro, M.; Scheiman, J.M.; Gralnek, I.M.; Campbell, H.E.; Rostom, A.; Villanueva, C.; Sung, J.J.Y. Non-variceal upper gastrointestinal bleeding. *Nat. Rev. Dis. Primers.* **2018**, *4*, 18020. [CrossRef] [PubMed]
14. Sakong, H.; Moon, H.S.; Choi, S.W.; Kang, S.H.; Sung, J.K.; Jeong, H.Y. ABC score is an effective predictor of outcomes in peptic ulcer bleeding. *Medicine* **2022**, *101*, e31541. [CrossRef] [PubMed]
15. Martin, T.A.; Tewani, S.; Clarke, L.; Aboubakr, A.; Palanisamy, S.; Lee, J.; Crawford, C.V.; Wan, D.W. Factors Associated With Emergency Department Discharge, Outcomes and Follow-Up Rates of Stable Patients With Lower Gastrointestinal Bleeding. *Gastroenterol. Res.* **2021**, *14*, 227–236. [CrossRef] [PubMed]
16. Redondo-Cerezo, E.; Ortega-Suazo, E.J.; Vadillo-Calles, F.; Valverde-Lopez, F.; Martínez-Cara, J.G.; Jimenez-Rosales, R. Upper gastrointestinal bleeding in patients 80 years old and over. A comparison with younger patients and risk factors analysis for in-hospital and delayed mortality. *Int. J. Clin. Pract.* **2021**, *75*, e14806. [CrossRef] [PubMed]

Disclaimer/Publisher's Note: The statements, opinions and data contained in all publications are solely those of the individual author(s) and contributor(s) and not of MDPI and/or the editor(s). MDPI and/or the editor(s) disclaim responsibility for any injury to people or property resulting from any ideas, methods, instructions or products referred to in the content.

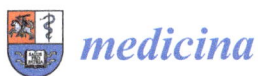

Article

Identification of Microbial Species and Analysis of Antimicrobial Resistance Patterns in Acute Cholangitis Patients with Malignant and Benign Biliary Obstructions: A Comparative Study

Bogdan Miuțescu [1,2], Deiana Vuletici [1,2,*], Călin Burciu [1,2], Adina Turcu-Stiolica [3], Felix Bende [1,2], Iulia Rațiu [1,2], Tudor Moga [1,2], Omar Sabuni [4], Adnan Anjary [5], Sami Dalati [6], Bogdan Silviu Ungureanu [7], Eyad Gadour [8,9], Florin George Horhat [10] and Alina Popescu [1,2]

1. Department of Gastroenterology and Hepatology, "Victor Babes" University of Medicine and Pharmacy Timisoara, Eftimie Murgu Square 2, 300041 Timisoara, Romania
2. Advanced Regional Research Center in Gastroenterology and Hepatology, "Victor Babes" University of Medicine and Pharmacy, 30041 Timisoara, Romania
3. Department of Pharmacoeconomics, University of Medicine and Pharmacy of Craiova, 200349 Craiova, Romania
4. Faculty of General Medicine, Altinbas University, Dilmenler Cd., 34217 Istanbul, Turkey
5. Faculty of General Medicine, Yeditepe University, Kayısdağı Cd., 34755 Istanbul, Turkey
6. Faculty of General Medicine, Baskent University, Fatih Sultan, 06790 Ankara, Turkey
7. Research Center of Gastroenterology and Hepatology, University of Medicine and Pharmacy of Craiova, 200349 Craiova, Romania
8. Department of Gastroenterology, King Abdulaziz Hospital-National Guard Health Affairs, Al Ahsa 31982, Saudi Arabia
9. Department of Medicine, Zamzam University College, Khartoum 11113, Sudan
10. Multidisciplinary Research Center on Antimicrobial Resistance (MULTI-REZ), Microbiology Department, "Victor Babes" University of Medicine and Pharmacy, 300041 Timisoara, Romania
* Correspondence: deiana.vuletici@umft.ro

Abstract: *Background and Objectives*: Acute cholangitis (AC) is still lethal if not treated promptly and effectively. Biliary drainage, also known as source control, has been acknowledged as the backbone treatment for patients with AC; nonetheless, antimicrobial therapy allows these patients to undergo non-emergent drainage procedures. This retrospective study aims to observe the bacterial species involved in AC and analyze the antimicrobial resistance patterns. *Materials and Methods*: Data were collected for four years, comparing patients with benign and malignant bile duct obstruction as an etiology for AC. A total of 262 patients were included in the study, with 124 cases of malignant obstruction and 138 cases of benign obstruction. *Results*: Positive bile culture was obtained in 192 (73.3%) patients with AC, with a higher rate among the benign group compared with malignant etiologies (55.7%.vs 44.3%). There was no significant difference between the Tokyo severity scores in the two study groups, identifying 34.7% cases of malignant obstruction with Tokyo Grade 1 (TG1) and 43.5% cases of TG1 among patients with benign obstruction. Similarly, there were no significant differences between the number of bacteria types identified in bile, most of them being monobacterial infections (19% in the TG1 group, 17% in the TG2 group, and 10% in the TG3 group). The most commonly identified microorganism in blood and bile cultures among both study groups was *E. coli* (46.7%), followed by *Klebsiella* spp. (36.0%) and *Pseudomonas* spp. (8.0%). Regarding antimicrobial resistance, it was observed that significantly more patients with malignant bile duct obstruction had a higher percentage of bacterial resistance for cefepime (33.3% vs. 11.7%, p-value = 0.0003), ceftazidime (36.5% vs. 14.5%, p-value = 0.0006), meropenem (15.4% vs. 3.6%, p-value = 0.0047), and imipenem (20.2% vs. 2.6%, p-value < 0.0001). *Conclusions*: The positive rate of biliary cultures is higher among patients with benign biliary obstruction, while the malignant etiology correlates with increased resistance to cefepime, ceftazidime, meropenem, and imipenem.

Keywords: acute cholangitis; antibiotic resistance; antimicrobial resistance; bile duct obstruction

1. Introduction

Acute cholangitis (AC) is a severe condition that affects the hepatobiliary system, with an associated mortality of 5–10% if treated with endoscopic biliary drainage [1,2] and approximately 50% if untreated [3]. The determining causes are diverse, with choledocholithiasis as the leading cause in 57% of cases [4], followed by malignant pathologies in 10–30% of patients [5]. The diagnosis is based on the pathognomonic signs of the dilated biliary tree, detected by diagnostic imaging [6]. The biological findings are correlated with alteration of complete blood count (CBC), increased aspartate aminotransferase (AST), alanine aminotransferase (ALT), bilirubin, gamma-glutamyl transferase (GGT), and alkaline phosphatase (ALP) [7].

The diagnosis of AC was based, until recently, on the Charcot triad, which uses as diagnostic criteria fever, abdominal pain, and jaundice [8]. However, despite its high specificity of 93–99%, its sensitivity is low (36–46%), thus making it a good confirmation test but a poor screening and diagnostic test [9,10]. All the efforts to increase the AC diagnosis were summarized in the first Tokyo Guideline from 2007 (TG07) [11], which was later updated to TG13 [6] and TG18 [12]. The Dutch Pancreatitis Study Group (DPSG) recently proposed new diagnostic criteria for AC in the presence of acute biliary pancreatitis [13].

The AC treatment is based on two management options that comprise antibiotic treatment (AT) and biliary drainage. According to TG18 [7], endoscopic retrograde cholangiopancreatography (ERCP) should be considered the first-line drainage procedure. For mild forms, the indication of drainage is correlated with the response to antibiotic treatment; however, for moderate AC, the drainage must be performed early, and for severe conditions, as soon as possible [7]. This indication is confirmed by multiple studies that concluded that early ERCP decreases the duration of hospitalization [14] and mortality [4,14]. The second management option for AC is antimicrobial treatment, where TG18 provides a large spectrum based on the three classifications of AC [15]. The importance of the administration of antibiotics has already been proven, but the duration of administration is a debated subject; some studies hypothesize that short-term AT has the same efficacy as long-term AT, with the condition that the biliary tree has been decompressed [16,17].

Cancer patients have a three-times higher risk of death from infection [18], which is a very common complication in this particular population [19]. Thus, increasing antibiotic resistance in patients with malignant diseases can lead to unfavorable outcomes after AC [20]. Although the incidence of bloodstream infection (BSI) in patients with solid tumors is lower than in hematological patients, the majority of studies have focused on patients with hematological malignancies, while the most frequent source of recurrent BSI seems to be cholangitis [21].

Multi-drug resistant (MDR) pathogens are an evolving problem in AC, especially in immunocompromised patients [22]. The factors that can lead to biliary MDR bacteria are male gender, nosocomial AC, prior antibiotic exposure, and prior biliary stenting; even so, the survival rate and hospital stay in AC patients with and without detected biliary MDR pathogens are similar [23]. Thus, in the current era of increasing antibiotic resistance, biliary cultures (BCs) are imperious, allowing for the proper adjustment of antibiotic treatment based on the antibiogram results. The positive rate of BC is directly correlated with the form of AC (80.4 vs. 82.2% vs. 88.6% in mild, moderate, and severe conditions, respectively [15], or, depending on the inclusion criteria, averaging 91.8% [24]). Studies have described that the positive rate of blood culture among patients with collected BC varies between 30% and 40%, where 87% of patients grew the same organism as their bile culture [24–26].

Although some studies have evaluated the microbiology of bile aspirates in patients with AC [27] and others have compared cholangitis patients with and without plastic biliary stents [28], there is still very limited information regarding bile culture and antibiotic susceptibility patterns in the malignant and benign etiologies of AC. Thus, one of the hypotheses raised by the current study assumes that there is a significant difference in the microbial species distribution between patients with AC caused by malignant biliary obstructions and those with benign biliary obstructions. Another hypothesis is that antimicrobial resistance patterns differ significantly between the microbial species isolated from patients with malignant biliary obstructions and those with benign biliary obstructions. Therefore, this study's primary purpose is to identify and compare the microbial species present in the bile aspirates of patients with acute cholangitis (AC) associated with malignant and benign biliary obstructions; to evaluate and compare the antimicrobial resistance patterns in the isolated microbial species from the bile aspirates of patients with malignant and benign biliary obstructions; and to provide evidence-based recommendations for the empirical antibiotic treatment of AC in patients with malignant and benign biliary obstructions.

2. Materials and Methods

2.1. Study Design and Ethics

A retrospective study was performed at the Emergency County Hospital Timisoara, a tertiary care center in Western Romania. All patients who underwent an ERCP for biliary drainage due to AC between June 2018 and June 2020 were included. All patients had a bile culture sample and a blood culture sample collected. Patients' medical data and personal information were collected from the medical records and patient files. The resistance of the bacteria to the antibiotics recommended by TG18 [15] was evaluated, and we attempted to identify the difference in antimicrobial resistance between malignant and benign bile duct obstruction causing AC. The study protocol conformed to the ethical guidelines of the 1975 Declaration of Helsinki. The internal review board approved it on 14 October 2022 (approval number I-27098).

2.2. Patients and Sampling

The diagnosis of AC was established using TG18 criteria 13. Patients were included in this study only once, on their first admission, despite some having more than one episode of AC during the data collection period. The exclusion criteria were: cholangitis secondary to ERCP, post-ERCP perforation, percutaneous or surgical drainage, or if the patient used antibiotic therapy (AT) for any other diseases when the AC was diagnosed.

All the patients received antibiotics according to their corresponding grade from TG18 recommendations [15] after admission, and the diagnosis of AC was established. In the department where the study was performed, the most common antibiotic schemes used for mild AC were ampicillin/sulbactam, ciprofloxacin, or levofloxacin for mild AC; ceftriaxone, cefepime, or piperacillin-tazobactam for moderate AC; and meropenem or imipenem for severe AC. Microorganisms from blood and bile samples were identified on culture media. The blood culture samples were collected at admission for the patients with moderate and severe forms of AC, according to TG18's recommendation. Because of our center's particularity as a tertiary endoscopy department, where patients are referred from different healthcare facilities, not all had a blood culture collected before initiating antibiotic therapy. Bile samples were obtained after cannulation via the sphincterotome before the therapeutic procedure. Firstly, at least 5 mL of bile that was collected was discarded; immediately after that, another 5 mL of bile was collected in a sterile tube containing a medium for anaerobic, aerobic bacterial cultures. The samples were incubated for at least seven days at 37 °C until microbial growth was detected. Antibiotic susceptibility testing (MIC) was performed using a VITEK® 2 system (bioMérieux, Marcy-l'Étoile, France) with the results interpreted according to the existing guidelines [29]. Clinical and Laboratory Standards Institute (CLSI) recommendations and criteria for all bacteria cultured were used to define susceptibility to antimicrobial agents [30].

On admission, B-mode ultrasonography was used to determine the cause of the obstruction. If a diagnosis could not be made, we performed an endoscopic ultrasound (EUS) procedure, contrast-enhanced computer tomography (CT), or CE magnetic resonance imaging (MRI), which are also used in the staging of malignant causes. In addition, we examined the tumor markers and histopathological findings from the ERCP or EUS biopsies to confirm the diagnosis. ERCP was used only as a therapeutic tool, performed with a therapeutic duodenoscope (Olympus Corp., Tokyo, Japan), and common bile duct cannulation was done using a guidewire. All ERCP procedures were performed under sedation using midazolam, propofol, and fentanyl by a team from anesthesia and intensive care; the drugs were combined according to their internal protocols. The timing of ERCP was established according to the severity of the disease and Tokyo Guidelines criteria by experienced endoscopists. The main goal of the ERCP for patients with choledocholithiasis was extracting the stones. In cases of complicated choledocholithiasis, which is difficult to extract, we placed plastic stents. For other cases, we placed plastic or metal stents, depending on the diagnosis.

2.3. Data Collection and Variables

Demographic data and the patient's medical history were collected from the patient's discharge reports. The variables considered for analysis comprised demographic data: the etiology of infection, the clinical characteristics of the study population (age, gender, age category, signs and symptoms, presence of bile duct stents, history of cholecystectomy, ERCP timing, hospitalization, Tokyo severity score), bacterial identification in bile (Gram-positive and Gram-negative organisms), and antimicrobial resistance patterns. The study included four antibiotics classes: penicillin, cephalosporins, fluoroquinolones, and carbapenems. These antibiotics were tested by the hospital per laboratory guidelines and are recommended by the Tokyo Guidelines 2018 for the treatment of AC until bile or blood culture validation.

2.4. Statistical Analysis

GraphPad Prism v9.2.0. (GraphPad, San Diego, CA, USA) and R statistical software version 4.0.3 (2021, GNU General Public License) were used for the statistical analysis. Continuous variables were given as mean (standard deviation) or median (interquartile range), while categorical variables were expressed as the number of subjects (n) and the percentage value (%). The distribution of continuous variables was tested by the D'Agostino–Pearson omnibus normality test, revealing the data to be nonparametrically distributed. Hence, nonparametric two-way analysis was performed using the Mann–Whitney U-test. Radar plots were designed using the Plotly package to distinguish the multidimensional data of antibiograms. Fisher's exact or chi-square test, two-sided, was used to compare categorical variables. The results were considered statistically significant, with a p-value of <0.05.

3. Results

3.1. Clinical Characteristics of the Study Population

A total number of 262 patients were included in this study. The etiology of cholangitis was analyzed in Table 1. Most patients in the benign group were diagnosed with choledochal lithiasis (48.5%). Forty-seven percent of patients (n = 124/262) were diagnosed with a malignant pathology, the leading cause being pancreatic cancer (24.8%). The mean age between the two groups had no statistical differences (p-value = 0.93); however, patients from the middle age category were more frequent in the malignant group and young patients in the benign group. No differences were found in gender between malignant and benign patients (p-value = 0.508), as seen in Table 2. Abdominal pain was more frequent in the benign group compared to the malignant group (80.4% vs. 58.1%, p-value < 0.0001). In patients presenting fever, no differences were observed between the two groups (p-value = 0.187). Prolonged hospital stay was more frequently associated with malignant diseases than benign ones (p-value = 0.04).

Table 1. Comparison of etiology between patients with malignant and benign disease.

Etiology	Total (n = 262)
Benign	Total 138 (52.7%)
Choledocholithiasis	127 (48.5%)
Vaterian ampulloma	5 (1.9%)
Benign coledochal stenosis	3 (1.1%)
Mirizzi syndrome	2 (0.8%)
Liver abscess	1 (0.4%)
Malignant	Total 124 (47.3%)
Pancreatic cancer	65 (24.8%)
Cholangiocarcinoma	35 (13.4%)
Malignant vaterian ampulloma	14 (5.3%)
Malignant extrinsic compression	7 (2.7%)
Gallbladder cancer	3 (1.1%)

Table 2. Clinical characteristics of the study population stratified by etiology of biliary obstruction.

Variables	Total (n = 262)	Malignant (n = 124)	Benign (n = 138)	Significance
Gender (male)	128 (48.9%)	61 (49.2%)	67 (48.6)	0.508
Age, mean (SD)	67.6 (14.1)	68.5 (11.3)	66.8 (16.2)	0.330
Age, median (IQR)	70.0 (19.0)	69.5 (16.8)	70.0 (22.2)	0.930
Age category				0.005
Young adults (18–39 years)	15 (5.7%)	2 (1.6%)	11 (8.0%)	
Middle age (40–65 years)	84 (32.1%)	50 (40.3%)	34 (24.6%)	
Older adults (>65 years)	159 (60.7%)	72 (58.1%)	87 (63.0%)	
Abdominal pain, yes	183 (69.8)	72 (58.1%)	111 (80.4%)	<0.001
Jaundice	234 (89.3%)	117 (94.4%)	117 (84.8%)	0.015
Fever	85 (32.4%)	35 (28.2%)	50 (36.2%)	0.187
Previous stent, yes	48 (18.3%)	41 (33.1%)	7 (5.1%)	<0.001
Cholecystectomy, yes	50 (19.1%)	19 (15.3%)	31 (22.5%)	0.158
ERCP timing				0.912
Emergent (<48 h)	176 (67.2%)	83 (66.9%)	93 (67.4%)	
Urgent (48–72 h)	44 (16.8%)	20 (16.1%)	24 (17.4%)	
Late (>72 h)	42 (16%)	21 (16.9%)	21 (15.2%)	
Hospitalization days	7 (4–10)	7 (5–10)	6 (4–10)	0.040
Weekend admission, yes	73 (27.9%)	29 (23.4%)	44 (31.9%)	0.132
Tokyo severity score,				0.075
Grade I	103 (39.3%)	43 (34.7%)	60 (43.5%)	
Grade II	95 (36.3%)	43 (34.7%)	52 (37.7%)	
Grade III	64 (24.4%)	38 (30.6%)	26 (18.8%)	

Data reported as n (%) and calculated using the chi-square test and Fisher's exact test unless specified differently; mean and SD values compared with Student's t-test; median and IQR values compared with Mann–Whitney U-test; IQR—interquartile range; SD—standard deviation.

3.2. Bacterial Identification

According to the Tokyo Guidelines of 2018, monomicrobial growth was found more in patients with mild severity (19%), followed by moderate severity (17%) and the severe grade (10%), as seen in Table 3. Monomicrobial growth was the most encountered (46%) in comparison with sterile (26%) or polymicrobial cultures (two bacteria—24% or three bacteria—3%). Cultures were positive in 192 of 262 bile specimens (73.3%), most of them (107/192, 55.7%) having a benign etiology for the acute obstruction of the main biliary duct; 44.3% of patients (85/192) had a malignant etiology of acute cholangitis.

Table 3. Bacterial presence in bile according to Tokyo Guidelines.

Tokyo Grade	Grade I ($n = 103$)	Grade II ($n = 95$)	Grade III ($n = 64$)	Significance
Sterile	26 (10%)	27 (10%)	17 (6%)	0.973
1 bacterium	50 (19%)	44 (17%)	27 (10%)	
2 bacteria	24 (9%)	21 (8%)	17 (6%)	
3 bacteria	3 (1%)	3 (1%)	3 (1%)	

Proportions evaluated with a chi-square test.

Table 4 describes a detailed comparison of isolated microorganisms from blood cultures and bile cultures between patients with malignant and benign obstruction causes. The most frequently encountered in bile cultures were Gram-negative bacteria, including *Escherichia coli* (*E. coli*) (37.6% for patients with malignant disease vs. 56.1% for patients with benign disease, $p = 0.003$), *Klebsiella* (29.4% for patients with malignant disease vs. 24.3% for patients with benign disease, $p = 0.876$), *Pseudomonas* (14.1% for patients with malignant disease vs. 10.3% for patients with benign disease, $p = 0.667$), and *Citrobacter* (7.1% for patients with malignant disease vs. 4.7% for patients with benign disease, $p = 0.760$). The most frequently encountered Gram-positive bacteria was *Enterococcus* (24.7% for patients with malignant disease vs. 18.7% for patients with benign disease, $p = 0.612$).

Table 4. Comparison of isolated microorganisms from bile cultures between patients with malignant and benign etiologies of obstruction.

Isolated Microorganisms from Bile Cultures No. of Patients (%)	Total ($n = 192$)	Malignant ($n = 85$)	Benign ($n = 107$)	Significance
Gram-negative organisms				
Escherichia coli	92/192 (47.9%)	32 (37.6%)	60 (56.1%)	0.003
Klebsiella spp.	51/192 (26.6%)	25 (29.4%)	26 (24.3%)	0.876
Pseudomonas spp.	25/192 (13%)	12 (14.1%)	11 (10.3%)	0.667
Enterobacter spp.	10/192 (5.2%)	4 (4.7%)	6 (5.6%)	0.752
Acinetobacter spp.	6/192 (3.1%)	5 (5.9%)	1 (0.9%)	0.104
Citrobacter spp.	11/192 (5.7%)	6 (7.1%)	5 (4.7%)	0.760
Gram-positive organisms				
Enterococcus spp.	41/192 (21.6%)	21 (24.7%)	20 (18.7%)	0.612
Streptococcus spp.	6/192 (3.1%)	1 (1.2%)	5 (4.8%)	0.217
Staphylococcus spp.	3/192 (1.6%)	2 (2.4%)	1 (0.9%)	0.604

Data reported as n (%) and calculated using the chi-square test and Fisher's exact test unless specified differently.

Of 262 patients with AC, 141 (53.8%) had a collected blood culture and 97 (68.8%) were sterile; from this amount, 67 (69%) had a positive bile culture. Bacterial growth in the blood culture was found in 31% of the patients. Of 44 patients with positive hemoculture, there was one bacterium grown in 41 (29%) patients and two bacteria grown in 3 (2%) patients. Of positive blood cultures, 29 (65%) had a similar germ with the bile culture, and 4 (9%) had negative bile culture. It was observed that the most frequent organism identified in blood cultures was *E. coli*, with 31.3% of all malignant obstructions and 55.2% in benign obstructions, respectively, and similarly in bile cultures, 50.0% in malignant cases vs. 40.9% in benign cases. The next-in-frequency organisms identified were *Klebsiella* spp. in approximately 20% of all blood cultures and *Pseudomonas* in about 5%. No statistical differences of isolated microorganisms were found in blood cultures comparing patients with malignant and benign diseases, as shown in Table 5.

Table 5. Comparison of isolated microorganisms from blood cultures between patients with malignant and benign causes of obstruction.

Isolated Microorganisms from Blood Cultures, n (%)	Malignant Disease (n = 16/127)	Benign Disease (n = 29/138)	Significance
Sterile	109 (85.8%)	111 (80.4%)	0.242
Gram-negative organisms			
Escherichia coli	5 (31.3%)	16 (55.2%)	0.123
Klebsiella spp.	4 (25.0%)	5 (17.2%)	0.533
Pseudomonas spp.	1 (6.3%)	1 (3.4%)	0.662
Enterobacter spp.	1 (6.3%)	3 (10.3%)	0.644
Acinetobacter spp.	1 (6.3%)	0 (0.0%)	0.173
Citrobacter spp.	0 (0.0%)	1 (3.4%)	0.452
Gram-positive organisms			
Enterococcus spp.	1 (6.3%)	1 (3.4%)	0.662
Staphylococcus spp.	3 (18.8%)	1 (3.4%)	0.084
Streptococcus spp.	0 (0.0%)	1 (3.4%)	0.452

Data reported as n (%) and calculated using the chi-square test and Fisher's exact test unless specified differently.

3.3. Antibiogram Study

A total of 266 antibiograms were analyzed, with 119 from patients with malignant obstruction and 147 from those with benign obstruction. The table summarizes the percentage of antibiotic resistance for each antibiotic in both groups, along with the statistical significance of the differences observed. Ampicillin/sulbactam showed resistance in 31.3% of the total cases (21/67), with 27.2% (6/22) resistance in malignant cases and 33.3% (15/45) in benign cases. The difference in resistance between the two groups was not statistically significant ($p = 0.780$). Piperacillin/tazobactam resistance was present in 17.3% of the total cases (36/207), with 19.7% (18/91) resistance in malignant cases and 15.6% (18/115) in benign cases. The difference was also not statistically significant ($p = 0.464$). According to the data from Table 6 and Figure 1, cefepime (p-value = 0.001), ceftazidime (p-value = 0.001), meropenem (p-value = 0.004), and imipenem (p-value < 0.001) had significantly higher resistance rates for the malignant group of patients than for the benign group. There were no significant differences in antibiotic resistance between the two groups for the other evaluated antibiotics recommended by the TG18.

Table 6. Evaluation of antibiotic resistance from bile culture, comparing malignant and benign obstructions in acute cholangitis patients.

Antibiotic Resistance n/Number of Antibiograms, %	Total (n = 266)	Malignant (n = 119)	Benign (n = 147)	Significance
Ampicillin/Sulbactam	21/67 (31.3%)	6/22 (27.2%)	15/45 (33.3%)	0.780
Piperacillin/Tazobactam	36/207 (17.3%)	18/91 (19.7%)	18/115 (15.6%)	0.464
Ciprofloxacin	45/225 (20.0%)	25/99 (25.2%)	20/125 (16.0%)	0.095
Levofloxacin	18/104 (17.3%)	6/37 (16.2%)	12/67 (17.9%)	0.999
Cefepime	41/196 (20.9%)	28/84 (33.3%)	13/111 (11.7%)	0.001
Ceftriaxone	11/73 (15.0%)	3/22 (13.6%)	8/51 (15.6%)	0.999
Ceftazidime	46/192 (23.9%)	30/82 (36.5%)	16/110 (14.5%)	0.001
Meropenem	17/194 (8.7%)	13/84 (15.4%)	4/110 (3.6%)	0.004
Imipenem	20/197 (10.1%)	17/84 (20.2%)	3/113 (2.6%)	<0.001

Data reported as n (%) and calculated using the chi-square test and Fisher's exact test unless specified differently. The percentage was computed from the number of patients with an antibiogram.

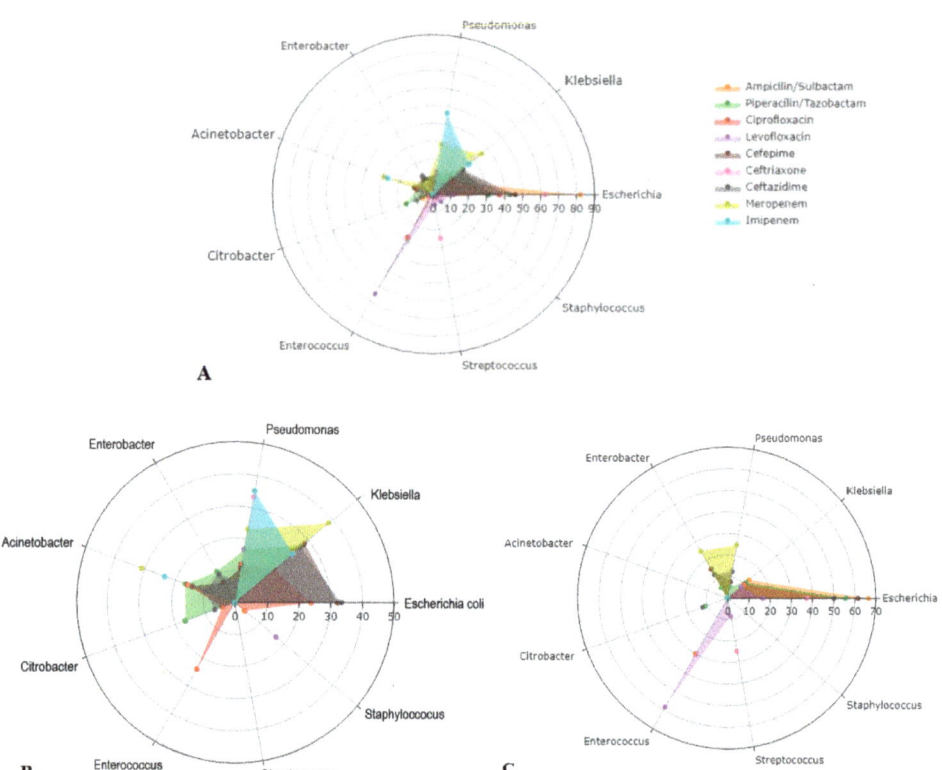

Figure 1. Radar plots reporting resistance microbial sensitivity of given antibiotics for patients with acute cholangitis. All patients (**A**), malignant (**B**), benign (**C**). Figures generated with Plotly data analytics and visualization tools.

A detailed breakdown of the bacterial resistance to antibiotics from bile culture is presented in Table 7, where the highest resistance profile was observed in samples positive with *Escherichia coli*. We observed a high resistance pattern of *E. coli* to ampicillin/sulbactam in benign (46.2%) and malignant (36.4%) cases. The second highest antimicrobial resistance of *E. coli* was identified for ceftazidime (33.3% in malignant cases and 22.6% in benign cases) and cefepime (31.0% in malignant cases and 16.7% in benign cases), respectively. The second most commonly identified bacteria was *Klebsiella* spp. in 27.1% of patients, having a high antimicrobial resistance pattern to ampicillin/sulbactam (33.3%) and ceftriaxone (22.2%) in patients with benign obstructions. *Klebsiella* spp. was also highly resistant to cefepime in malignant cases (34.8%) and piperacillin/tazobactam in 18.5% of benign cases, respectively. The third most commonly involved bacteria was *Enterococcus* spp. in 21.4% of patients, equally between the malignant and benign causes of obstruction. *Enterococcus* was resistant to ciprofloxacin in 50% of benign cases and 40% of malignant cases and to levofloxacin in 50% of benign cases and 26.7% of malignant patients.

Table 7. Evaluation of bacterial resistance to antibiotics from bile culture in patients with acute cholangitis.

Isolated Microorganisms from Bile Cultures No. of Patients (%)	Escherichia coli n = 92/192 (47.9%)		Klebsiella spp. n = 52/192 (27.1%)		Pseudomonas spp. n = 23/192 (11.9%)		Enterococcus spp. n = 41/192 (21.4%)	
	Malignant 34.8% (32/92)	Benign 64.2% (60/92)	Malignant 48.1% (25/52)	Benign 51.9% (27/52)	Malignant 52.2% (12/23)	Benign 47.8% (11/23)	Malignant 51.2% 21/41	Benign 48.8% 20/41
Ampicillin/Sulbactam	36.4% (4/11)	46.7% (14/30)	0% (0/6)	33.3% (3/9)	0% (0/0)	0% (0/0)	0% (0/2)	0% (0/0)
Piperacillin/Tazobactam	9.4% (3/32)	25.9% (15/58)	20% (5/25)	18.5% (5/27)	33.3% (4/12)	22.2% (2/9)	0% (0/0)	0% (0/0)
Ciprofloxacin	25% (7/28)	19.2% (10/52)	19% (4/21)	11.5 (3/26)	25 (3/12)	10% (1/10)	40% (6/15)	50% (9/18)
Levofloxacin	0% (0/7)	8% (2/25)	0% (0/2)	11.1% (1/9)	20% (1/5)	0.5% (0/4)	26.7% (4/15)	50% (9/18)
Cefepime	31% (9/29)	16.7% (9/54)	34.8% (8/23)	0% (0/27)	27.3% (3/11)	20% (2/10)	0% (0/0)	0% (0/0)
Ceftriaxone	18.2% (2/11)	17.2% (5/29)	0% (0/5)	22.2% (2/9)	100% (1/1)	0% (0/1)	0% (0/0)	0% (0/0)
Ceftazidime	33.3% (10/30)	22.6% (12/53)	34.8% (8/23)	7.7% (2/26)	20% (2/10)	30% (3/10)	0% (0/0)	0% (0/0)
Meropenem	0% (0/29)	0% (0/53)	16.7% (4/24)	3.8% (1/26)	40% (4/10)	22.2% (2/9)	0% (0/0)	0% (0/0)
Imipenem	0% (0/30)	1.8% (1/55)	17.4% (4/23)	3.7% (1/27)	60% (6/10)	20% (2/10)	0% (0/0)	0% (0/0)

4. Discussion

4.1. Current Findings and Published Data

Based on the findings, the current study carries significant implications for the clinical management of acute cholangitis patients with malignant and benign biliary obstructions by providing valuable insights into the microbial species and their antimicrobial resistance patterns in these patient groups. Among the study's key findings, it was observed that *E. coli* was the most frequently encountered bacteria in bile cultures, with a higher prevalence in patients with benign disease than malignant disease (56.1% vs. 37.6%, $p = 0.003$). Moreover, cefepime, ceftazidime, meropenem, and imipenem had significantly higher resistance rates in the malignant group compared to the benign group (p-values < 0.05). These results are important because they can help guide appropriate empirical antibiotic therapy selection for acute cholangitis patients based on their underlying biliary obstruction etiology. For instance, the higher resistance rates observed for certain antibiotics in the malignant group may warrant the use of alternative antibiotics in these patients. Furthermore, identifying the most frequently encountered microorganisms in bile cultures, such as *E. coli*, can help develop targeted therapies.

The choice of antimicrobial treatment depends on the severity of cholangitis and local resistance to antibiotics. Therefore, updates for local antibiograms are necessary to provide efficient therapy in clinical practice. Previously published data show a positive rate of bile cultures for patients with AC, ranging from 28% to 93% [27,31]. In the present study, a positive bile culture was obtained in 192 patients with AC, representing 73.3% of the entire cohort, with a higher rate among the benign group than the malignant one (55.7% vs. 44.3%). On the other hand, 69% of blood cultures were sterile, compared with only 26.7% of sterile bile cultures. It was previously observed in other studies that positive rates of blood cultures among patients with AC range from 21% to 71% [32].

Our study confirmed the benefit of bile culture over blood culture since the positive rate was much higher in BC compared with blood culture. However, in the cases of positive blood culture, the same germ in BC was found in 65% of cases, lower than the data presented by Chandra [26]. The superiority of BC was proven by a lower number of false-negative bile cultures compared with false-negative blood cultures. The high sensitivity and low specificity of TG18, as opposed to Charco's triad, which has low sensitivity but very high specificity, can explain the number of false-negative AC cases [10]. Recent data published by Gromski et al., where the AC diagnostic criteria were similar to Charcot's triad, showed a positive BC rate of 91.8% [24], higher than our study's rate.

In this study, *E. coli* was the predominant isolate in both groups. However, it was statistically more present in patients with benign disease (37.6% vs. 56.1%, p-value = 0.003). *Klebsiella* spp. was the second most commonly identified germ, which was more frequent in malignant etiologies (29.4% vs. 24.3%). The main findings of the present study are consistent with the Study for Monitoring Antimicrobial Resistance Trends (SMART) results, which reported culture and antimicrobial susceptibility data from intra-abdominal collections. Gomi et al. published a large-cohort multicenter observational study in 2017 among patients with AC, where the most frequent organism found in bile culture was *Escherichia coli* [33]. Similarly, review studies reported that coliform organisms such as *Escherichia coli* (25–50%), *Klebsiella* spp. (15–20%), and *Enterobacter* species (5–10%) are among the most commonly identified bacteria [34,35], while Enterococcus species were identified in 10–20% of infections. Occasionally, anaerobic bacteria such as *Bacteroides fragilis* and *Clostridium perfringens* may also induce AC, especially in individuals with a history of biliary operations and the geriatric population. However, these pathogens were not identified in our research, likely due to insufficient sample size or due to the high number of false-negative results that are often found in anaerobic bacteria [36,37].

The Tokyo Guidelines suggest using beta-lactamase or cephalosporine-based antimicrobial therapy in mild cholangitis. In our study, the resistance to ampicillin/sulbactam was above 20%, consistent with the information found in the Tokyo Guidelines, without significant differences between malignant and benign etiologies of cholangitis (22.2% vs. 33.3%). It was observed that the overall increased resistance rate of *E. coli* has an increasing trend for ampicillin/sulbactam [38]. Similar findings were seen in our study, where resistance was higher in benign cases than in malignant cases. These findings prompted us to change the current antibiotic therapy protocol so that empirical ampicillin/sulbactam treatment is no longer given in AC, except in cases where a previous bile culture was sensitive to this antibiotic. The treatment will then be modified based on the results of the bile culture from the current hospitalization.

In addition, in benign cases, *Klebsiella* spp. susceptibility to ampicillin/sulbactam was reduced. This could be due to the extensive use of this antibiotic in the absence of studies demonstrating local susceptibility to ampicillin/sulbactam. Furthermore, the proportion of mild forms of benign AC is greater than the proportion of malignant AC; in this case, over-exposure to ampicillin/sulbactam can lead to decreased susceptibility. For fluoroquinolones, also recommended in mild forms of AC, the resistance is around 20%, without differences between etiologies. For moderate cholangitis, TG18 suggests using cephalosporine; in our study, the resistance to ceftriaxone was similar in both etiologies.

However, we found that patients with cancer have greater levels of cefepime and ceftazidime resistance. This discrepancy can be attributed to the increasing resistance of *E. coli* and *Klebsiella* spp., the two most prevalent germs identified in patients with cancer in our study. *Klebsiella* spp. is part of the ESKAPE group, commonly associated with antibiotic resistance in hospital settings. Knowing the increased risk of infection in cancer patients, a possible causality can be linked to the intensive use of this antibiotic in other infections [39]. However, the possibility of other confounding factors cannot be ruled out. Meropenem and imipenem, prescribed for severe types of AC, have shown higher resistance in malignant patients compared to benign cases (15.4% vs. 3.6% and 20.2% vs. 2.6%, respectively). These findings can be explained by the significant carbapenem resistance of *Klebsiella* spp. in malignant patients due to biofilm production, as described by other studies [40]. The molecular mechanisms of carbapenem resistance in *Enterobacteriaceae* are represented by two major mechanisms: β-lactamase activity combined with structural mutations and the production of carbapenemases, enzymes that hydrolyze carbapenem antibiotics [41]. Carbapenemase-producing *Klebsiella pneumoniae* isolated from pediatric cancer patients has been reported [42]. Other studies have reported the capability of *Klebsiella* spp. to acquire resistance to fourth-generation cephalosporins, information that can be correlated with our findings in antimicrobial resistance [43]. However, the resistance and susceptibility of *Klebsiella* spp. to sulbactam and associated combinations remain a debate [44,45].

4.2. Study Strengths and Limitations

As a retrospective and descriptive study, doubts can be raised about the extent of the result's applicability to other settings. This study was not intended to be a final work but, rather, only an initial work documenting the antimicrobial susceptibilities of biliary pathogens. At this time, the study is best when limited to the area where the study facility is located and to the population of the country. Being a tertiary hospital that assures ERCP for four counties, not all patients had blood cultures collected; therefore, selection bias can occur. Other biases can happen due to missing data. Another limitation is that not all the antibiotics evaluated had been tested for all germs, a condition generated by the study's retrospective design. In the future, we need prospective studies that will test TG-recommended antibiotics for all germs and can validate the results of this study. Aside from the limitations mentioned above, the current study adds to the existing literature by providing new evidence on bacterial identification in biliary tract infections and the spectrum of antimicrobial resistance in the context of alarmingly increasing resistant infections, particularly in malignant patients. Nevertheless, based on our findings, future studies can explore in-depth specific classes of antibiotics with a potential application in treating AC as well as include the detection of beta-lactamase and carbapenemase in the tested samples. Because very few studies on acute cholangitis have been published with the same goals, more multicentric studies are needed to gain a better understanding of the bacteria involved and the spectrum of antimicrobial resistance.

5. Conclusions

In conclusion, the positive rate of biliary culture was higher in patients with acute cholangitis of a benign cause. Overall, patients with malignant causes of obstruction showed a higher rate of antimicrobial resistance and exhibited a different spectrum of pathogens. Our findings could help in establishing empiric antibiotic therapy in complicated cases of AC, providing a higher success rate of the empiric treatment. A multidisciplinary approach might be beneficial to the discussion and provision of appropriate antimicrobial agents in the institution, region, and country.

Author Contributions: Conceptualization, B.M., and D.V.; methodology, C.B. and F.G.H.; software, A.T.-S.; validation, I.R., A.P., T.M. and B.S.U.; formal analysis, B.M.; investigation, B.M., I.R. and T.M.; resources, F.B.; data curation, D.V. and C.B.; writing—original draft preparation, B.M.; writing—review and editing, A.P., T.M., F.B., B.S.U., I.R., O.S., A.A., S.D., F.G.H. and E.G.; visualization, A.T.-S.; supervision, B.M., I.R., A.P., F.B., T.M. and C.B.; project administration, B.M. All authors have read and agreed to the published version of the manuscript.

Funding: This research received no external funding.

Institutional Review Board Statement: The study was conducted according to the guidelines of the Declaration of Helsinki and approved by the Ethics Committee of Victor Babes' University of Medicine and Pharmacy in Timisoara (approval number I-27098 from 14 October 2022).

Informed Consent Statement: Written informed consent has been obtained from the patients to publish this paper.

Data Availability Statement: Data are available on request.

Conflicts of Interest: The authors declare no conflict of interest.

References

1. Lai, E.C.; Mok, F.P.; Tan, E.S.; Lo, C.-M.; Fan, S.-T.; You, K.-T.; Wong, J. Endoscopic Biliary Drainage for Severe Acute Cholangitis. *N. Engl. J. Med.* **1992**, *326*, 1582–1586. [CrossRef] [PubMed]
2. Sokal, A.; Sauvanet, A.; Fantin, B.; de Lastours, V. Acute cholangitis: Diagnosis and management. *J. Visc. Surg.* **2019**, *156*, 515–525. [CrossRef]
3. Andrew, D.J.; Johnson, S.E. Acute suppurative cholangitis, a medical and surgical emergency. A review of ten years experience emphasizing early recognition. *Am. J. Gastroenterol.* **1970**, *54*, 141–154. [PubMed]
4. Du, L.; Cen, M.; Zheng, X.; Luo, L.; Siddiqui, A.; Kim, J.J. Timing of Performing Endoscopic Retrograde Cholangiopancreatography and Inpatient Mortality in Acute Cholangitis: A Systematic Review and Meta-Analysis. *Clin. Transl. Gastroenterol.* **2020**, *11*, e00158. [CrossRef]
5. Kimura, Y.; Takada, T.; Kawarada, Y.; Nimura, Y.; Hirata, K.; Sekimoto, M.; Yoshida, M.; Mayumi, T.; Wada, K.; Miura, F.; et al. Definitions, pathophysiology, and epidemiology of acute cholangitis and cholecystitis: Tokyo Guidelines. *J. Hepato-Biliary-Pancreat. Surg.* **2007**, *14*, 15–26. [CrossRef] [PubMed]
6. Kiriyama, S.; Takada, T.; Strasberg, S.M.; Solomkin, J.; Mayumi, T.; Pitt, H.A.; Gouma, D.J.; Garden, O.J.; Büchler, M.W.; Yokoe, M.; et al. TG13 guidelines for diagnosis and severity grading of acute cholangitis (with videos). *J. Hepato-Biliary-Pancreat. Sci.* **2013**, *20*, 24–34. [CrossRef]
7. Miura, F.; Okamoto, K.; Takada, T.; Strasberg, S.M.; Asbun, H.J.; Pitt, H.A.; Gomi, H.; Solomkin, J.; Schlossberg, D.; Han, H.-S.; et al. Tokyo Guidelines 2018: Initial management of acute biliary infection and flowchart for acute cholangitis. *J. Hepato-Biliary-Pancreat. Sci.* **2018**, *25*, 31–40. [CrossRef]
8. Charcot, M. De la fievre hepatique symptomatique—Comparison avec la fievre uroseptique. In *Lecons sur les Maladies du Foie des Voies Biliares et des Reins*; Bourneville et Sevestre: Paris, France, 1877; pp. 176–185.
9. Rumsey, S.; Winders, J.; MacCormick, A.D. Diagnostic accuracy of Charcot's triad: A systematic review. *ANZ J. Surg.* **2017**, *87*, 232–238. [CrossRef]
10. Weiland, C.J.S.; Busch, C.B.E.; Bhalla, A.; Bruno, M.J.; Fockens, P.; Hooft, J.E.; Poen, A.C.; Timmerhuis, H.C.; Umans, D.S.; Venneman, N.G.; et al. Performance of diagnostic tools for acute cholangitis in patients with suspected biliary obstruction. *J. Hepato-Biliary-Pancreat. Sci.* **2021**, *29*, 479–486. [CrossRef]
11. Wada, K.; Takada, T.; Kawarada, Y.; Nimura, Y.; Miura, F.; Yoshida, M.; Mayumi, T.; Strasberg, S.; Pitt, H.A.; Gadacz, T.R.; et al. Diagnostic criteria and severity assessment of acute cholangitis: Tokyo Guidelines. *J. Hepato-Biliary-Pancreat. Surg.* **2007**, *14*, 52–58. [CrossRef]
12. Yokoe, M.; Hata, J.; Takada, T.; Strasberg, S.M.; Bun, T.A.Y.; Wakabayashi, G.; Kozaka, K.; Endo, I.; DeZiel, D.J.; Miura, F.; et al. Tokyo Guidelines 2018: Diagnostic criteria and severity grading of acute cholecystitis (with videos). *J. Hepato-Biliary-Pancreat. Sci.* **2018**, *25*, 41–54. [CrossRef] [PubMed]
13. Schepers, N.J.; Hallensleben, N.D.L.; Besselink, M.G.; Anten, M.-P.G.F.; Bollen, T.L.; da Costa, D.W.; van Delft, F.; van Dijk, S.M.; van Dullemen, H.M.; Dijkgraaf, M.G.W.; et al. Urgent endoscopic retrograde cholangiopancreatography with sphincterotomy versus conservative treatment in predicted severe acute gallstone pancreatitis (APEC): A multicentre randomised controlled trial. *Lancet* **2020**, *396*, 167–176. [CrossRef] [PubMed]
14. Mulki, R.; Shah, R.; Qayed, E. Early *vs* late endoscopic retrograde cholangiopancreatography in patients with acute cholangitis: A nationwide analysis. *World J. Gastrointest. Endosc.* **2019**, *11*, 41–53. [CrossRef]
15. Gomi, H.; Solomkin, J.; Schlossberg, D.; Okamoto, K.; Takada, T.; Strasberg, S.M.; Ukai, T.; Endo, I.; Iwashita, Y.; Hibi, T.; et al. Tokyo Guidelines 2018: Antimicrobial therapy for acute cholangitis and cholecystitis. *J. Hepato-Biliary-Pancreat. Sci.* **2018**, *25*, 3–16. [CrossRef] [PubMed]
16. Tinusz, B.; Szapáry, L.; Páládi, B.; Tenk, J.; Rumbus, Z.; Pécsi, D.; Szakács, Z.; Varga, G.; Rakonczay, Z.; Szepes, Z.; et al. Short-Course Antibiotic Treatment Is Not Inferior to a Long-Course One in Acute Cholangitis: A Systematic Review. *Dig. Dis. Sci.* **2019**, *64*, 307–315. [CrossRef]
17. Haal, S.; Böhmer, B.T.; Balkema, S.; Depla, A.C.; Fockens, P.; Jansen, J.M.; Kuiken, S.D.; Liberov, B.I.; Van Soest, E.; Hooft, J.E.; et al. Antimicrobial therapy of 3 days or less is sufficient after successful ERCP for acute cholangitis. *United Eur. Gastroenterol. J.* **2020**, *8*, 481–488. [CrossRef]
18. Zheng, Y.; Chen, Y.; Yu, K.; Yang, Y.; Wang, X.; Yang, X.; Qian, J.; Liu, Z.-X.; Wu, B. Fatal Infections Among Cancer Patients: A Population-Based Study in the United States. *Infect. Dis. Ther.* **2021**, *10*, 871–895. [CrossRef]
19. Rolston, K.V.I. Infections in Cancer Patients with Solid Tumors: A Review. *Infect. Dis. Ther.* **2017**, *6*, 69–83. [CrossRef]
20. Teillant, A.; Gandra, S.; Barter, D.; Morgan, D.J.; Laxminarayan, R. Potential burden of antibiotic resistance on surgery and cancer chemotherapy antibiotic prophylaxis in the USA: A literature review and modelling study. *Lancet Infect. Dis.* **2015**, *15*, 1429–1437. [CrossRef]
21. Gudiol, C.; Aguado, J.M.; Carratala, J. Bloodstream infections in patients with solid tumors. *Virulence* **2016**, *7*, 298–308. [CrossRef]
22. Rupp, C.; Bode, K.; Weiss, K.H.; Rudolph, G.; Bergemann, J.; Kloeters-Plachky, P.; Chahoud, F.; Stremmel, W.; Gotthardt, D.N.; Sauer, P. Microbiological Assessment of Bile and Corresponding Antibiotic Treatment: A Strobe-Compliant Observational Study of 1401 Endoscopic Retrograde Cholangiographies. *Medicine* **2016**, *95*, e2390. [CrossRef]
23. Reuken, P.A.; Torres, D.; Baier, M.; Löffler, B.; Lübbert, C.; Lippmann, N.; Stallmach, A.; Bruns, T. Risk Factors for Multi-Drug Resistant Pathogens and Failure of Empiric First-Line Therapy in Acute Cholangitis. *PLoS ONE* **2017**, *12*, e0169900. [CrossRef]

24. Gromski, M.A.; Gutta, A.; Lehman, G.A.; Tong, Y.; Fogel, E.L.; Watkins, J.L.; Easler, J.J.; Bick, B.L.; McHenry, L.; Beeler, C.; et al. Microbiology of bile aspirates obtained at ERCP in patients with suspected acute cholangitis. *Endoscopy* **2022**, *54*, 1045–1052. [CrossRef]
25. Otani, T.; Ichiba, T.; Seo, K.; Naito, H. Blood cultures should be collected for acute cholangitis regardless of severity. *J. Infect. Chemother.* **2022**, *28*, 181–186. [CrossRef]
26. Chandra, S.; Klair, J.S.; Soota, K.; Livorsi, D.J.; Johlin, F.C. Endoscopic Retrograde Cholangio-Pancreatography-Obtained Bile Culture Can Guide Antibiotic Therapy in Acute Cholangitis. *Dig. Dis.* **2019**, *37*, 155–160. [CrossRef]
27. Zhao, C.; Liu, S.; Bai, X.; Song, J.; Fan, Q.; Chen, J. A Retrospective Study on Bile Culture and Antibiotic Susceptibility Patterns of Patients with Biliary Tract Infections. *Evid.-Based Complement. Altern. Med.* **2022**, *2022*, 9255444. [CrossRef] [PubMed]
28. Rerknimitr, R.; Fogel, E.L.; Kalayci, C.; Esber, E.; Lehman, G.A.; Sherman, S. Microbiology of bile in patients with cholangitis or cholestasis with and without plastic biliary endoprosthesis. *Gastrointest. Endosc.* **2002**, *56*, 885–889. [CrossRef] [PubMed]
29. Ligozzi, M.; Bernini, C.; Bonora, M.G.; de Fatima, M.; Zuliani, J.; Fontana, R. Evaluation of the VITEK 2 System for Identification and Antimicrobial Susceptibility Testing of Medically Relevant Gram-Positive Cocci. *J. Clin. Microbiol.* **2002**, *40*, 1681–1686. [CrossRef] [PubMed]
30. Clinical and Laboratory Standards Institute (CLSI). *Performance Standards for Antimicrobial Susceptibility Testing*; Twenty-Second Informational Supplement; CLSI Document M100-S22; Clinical and Laboratory Standards Institute: Wayne, PA, USA, 2013.
31. Rehman, S.; Ahmed, S.; Metry, M.; Canelo, R. Significance of Bile Culture and Biliary Tract Pathology in Determining Severity of Cholangitis; Review of Current Literature. *Ann. Emerg. Surg.* **2017**, *2*, 1009.
32. Tanaka, A.; Takada, T.; Kawarada, Y.; Nimura, Y.; Yoshida, M.; Miura, F.; Hirota, M.; Wada, K.; Mayumi, T.; Gomi, H.; et al. Antimicrobial therapy for acute cholangitis: Tokyo Guidelines. *J. Hepato-Biliary-Pancreat. Surg.* **2007**, *14*, 59–67. [CrossRef]
33. Melzer, M.; Toner, R.; Lacey, S.; Bettany, E.; Rait, G. Biliary tract infection and bacteraemia: Presentation, structural abnormalities, causative organisms and clinical outcomes. *Postgrad. Med. J.* **2007**, *83*, 773–776. [CrossRef] [PubMed]
34. Lee, C.-C.; Chang, I.-J.; Lai, Y.-C.; Chen, S.-Y.; Chen, S.-C. Epidemiology and Prognostic Determinants of Patients with Bacteremic Cholecystitis or Cholangitis. *Am. J. Gastroenterol.* **2007**, *102*, 563–569. [CrossRef] [PubMed]
35. Rhodes, A.; Evans, L.E.; Alhazzani, W.; Levy, M.M.; Antonelli, M.; Ferrer, R.; Kumar, A.; Sevransky, J.E.; Sprung, C.L.; Nunnally, M.E.; et al. Surviving Sepsis Campaign: International Guidelines for Management of Sepsis and Septic Shock: 2016. *Intensive Care Med.* **2017**, *43*, 304–377. [CrossRef] [PubMed]
36. Sacks, D.; Baxter, B.; Campbell, B.C.V.; Carpenter, J.S.; Cognard, C.; Dippel, D.; Eesa, M.; Fischer, U.; Hausegger, K.; Hirsch, J.A.; et al. Multisociety Consensus Quality Improvement Revised Consensus Statement for Endovascular Therapy of Acute Ischemic Stroke. *Int. J. Stroke* **2018**, *13*, 612–632. [CrossRef]
37. Kwan, K.E.L.; Shelat, V.G.; Tan, C.H. Recurrent pyogenic cholangitis: A review of imaging findings and clinical management. *Abdom. Radiol.* **2017**, *42*, 46–56. [CrossRef]
38. Li, M.; Liu, Q.; Teng, Y.; Ou, L.; Xi, Y.; Chen, S.; Duan, G. The resistance mechanism of Escherichia coli induced by ampicillin in laboratory. *Infect. Drug Resist.* **2019**, *12*, 2853–2863. [CrossRef]
39. Rice, L.B. Federal Funding for the Study of Antimicrobial Resistance in Nosocomial Pathogens: No ESKAPE. *J. Infect. Dis.* **2008**, *197*, 1079–1081. [CrossRef]
40. Di Domenico, E.G.; Cavallo, I.; Sivori, F.; Marchesi, F.; Prignano, G.; Pimpinelli, F.; Sperduti, I.; Pelagalli, L.; Di Salvo, F.; Celesti, I.; et al. Biofilm Production by Carbapenem-Resistant Klebsiella pneumoniae Significantly Increases the Risk of Death in Oncological Patients. *Front. Cell. Infect. Microbiol.* **2020**, *10*, 561741. [CrossRef]
41. Logan, L.K.; Weinstein, R.A. The Epidemiology of Carbapenem-Resistant Enterobacteriaceae: The Impact and Evolution of a Global Menace. *J. Infect. Dis.* **2017**, *215* (Suppl. 1), S28–S36. [CrossRef]
42. Osama, D.; El-Mahallawy, H.; Mansour, M.T.; Hashem, A.; Attia, A.S. Molecular Characterization of Carbapenemase-Producing Klebsiella pneumoniae Isolated from Egyptian Pediatric Cancer Patients Including a Strain with a Rare Gene-Combination of β-Lactamases. *Infect. Drug Resist.* **2021**, *14*, 335–348. [CrossRef]
43. Bouza, E.; Cercenado, E. *Klebsiella* and *Enterobacter*: Antibiotic resistance and treatment implications. *Semin. Respir. Infect.* **2002**, *17*, 215–230. [CrossRef] [PubMed]
44. Nirwati, H.; Sinanjung, K.; Fahrunissa, F.; Wijaya, F.; Napitupulu, S.; Hati, V.P.; Hakim, M.S.; Meliala, A.; Aman, A.T.; Nuryastuti, T. Biofilm formation and antibiotic resistance of Klebsiella pneumoniae isolated from clinical samples in a tertiary care hospital, Klaten, Indonesia. *BMC Proc.* **2019**, *13* (Suppl. 11), 20. [CrossRef] [PubMed]
45. Chen, K.-J.; Chen, Y.-P.; Chen, Y.-H.; Liu, L.; Wang, N.-K.; Chao, A.-N.; Wu, W.-C.; Hwang, Y.-S.; Chou, H.-D.; Kang, E.Y.-C.; et al. Infection Sources and *Klebsiella pneumoniae* Antibiotic Susceptibilities in Endogenous *Klebsiella* Endophthalmitis. *Antibiotics* **2022**, *11*, 866. [CrossRef] [PubMed]

Disclaimer/Publisher's Note: The statements, opinions and data contained in all publications are solely those of the individual author(s) and contributor(s) and not of MDPI and/or the editor(s). MDPI and/or the editor(s) disclaim responsibility for any injury to people or property resulting from any ideas, methods, instructions or products referred to in the content.

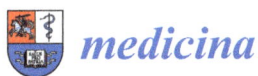

Article

Initial Experience of Robot-Assisted Transabdominal Preperitoneal (TAPP) Inguinal Hernia Repair by a Single Surgeon in South Korea

Yun Suk Choi, Kyeong Deok Kim, Moon Suk Choi, Yoon Seok Heo, Jin Wook Yi *,† and Yun-Mee Choe *,†

Department of Surgery, Inha University Hospital & College of Medicine, Incheon 22332, Republic of Korea
* Correspondence: jinwook.yi@inha.ac.kr (J.W.Y.); gsmee@inha.ac.kr (Y.-M.C.);
  Tel.: +82-32-890-3437 (J.W.Y. & Y.-M.C.); Fax: +82-32-890-3549 (J.W.Y. & Y.-M.C.)
† These authors contributed equally to this work.

Abstract: *Background and Objectives*: Inguinal hernia is a common surgical disease. Traditional open herniorrhaphy has been replaced by laparoscopic herniorrhaphy. Nowadays, many attempts at robotic herniorrhaphy have been reported in western countries, but there have been no reports in South Korea. The purpose of this study is to report our initial experience with robotic inguinal hernia surgery, compared to laparoscopic inguinal hernia surgery. *Materials and Methods*: We analyzed the clinical data from 100 patients who received inguinal hernia surgery in our hospital from November 2020 to June 2022. Fifty patients underwent laparoscopic surgery, and 50 patients underwent robotic surgery using the da Vinci Xi system. All hernia surgeries were performed by a single surgeon using the transabdominal preperitoneal (TAPP) method. *Results*: The mean operation time and hospital stay were not statistically different. On the first postoperative day, the visual analog scale (VAS) pain score was significantly lower in the robotic surgery group (2.9 ± 0.5 versus 2.5 ± 0.7, $p = 0.015$). Cumulative sum analysis revealed an approximately 12-case learning curve for robotic-assisted TAPP hernia surgery. *Conclusions*: Robotic-assisted TAPP inguinal hernia surgery is technically acceptable to surgeons who have performed laparoscopic inguinal hernia surgery, and the learning curve is relatively short. It is thought to be a good step toward learning other robot-assisted operations.

Keywords: inguinal hernia; robotic surgery; hernia surgery

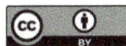

1. Introduction

Inguinal hernias have a lifetime incidence of 25% among men and 3% among women [1,2]. In the United States, 700,000 to 800,000 hernia repairs are performed annually. In South Korea, about 34,000 such annual repairs are performed out of about 50,000 patients treated for inguinal hernias. [1–5] Inguinal hernia causes discomfort to the patient as it progresses, and bowel strangulation may occur in severe cases. Hernia is a problem caused by a structural defect in the human body, and surgery to correct it is performed as the gold standard of treatment.

Open hernia surgery was the mainstay of hernia repair until the late 1990s. The tension-free and Lichtenstein methods of open hernia repair were introduced to reduce postoperative pain and recurrence. [1] After the development of endoscopic surgery, laparoscopic inguinal hernia surgery was first reported in 1991 by Ger et al. [6] The rate of laparoscopic hernia surgery has been gradually increasing recently, and it is considered the primary operation choice by some surgeons. In South Korea, more than 40% of inguinal hernia operations are performed laparoscopically. [4,5] The advantages of laparoscopic hernia repair include the following: it is associated with less pain, smaller wounds, lower recurrence rates, earlier returns to work, school, and activities of daily living, and lower complication rates. Also, bilateral hernia surgery is possible with the same incision with a laparoscopic approach [7,8].

Several studies have demonstrated the advantages of robotic surgery, such as 3-dimensional visualization, the elimination of tremor, EndoWrist's precise and free movement, and improved surgeon comfort and performance. [7–10] Given these advantages, robotic surgery has been applied to a variety of surgical contexts, and this has further confirmed its safety and efficacy. [11–14] The first report of robot-assisted hernia surgery was of a repair performed together with urologic procedures in 2014, and Dominguez et al. reported the first robotic hernia surgery results. [1,15] Since then, robotic hernia surgery has been reported to reduce postoperative pain and facilitate ergonomic optimization for surgeons, and it has been attempted and adopted by surgeons worldwide [1,15–17].

Our institution has performed the most robotic inguinal hernia surgeries in South Korea. This study aimed to evaluate the safety and effectiveness of robotic inguinal hernia surgery compared with laparoscopic inguinal hernia surgery and the learning curve for robotic inguinal hernia surgery.

2. Materials and Methods

2.1. Study Design

We retrospectively analyzed the electronic medical data of patients who underwent laparoscopic or robot-assisted inguinal hernia surgery at our hospital between November 2020 and June 2022. The surgical candidates for robotic inguinal hernia surgery were the same as those for laparoscopic hernia surgery. The choice was left to the patients after they were provided with detailed information about both options. Robotic inguinal hernia surgery was chosen when the patient agreed to the procedure despite its higher expense compared to laparoscopic surgery. We reviewed clinical data, including age, gender, body mass index (BMI), preoperative clinical diagnosis, preoperative morbidity, preoperative hernia surgery history, hernia type, operation time, postoperative pain, hospital stay, postoperative complications, and cost of surgery. All surgical videos were recorded, and we reviewed all of these videos. We captured video clips of important moments and determined actual operation times using the surgical videos. In cases of combined other operations, operation time and cost of surgery data were only evaluated for the hernia surgery. The cost of surgery variable only took into account the fees paid for surgery and excluded extra expenses, such as hospitalization fees and others.

2.2. Patients

From November 2020 through June 2022, 100 cases of robotic and laparoscopic inguinal hernia surgery were performed by a single surgeon (YS Choi) at the authors' hospital. All patients underwent inguinal hernia surgery using the transabdominal preperitoneal (TAPP) approach. The analysis considered two groups: the laparoscopic inguinal hernia repair (LIHR) group and the robotic inguinal hernia repair (RIHR) group. There were 50 patients in each group.

The surgeon for all of the cases is a gastrointestinal surgeon who has performed more than 100 cases of LIHR using totally extraperitoneal (TEP) and TAPP approaches. After the introduction of robotic-assisted TAPP hernia surgery at our hospital. This was the main technique of choice except when there were contraindications such as previous abdominal surgery history, previous laparoscopic hernia surgery history, or a poor condition for general anesthesia.

2.3. Statistics and Ethical Considerations

All statistical analyses were performed using SPSS Statistics for Windows, version 28 (IBM Corp., Armonk, NY, USA). Continuous variables are presented as means ± standard deviations. Unpaired t-tests were used to compare means. The chi-square test, or Fisher's exact test, was applied to the cross-table analysis according to the sample size.

The ethics of this study were approved by the Institutional Review Board of Inha University Hospital (IRB number: INHAUH 2022-11-024).

2.4. Cumulative Sum (CUSUM) Analysis

The operation times of robotic-assisted TAPP operations were analyzed from the start of 50 cases. All surgical videos were reviewed, and the console times of all robotic procedures were determined. In the case of bilateral hernias, we considered the need for surgery only on the more severe side. The learning curve was assessed based on the console times. Inflection points were based on each set of three or more consecutive negative values. Based on these inflection points, the learning curve was divided into pre-adapted and post-adapted phases.

2.5. Surgical Procedure for Robotic-Assisted TAPP Inguinal Hernia Repair

All operations were performed via the TAPP approach. Under general anesthesia, patients were placed in the supine position. Three trocars were inserted (Figure 1). The trocar locations were as follows: a camera port was inserted through the umbilicus, and two operating ports were inserted at both lateral aspects of the rectus abdominis muscle. A 12-mm trocar was used to insert mesh or gauze through the umbilicus. We tried to hide a 12-mm trocar wound using the umbilicus. The same locations were used for the robotic and laparoscopic groups. A distance of about 10 cm was maintained between the trocars.

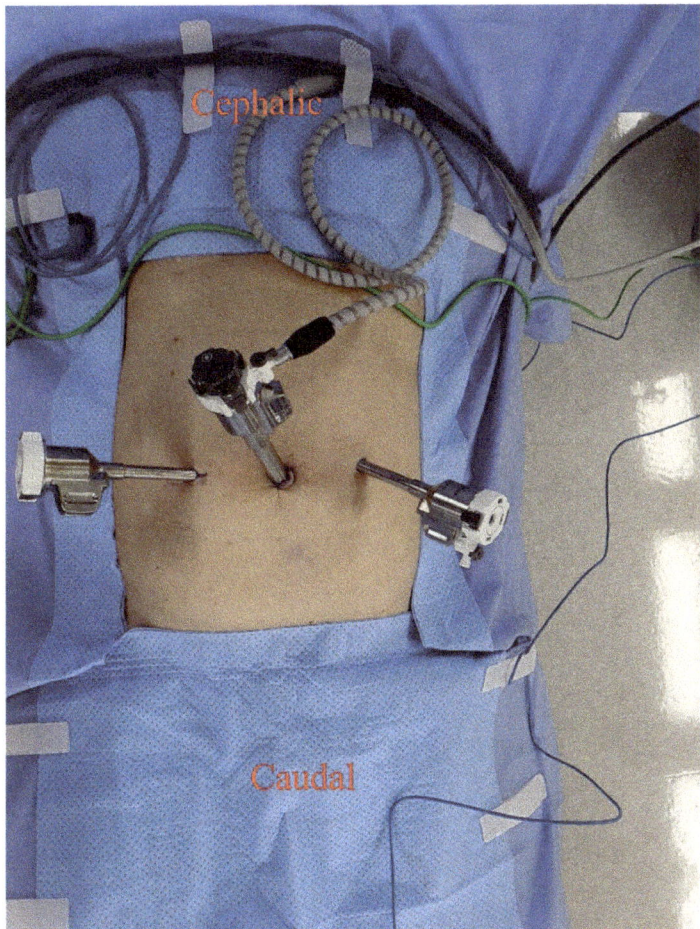

Figure 1. Robotic-assisted TAPP inguinal hernia surgery trocar placement.

In the RIHR group, the camera was first inserted, and then targeting was performed on the hernia site. In bilateral hernia repairs, targeting was performed in the middle of both hernias. To prevent collision of the robot arms, we spaced the robotic arms as far apart as possible, and we performed robotic machine docking (Figure 2). We use three types of robotic EndoWrist instruments: prograsp forceps for tissue grasping, monopolar curved scissors for dissecting the peritoneum, and mega needle holders for dissecting the hernia sac and suturing the peritoneum.

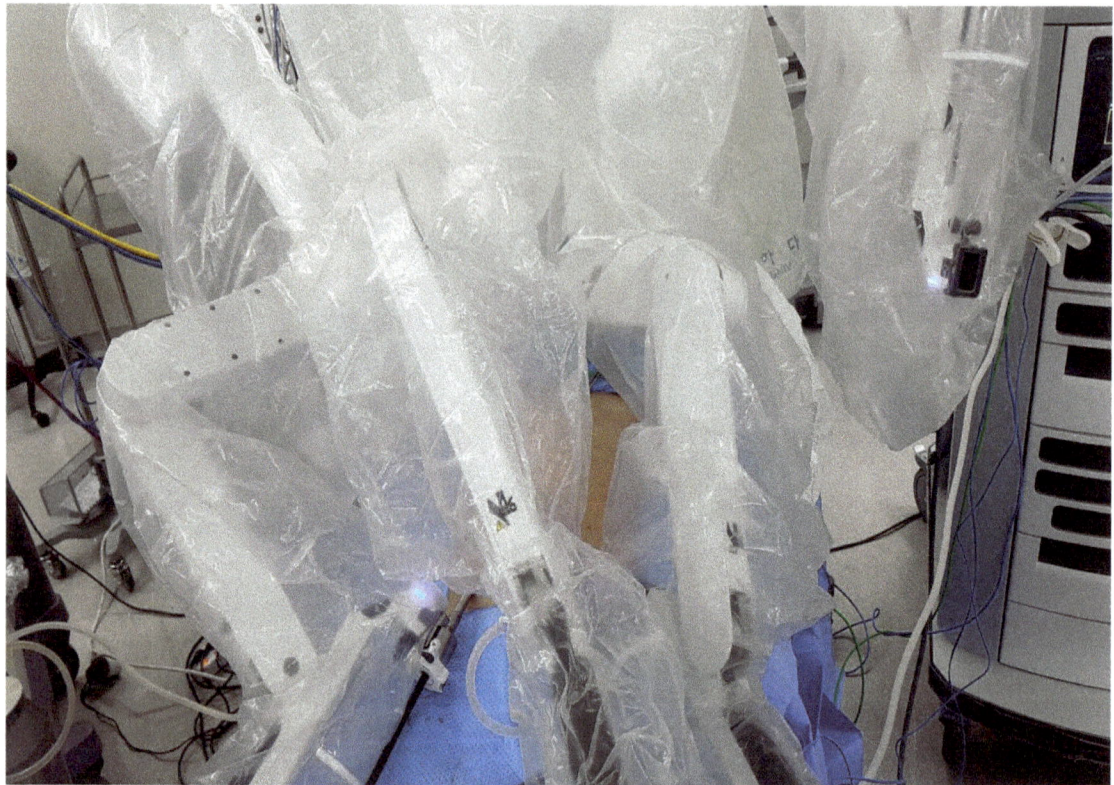

Figure 2. Robotic-assisted TAPP inguinal hernia surgery docking status.

The steps of RIHR are shown in Figure 3. The peritoneum was dissected using monopolar curved scissors (Figure 3A). At this time, we were careful to avoid damage to the inferior epigastric vessels, and we started peritoneal dissection adjacent to the vessels. We performed a sufficiently wide area dissection that included the hernia site and inserted a 15.7 X 10.3 cm large size mesh (3DMax™ Light Mesh,1 Becton drive Franklin Lakes, NJ 07417, USA) without wrinkles. In the case where there were adhesions of the omentum or bowel around the hernia site during surgery, we performed adhesiolysis before peritoneal dissection.

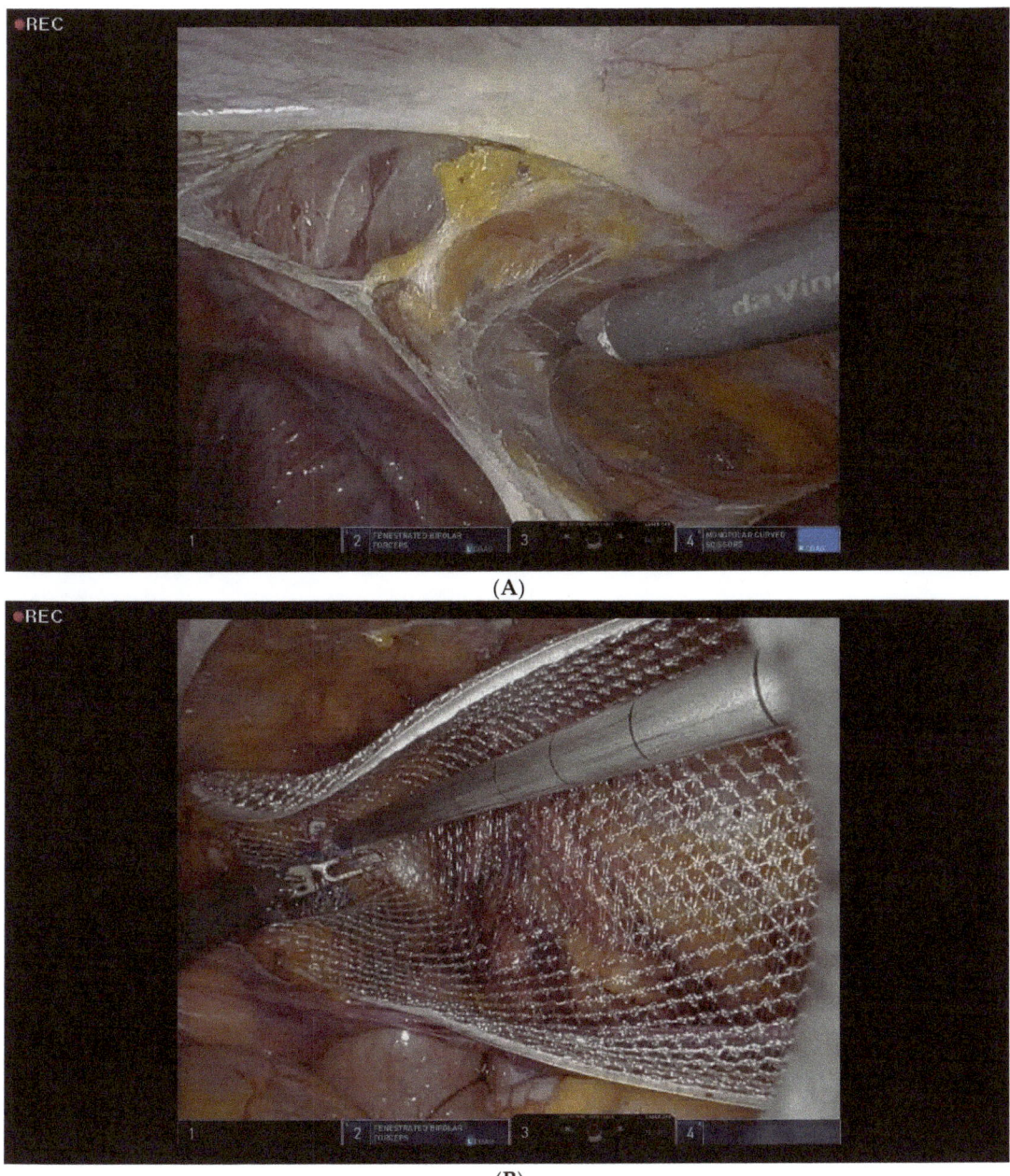

Figure 3. *Cont.*

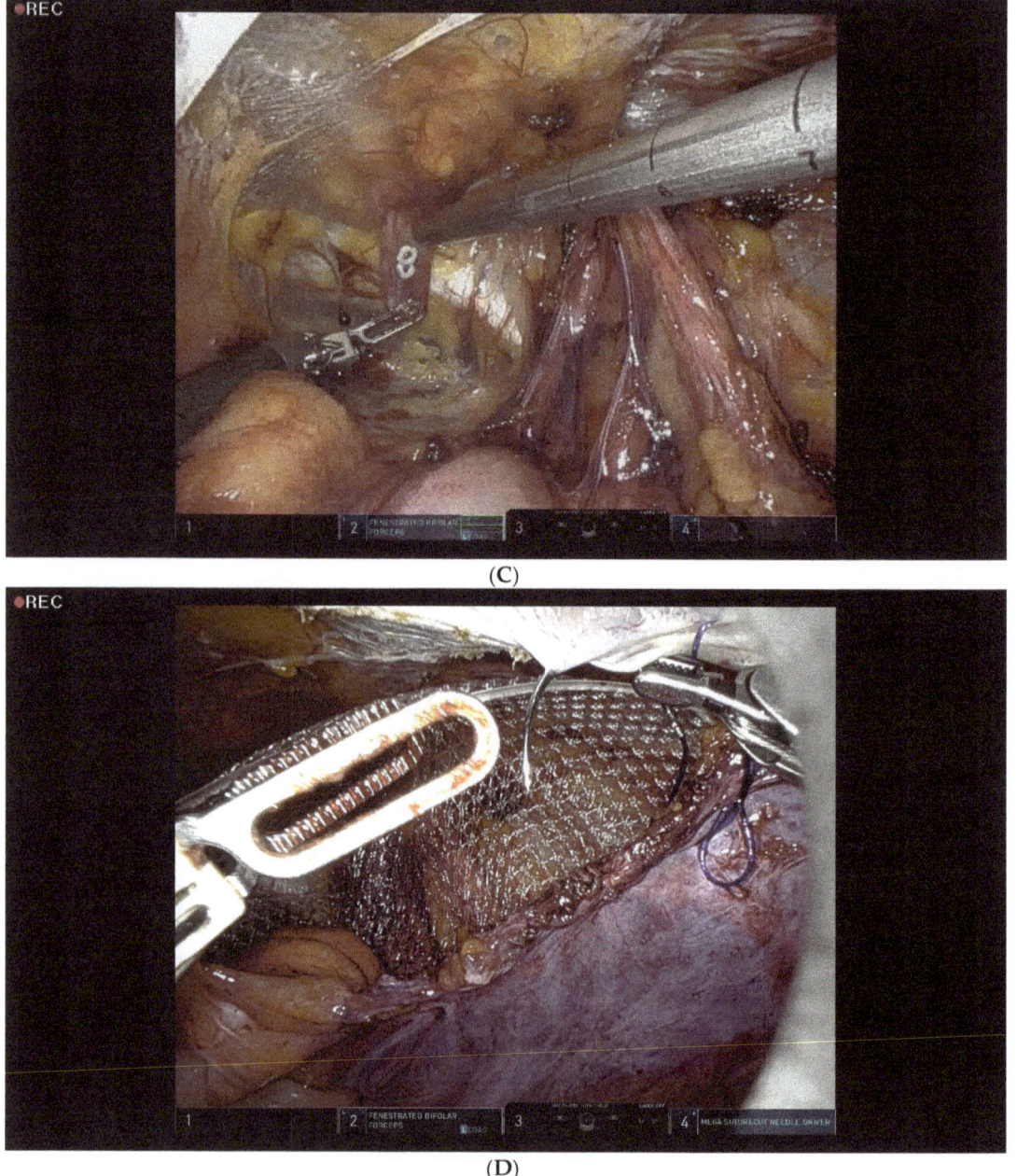

Figure 3. Robotic-assisted TAPP hernia repair procedure. (**A**). Peritoneum dissection using monopolar curved scissors. (**B**). Mesh application using a tack on the pubic bone. (**C**). Hernia sac fixation using a tack on the pubic bone. (**D**). Reperitonization using a robotic arm.

After peritoneal dissection, we identified the hernia sac and dissected the hernia sac from the vas deferens and testicular vessels. A large-sized mesh was applied to a large enough area to include the entire hernia site, and we fixed the mesh onto the pubic bone using a tacker. To prevent injury by tacker slippage during fixation, we immobilized the tacker with a robot arm before firing the tacker (Figure 3B).

For indirect hernia cases, we performed hernia sac inversion after hernia sac dissection, and we sutured the hernia sac together during reperitonization. For direct hernia cases, we fixed the hernia sac to the pubic bone using a tacker to flatten the hernia site (Figure 3C), and we applied a large-size mesh to the pubic bone with a tacker. After reperitonization, we confirmed that there were no defects in the peritoneum without exposure to mesh, and we completed the operation (Figure 3D).

3. Results

Table 1 summarizes the clinical characteristics of the 50 patients who underwent LIHR and the 50 patients who underwent RIHR. The mean age of the LIHR group was significantly higher than that of the RHIR group (64.40 ± 14.83 versus 54.40 ± 13.97 years; $p = 0.001$). There were no differences in gender ratio or mean BMI between the two groups. The mean American Society of Anesthesiology (ASA) score indicating preoperative condition was significantly higher in the LIHR group. (2.32 ± 0.55 versus 2.02 ± 0.38; $p = 0.002$). The proportion of patients with ASA III (indicating patients with severe systemic disease) was significantly higher in the LIHR group (18/50 (36.0%) versus 4/50 (8.0%); $p = 0.003$). The LIHR group had significantly more patients with hypertension (HTN) than the RIHR group, but there were no significant differences in terms of other underlying diseases and lifestyle factors between the two groups.

Table 1. Clinical characteristics of hernia patients.

Variables	All (n = 100)	Laparoscopic TAPP (n = 50)	Robotic TAPP (n = 50)	p-Value
Age (years, mean ± SD)	59.4 ± 15.2	64.4 ± 14.8	54.4 ± 14.0	0.001
BMI [a]	24.3 ± 2.9	23.8 ± 2.9	24.8 ± 3.0	0.116
Gender (%)				
Male	99 (99%)	49 (98%)	50 (100%)	0.315
Female	1 (1%)	1 (2%)	0 (0%)	
ASA [b] score	2.2 ± 0.5	2.3 ± 0.6	2.0 ± 0.4	0.002
CLASS I (%)	5 (5%)	2 (2%)	3 (6%)	0.003
CLASS II (%)	73 (60%)	30 (60%)	43 (86%)	
CLASS III (%)	22 (100%)	18 (36%)	4 (8%)	
Comorbidities (%)				
HTN [c]	44 (43%)	30 (60%)	14 (28%)	0.001
DM [d]	14 (13%)	9 (18%)	5 (10%)	0.249
Cardiovascular	15 (15%)	10 (20%)	5 (10%)	0.161
Pulmonary	10 (10%)	7 (14%)	3 (6%)	0.182
Renal	0 (0%)	0 (0%)	0 (0%)	1
Liver	6 (6%)	3 (6%)	3 (6%)	1
Cerebral	4 (4%)	3 (6%)	1 (2%)	0.307
Other cancer history	10 (10%)	6 (12%)	4 (8%)	0.505
BPH [e]	20 (20%)	12 (24%)	8 (16%)	0.317
Smoking	34 (34%)	15 (30%)	19 (38%)	0.398
Alcohol	42 (42%)	20 (40%)	22 (44%)	0.685
Steroid use	0 (0%)	0 (0%)	0 (0%)	1

[a] Body mass index; [b] American Society of Anesthesiology; [c] Hypertension; [d] Diabetes mellitus; [e] Benign prostate hyperplasia.

Table 2 summarizes the operational details of the two groups. There was no significant difference in mean operation time between the LIHR and RIHR groups (31.52 ± 10.31 versus 30.22 ± 11.87 min; $p = 0.56$). The mean cost of surgery was significantly higher in the RIHR group (209.61 ± 27.52 US dollars versus 3814.75 ± 172.97 US dollars; $p < 0.001$). The RIHR group's cost of surgery includes the cost of several consumables, including a $400 laparoscopic tacker. All operations were completed according to the existing planned surgical method, without open or laparoscopic conversion. There was no significant difference in hernia type between the 2 groups. Indirect hernias were the most common, followed by direct hernias. There were 2 cases of combined hernias in the RIHR group and 1 case in the LIHR group. There was 1 case of femoral hernia in the RIHR group and 1 case of spigelian hernia in the LIHR group. Right-sided inguinal hernias were more common than left-sided inguinal hernias in both groups. There were 5 cases of bilateral inguinal hernias in the LIHR group and 3 cases in the RIHR group, respectively.

Table 2. Intraoperative details.

Variables	All (n = 100)	Laparoscopic TAPP (n = 50)	Robotic TAPP (n = 50)	*p*-Value
Operation time (minutes, mean ± SD)	30.8 ± 11.1	31.5 ± 10.3	30.2 ± 11.9	0.56
Conversion rate (%) (Open or Laparoscopic)	0 (0%)	0 (0%)	0 (0%)	1
Cost of surgery (USD [a])		209.6 ± 27.5	3814.8 ± 172.9	<0.001
Type of hernia (%)				0.829
Indirect only	87 (87%)	44 (88%)	43 (86%)	
Direct only	7 (7%)	3 (6%)	4 (8%)	
Combined direct and indirect	3 (3%)	1 (2%)	2 (4%)	
Femoral	1 (1%)	0 (0%)	1 (2%)	
Spigelian	1 (1%)	1 (2%)	0 (0%)	
Hernia site (%)				0.483
Right	61 (61%)	32 (64%)	29 (58%)	
Left	31 (31%)	13 (26%)	18 (36%)	
Bilateral	8 (8%)	5 (10%)	3 (6%)	
Previous contralateral hernia (%)	10 (10%)	4 (8%)	6 (12%)	0.505
Complex hernia (%)				
Recurrent hernia	8 (8%)	5 (10%)	3 (6%)	0.461
Incarceration	9 (9%)	4 (8%)	5 (10%)	0.727
Prostatectomy history	8 (8%)	6 (12%)	2 (4%)	0.14

[a] United States dollar.

The postoperative outcomes are summarized in Table 3. There were no significant intergroup differences in hospital stays, readmission rates within 30 days, or hernia recurrence rates. Postoperative pain was evaluated using a visual analog scale (VAS). There was no difference in VAS pain scores on operation day. On postoperative day 1, the VAS pain score was statistically significantly lower in the RIHR group (2.86 ± 0.54 versus 2.54 ± 0.73; $p = 0.015$). Postoperative seroma and hematoma formation occurred more frequently in the LIHR group, but there was no significant difference. Urinary retention was also more common in the LIHR group, but again, there was no significant difference between the groups (5/50 (10.0%) versus 3/50 (6.0%); $p = 0.461$).

Table 3. Postoperative outcomes.

Variables	All (n = 100)	Laparoscopic TAPP (n = 50)	Robotic TAPP (n = 50)	p-Value
Hospital stay (days, mean ± SD)	3.4 ± 1.6	3.5 ± 2.2	3.4 ± 0.6	0.658
VAS [a] score				
Operation day (0–10, mean ± SD)	4.7 ± 1.0	4.6 ± 1.1	4.8 ± 0.9	0.243
Postoperative 1 day (0–10, mean ± SD)	2.7 ± 0.7	2.9 ± 0.5	2.5 ± 0.7	0.015
Readmission within 30 days (%)	0 (0%)	0 (0%)	0 (0%)	1
Hernia recurrence (%)	1 (1%)	1 (2%)	0 (0%)	0.315
Postoperative outcome (%)				
Infection (Surgical site, Mesh)	0 (0%)	0 (0%)	0 (0%)	1
Seroma	2 (2%)	2 (4%)	0 (0%)	0.153
Hematoma	4 (4%)	3 (6%)	1 (2%)	0.307
Prolonged ileus	0 (0%)	0 (0%)	0 (0%)	1
Bowel obstruction	0 (0%)	0 (0%)	0 (0%)	1
Bladder injury	0 (0%)	0 (0%)	1 (2%)	0.315
Urinary retention	8 (8%)	5 (10%)	3 (6%)	0.461

[a] visual analog scale.

The console time of robotic inguinal hernia surgery was analyzed using CUSUM analysis (Figure 4). The inflection point was measured at approximately 12 cases. After the inflection point, it was confirmed that the CUSUM score decreased continuously. We compared the operation times between the pre-adapted phase and the post-adapted phase based on the inflection point. The mean operation time was shorter in the post-adaptation phase than in the pre-adaptation phase, but this difference was not statistically significant (35.50 ± 17.01 versus 28.55 ± 9.41 min; p = 0.077).

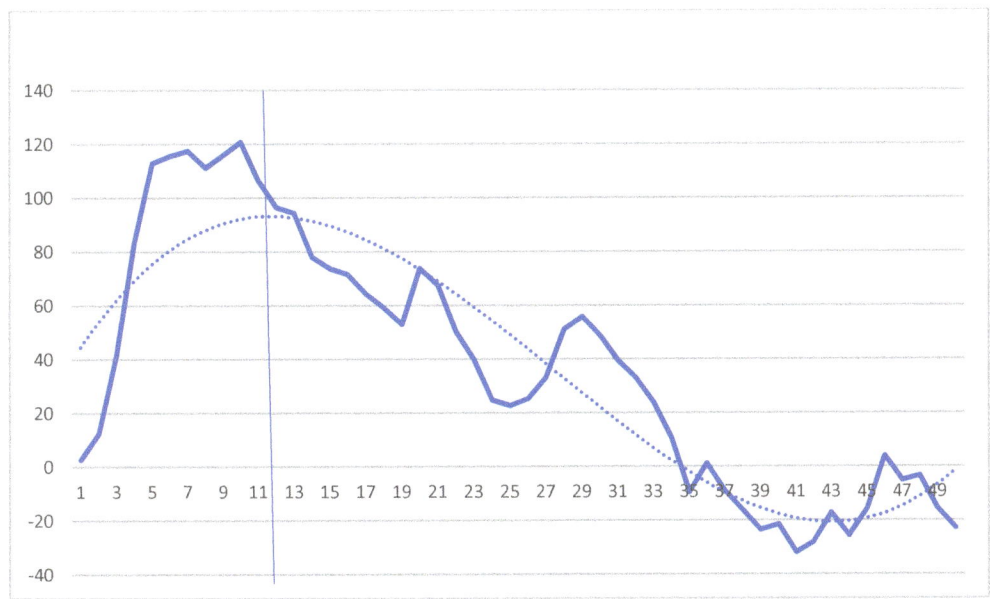

Figure 4. Cumulative sum (CUSUM) analysis of console times for robotic-assisted TAPP inguinal hernia surgery. The x-axis indicates consecutive cases, and the y-axis indicates the CUSUM score for robot console times. The vertical line represents the inflection point that divides between the early and late phases.

4. Discussion

Many studies have evaluated the advantages and disadvantages of robotic inguinal hernia surgery. Robotic inguinal hernia surgery is more expensive and takes longer than conventional laparoscopic inguinal hernia surgery, and it is not conducive to operator ergonomics. [18] Several articles have reported relatively long operation times but low postoperative complication rates and pain levels associated with robotic inguinal surgery. [16,17,19,20] The Da Vinci Xi system dramatically reduced robot docking time compared with the previous Si system. In our study, the actual docking time was about 2 min. Considering that there was little difference between the laparoscopic operation time and the robot console time (31.5 ± 10.3 versus 30.2 ± 11.9 min; p = 0.56), the mean total operation time was not different between the two groups. After passing the learning curve, the mean operation time decreased to 28 min, and there was no statistically significant difference in operation time between the pre-adaptation phase and the post-adaptation phase. (31.52 ± 10.31 versus 28.55 ± 9.41 min; p = 0.169). The long operation times mentioned in previous publications did not apply to our study. In our study, the mean pain score on the first postoperative day was lower in the RIHR group. Postoperative complication rates were lower in the RIHR group, but there was no statistical difference.

The learning curve for robotic inguinal hernia surgery was about 12 cases in our study, which was similar to what has been reported elsewhere. [20] However, longer learning curves have also been reported. [21] Laparoscopic inguinal hernia surgery is a frequently performed operation. [1–5] Robotic inguinal hernia surgery has favorable characteristics, such as short operation times, a short learning curve, a relatively fixed view, and minimal equipment requirements. Considering this, robotic inguinal hernia surgery is thought to be a good option for a first procedure for surgeons learning robotic surgery.

The 3-dimensional augmented view of the robotic surgery system is helpful for protecting the vas deferens and testicular vessels. The EndoWrist movement of the robotic arm facilitates efficient removal of the hernia sac without damaging these structures. Old and severe hernias are associated with difficult hernia sac dissections due to severe adhesions. The free movement and strong force of the robotic arm make this easier, and these features are very useful for the excision of huge cord lipomas. The robotic surgery system is helpful for reperitonization after mesh application. The free movement of the robotic arm facilitates reverse suturing and complete reperitonization of the injured peritoneum during hernia sac dissection without mesh exposure. The conventional laparoscopic TAPP approach is inconvenient for human ergonomics due to the surgeon's posture being very uncomfortable; however, this ergonomic inconvenience has been improved, and the operator is now able to perform the operation in a more comfortable position. We plan to conduct a study investigating surgical ergonomics in this context using intraoperative surgeon electromyography (EMG) in the future [22–25].

The central camera port was inserted transumbilically to minimize scarring, and the two ports for the remaining robotic arm were inserted into the lateral aspects of the rectus abdominis muscle. Using these port locations, it is easy to operate on incidentally discovered contralateral hernias. In addition, surgeries such as cholecystectomy can be performed only by changing the direction of the robot docking without changing the port site. We performed robotic-assisted TAPP inguinal repair on 2 patients with morbid obesity (BMI ≥35). In such cases, it is difficult to secure the operative field because of the severe visceral obesity, so an additional assist port is used. The intuitive guideline recommended that an assist port be inserted at the level of the epigastric area between the two robot arms. In this situation, an assistant must be placed between the robot arms, which can lead to frequent extracorporeal fighting between the robot arm and the assistant. In our experience, insertion of the assistant on the lateral side of the arm opposite the hernia site reduces this extracorporeal fighting. The para-umbilical camera port is considered to move toward the hernia site in morbidly obese patients. This can help further centralize the target anatomy and avoid a thick pannus and preperitoneal fat layer over the median umbilical ligament in obese patients. This may be helpful in reducing the use of additional ports.

There was no significant difference in the rates of hematoma formation, but hematomas were more frequently encountered in the LIHR group (n = 3) than the RIHR group (n = 1). For mesh fixation during inguinal hernia surgery, the mesh is usually fixed to the pubic bone or rectus muscle using a tacker. The assistant uses the tacker in robotic hernia surgery, and tacker misfires can cause bleeding and injury to surrounding organs. In our study, one tacker misfire occurred due to slipping during tacker fire, and we performed prolonged gauze compression to induce and confirm hemostasis. Given this concern, some surgeons prefer to use fibrin glue for mesh fixation or do not perform mesh fixation. However, it is necessary to pull the hernia sac and fix it to the pubic bone with a tacker to flatten the hernia sac in direct and other hernias. To prevent misfire, it is helpful to immobilize the assistant's tacker with the opposite robot arm and guide positioning to prevent tacker slipping (Figure 3B).

Our study had some limitations, including the relatively small sample size (50 cases per group) and the fact that selection bias cannot be excluded in retrospective studies. Because robotic surgery is expensive, it was mainly chosen by people with personal health insurance. In South Korea, these people are relatively young and have a lot of interest in health. This selection bias occurred because a randomized control trial was impossible due to cost differences. However, our study was meaningful in that it was the first study on robotic inguinal hernia surgery conducted in South Korea. Recently, interest in robotic inguinal hernia surgery has increased in South Korea. Surgeons at various hospitals are introducing robotic inguinal hernia surgery into their practices, and a large number of multicenter studies on the effectiveness and safety of robotic inguinal hernia surgery are planned.

The authors should discuss the results and how they can be interpreted from the perspective of previous studies and the working hypotheses. The findings and their implications should be discussed in the broadest possible context. Future research directions may also be highlighted.

5. Conclusions

Robotic-assisted TAPP inguinal hernia surgery is a safe and efficient minimally invasive surgical procedure associated with a short learning curve. It can be learned without difficulty by surgeons who are proficient at laparoscopic inguinal hernia surgery. Also, robot inguinal hernia surgery is acceptable as a bridge operation for other, more complex robot surgeries.

Author Contributions: Conceptualization, Y.S.C.; methodology, Y.S.C.; formal analysis, Y.S.C. and M.S.C.; investigation, Y.S.C.; resources, Y.S.C.; data curation, Y.S.C. and K.D.K.; writing—original draft preparation, Y.S.C.; writing—review and editing, J.W.Y. and Y.-M.C.; visualization, Y.S.C.; supervision, Y.S.H., J.W.Y. and Y.-M.C.; project administration, Y.S.C. All authors have read and agreed to the published version of the manuscript.

Funding: This research received no external funding.

Institutional Review Board Statement: The study was conducted in accordance with the Declaration of Helsinki and approved by the Institutional Review Board of Inha University Hospital & College of Medicine (protocol code INHAUH 2022-11-024 and date of approval 28 November 2022).

Informed Consent Statement: Patient consent was waived due to a retrospective study of the medical record.

Data Availability Statement: No new data were created or analyzed in this study from medical records.

Acknowledgments: This study was supported by a research grant from Inha University Hospital.

Conflicts of Interest: The authors declare no conflict of interest.

References

1. International guidelines for groin hernia management. *Hernia* **2018**, *22*, 1–165. [CrossRef] [PubMed]
2. Kingsnorth, A.; LeBlanc, K. Hernias: Inguinal and incisional. *Lancet* **2003**, *362*, 1561–1571. [CrossRef] [PubMed]
3. Schumpelick, V.; Treutner, K.H.; Arlt, G. Inguinal hernia repair in adults. *Lancet* **1994**, *344*, 375–379. [CrossRef] [PubMed]
4. Han, S.R.; Kim, H.J.; Kim, N.H.; Shin, S.; Yoo, R.N.; Kim, G.; Cho, H.M. Inguinal hernia surgery in Korea: Nationwide data from 2007–2015. *Ann. Surg. Treat. Res.* **2019**, *97*, 41–47. [CrossRef] [PubMed]
5. Health Insurance Review and Assessment Service. *Korea Healthcare Bigdata Hub [Internet]*; Health Insurance Review and Assessment Service: Wonju, Republic of Korea, 2021. Available online: http://opendata.hira.or.kr/ (accessed on 6 January 2020).
6. Ger, R. Laparoscopic hernia operation. *Der Chirurg; Zeitschrift fur alle Gebiete der Operativen Medizen* **1991**, *62*, 266–270. [PubMed]
7. Aiolfi, A.; Cavalli, M.; Micheletto, G.; Lombardo, F.; Bonitta, G.; Morlacchi, A.; Bruni, P.G.; Campanelli, G.; Bona, D. Primary inguinal hernia: Systematic review and Bayesian network meta-analysis comparing open, laparoscopic transabdominal preperitoneal, totally extraperitoneal, and robotic preperitoneal repair. *Hernia* **2019**, *23*, 473–484. [CrossRef] [PubMed]
8. Pirolla, E.H.; Patriota, G.P.; Pirolla, F.J.C.; Ribeiro, F.P.G.; Rodrigues, M.G.; Ismail, L.R.; Ruano, R.M. Inguinal Repair via Robotic Assisted Technique: Literature Review. *Arq. Bras. Cir. Dig. ABCD Braz. Arch. Dig. Surg.* **2018**, *31*, e1408. [CrossRef]
9. Aiolfi, A.; Cavalli, M.; Micheletto, G.; Bruni, P.G.; Lombardo, F.; Perali, C.; Bonitta, G.; Bona, D. Robotic inguinal hernia repair: Is technology taking over? Systematic review and meta-analysis. *Hernia* **2019**, *23*, 509–519. [CrossRef]
10. Ishii, H.; Rai, B.P.; Stolzenburg, J.U.; Bose, P.; Chlosta, P.L.; Somani, B.K.; Nabi, G.; Qazi, H.A.; Rajbabu, K.; Kynaston, H.; et al. Robotic or open radical cystectomy, which is safer? A systematic review and meta-analysis of comparative studies. *J. Endourol.* **2014**, *28*, 1215–1223. [CrossRef]
11. Escobar Dominguez, J.E.; Ramos, M.G.; Seetharamaiah, R.; Donkor, C.; Rabaza, J.; Gonzalez, A. Feasibility of robotic inguinal hernia repair, a single-institution experience. *Surg. Endosc.* **2016**, *30*, 4042–4048. [CrossRef]
12. Oviedo, R.J.; Robertson, J.C.; Alrajhi, S. First 101 Robotic General Surgery Cases in a Community Hospital. *JSLS J. Soc. Laparoendosc. Surg.* **2016**, *20*, e2016.00056. [CrossRef] [PubMed]
13. Arcerito, M.; Changchien, E.; Bernal, O.; Konkoly-Thege, A.; Moon, J. Robotic Inguinal Hernia Repair: Technique and Early Experience. *Am. Surg.* **2016**, *82*, 1014–1017. [CrossRef]
14. Kudsi, O.Y.; McCarty, J.C.; Paluvoi, N.; Mabardy, A.S. Transition from Laparoscopic Totally Extraperitoneal Inguinal Hernia Repair to Robotic Transabdominal Preperitoneal Inguinal Hernia Repair: A Retrospective Review of a Single Surgeon's Experience. *World J. Surg.* **2017**, *41*, 2251–2257. [CrossRef] [PubMed]
15. Escobar Dominguez, J.E.; Gonzalez, A.; Donkor, C. Robotic inguinal hernia repair. *J. Surg. Oncol.* **2015**, *112*, 310–314. [CrossRef] [PubMed]
16. Qabbani, A.; Aboumarzouk, O.M.; ElBakry, T.; Al-Ansari, A.; Elakkad, M.S. Robotic inguinal hernia repair: Systematic review and meta-analysis. *ANZ J. Surg.* **2021**, *91*, 2277–2287. [CrossRef]
17. Morrell, A.L.G.; Morrell Junior, A.C.; Mendes, J.M.F.; Morrell, A.G.; Morrell, A. Robotic TAPP inguinal hernia repair: Lessons learned from 97 cases. *Rev. Col. Bras. Cir.* **2021**, *48*, e20202704. [CrossRef]
18. Prabhu, A.S.; Carbonell, A.; Hope, W.; Warren, J.; Higgins, R.; Jacob, B.; Blatnik, J.; Haskins, I.; Alkhatib, H.; Tastaldi, L.; et al. Robotic Inguinal vs. Transabdominal Laparoscopic Inguinal Hernia Repair: The RIVAL Randomized Clinical Trial. *JAMA Surg.* **2020**, *155*, 380–387. [CrossRef]
19. Tatarian, T.; Nie, L.; McPartland, C.; Brown, A.M.; Yang, J.; Altieri, M.S.; Spaniolas, K.; Docimo, S.; Pryor, A.D. Comparative perioperative and 5-year outcomes of robotic and laparoscopic or open inguinal hernia repair: A study of 153,727 patients in the state of New York. *Surg. Endosc.* **2021**, *35*, 7209–7218. [CrossRef]
20. Tam, V.; Rogers, D.E.; Al-Abbas, A.; Borrebach, J.; Dunn, S.A.; Zureikat, A.H.; Zeh, H.J., 3rd; Hogg, M.E. Robotic Inguinal Hernia Repair: A Large Health System's Experience With the First 300 Cases and Review of the Literature. *J. Surg. Res.* **2019**, *235*, 98–104. [CrossRef]
21. Kudsi, O.Y.; Bou-Ayash, N.; Gokcal, F.; Crawford, A.S.; Chung, S.K.; Chudner, A.; Litwin, D. Learning curve of robot-assisted transabdominal preperitoneal (rTAPP) inguinal hernia repair: A cumulative sum (CUSUM) analysis. *Surg. Endosc.* **2022**, *36*, 1827–1837. [CrossRef]
22. González-Sánchez, M.; González-Poveda, I.; Mera-Velasco, S.; Cuesta-Vargas, A.I. Comparison of fatigue accumulated during and after prolonged robotic and laparoscopic surgical methods: A cross-sectional study. *Surg. Endosc.* **2017**, *31*, 1119–1135. [CrossRef] [PubMed]
23. Armijo, P.R.; Huang, C.K.; High, R.; Leon, M.; Siu, K.C.; Oleynikov, D. Ergonomics of minimally invasive surgery: An analysis of muscle effort and fatigue in the operating room between laparoscopic and robotic surgery. *Surg. Endosc.* **2019**, *33*, 2323–2331. [CrossRef] [PubMed]

24. Yoon, S.H.; Jung, M.C.; Park, S.Y. Evaluation of surgeon's muscle fatigue during thoracoscopic pulmonary lobectomy using interoperative surface electromyography. *J. Thorac. Dis.* **2016**, *8*, 1162–1169. [CrossRef] [PubMed]
25. Choi, Y.; Joo, H.-j.; Ahn, J.-H.; Kong, H.-J.; Yi, J. Forearm Muscle Activity Patterns during Open Thyroidectomy Using 8-Channel Surface Electromyography. *J. Endocr. Surg.* **2021**, *21*, 27–37. [CrossRef]

Disclaimer/Publisher's Note: The statements, opinions and data contained in all publications are solely those of the individual author(s) and contributor(s) and not of MDPI and/or the editor(s). MDPI and/or the editor(s) disclaim responsibility for any injury to people or property resulting from any ideas, methods, instructions or products referred to in the content.

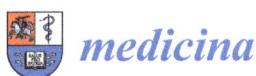

Article

Atherosclerotic Cardiovascular Disease in Inflammatory Bowel Disease: The Role of Chronic Inflammation and Platelet Aggregation

Sofija I. Lugonja [1], Ivana L. Pantic [2], Tamara M. Milovanovic [2,3], Vesna M. Grbovic [4,5], Bojana M. Djokovic [6,7,*], Željko D. Todorovic [6,8], Stefan M. Simovic [6,7], Raša H. Medovic [9,10], Nebojsa D. Zdravkovic [11] and Natasa D. Zdravkovic [6,12]

1. Division of Gastroenterology, Department of Internal Medicine, General Hospital "Djordje Joanovic", 5 Dr. Vase Savica Street, 23000 Zrenjanin, Serbia
2. Clinic of Gastroenterology and Hepatology, University Clinical Center of Serbia, 2 Dr. Koste Todorovica Street, 11000 Belgrade, Serbia
3. Faculty of Medicine, University of Belgrade, 8 Dr. Subotica Starijeg Street, 11000 Belgrade, Serbia
4. Department of Physical Medicine and Rehabilitation, Faculty of Medical Sciences, University of Kragujevac, 69 Svetozar Markovic Street, 34000 Kragujevac, Serbia
5. Center for Physical Medicine and Rehabilitation, University Clinical Center Kragujevac, 30 Zmaj Jovina Street, 34000 Kragujevac, Serbia
6. Department of Internal Medicine, Faculty of Medical Sciences, University of Kragujevac, 69 Svetozar Markovic Street, 34000 Kragujevac, Serbia
7. Clinic for Cardiology, University Clinical Center Kragujevac, 30 Zmaj Jovina Street, 34000 Kragujevac, Serbia
8. Clinic for Hematology, University Clinical Center Kragujevac, 30 Zmaj Jovina Street, 34000 Kragujevac, Serbia
9. Department of Pediatrics, Faculty of Medical Sciences, University of Kragujevac, 69 Svetozar Markovic Street, 34000 Kragujevac, Serbia
10. Pediatric Clinic, University Clinical Center Kragujevac, 30 Zmaj Jovina Street, 34000 Kragujevac, Serbia
11. Department of Medical Statistics and Informatics, Faculty of Medical Sciences, University of Kragujevac, 69 Svetozar Markovic Street, 34000 Kragujevac, Serbia
12. Clinic for Gastroenterology and Hepatology, University Clinical Center Kragujevac, 30 Zmaj Jovina Street, 34000 Kragujevac, Serbia
* Correspondence: bojanadjokovic86@yahoo.com; Tel.: +381643376566

Abstract: *Background and Objectives*: Atherosclerosis is one of inflammatory bowel disease's most significant cardiovascular manifestations. This research aimed to examine the relationship between biochemical, haemostatic, and immune parameters of atherosclerosis and ulcerative colitis patients and its relationship to platelet aggregation. *Materials and Methods*: A clinical, observational cross-sectional study was performed, during which the tested parameters were compared in the experimental and control groups. The patients were divided into four groups. The first group had 25 patients who had ulcerative colitis and atherosclerosis. The second group included 39 patients with ulcerative colitis without atherosclerosis. The third group comprised 31 patients suffering from atherosclerosis without ulcerative colitis, and the fourth group comprised 25 healthy subjects. *Results*: In our study, we registered statistically higher levels of inflammatory markers like SE, CRP, Le, fecal calprotectin, TNF-α, and IL-6, as well as the higher value of thrombocytes and thrombocyte aggregation in the group of patients with ulcerative colitis compared to the control group. Lower levels of total cholesterol and LDL were also recorded in patients with ulcerative colitis and atherosclerosis and ulcerative colitis without atherosclerosis compared to healthy control. Triglyceride and remnant cholesterol were higher in patients with ulcerative colitis and atherosclerosis when compared to patients with ulcerative colitis and healthy control but lower than in patients with atherosclerosis only. *Conclusions*: Several inflammatory markers and platelet aggregation could be good discrimination markers for subjects with ulcerative colitis with the highest risk of atherosclerosis.

Keywords: atherosclerosis; ulcerative colitis; inflammation

1. Introduction

Inflammatory bowel diseases are chronic idiopathic gastrointestinal tract diseases, primarily Crohn's disease and ulcerative colitis, with 5–15% of patients presenting as indeterminate colitis [1,2]. Ulcerative colitis is a chronic immune-mediated inflammation that can affect the mucosa of any part of the colon, with a tendency to spread from the rectum proximally in continuity [3–5]. Ulcerative colitis is characterized by periods of relapse and remission. The typical clinical presentation includes bloody diarrhea with or without mucus, abdominal pain, rectal urgency, tenesmus, weight loss, and asthenia [6,7]. Inflammatory bowel diseases (IBD) can give a wide range of extraintestinal manifestations: hepatobiliary, genitourinary, musculoskeletal, respiratory, ophthalmic, skin, and cardiovascular [8,9]. One of the IBD's most significant cardiovascular manifestations is atherosclerosis, the most common and important cause of coronary, cerebral, and peripheral artery diseases and the aorta. It is a pathological process that most often affects the tunica intima of the arteries, causing later changes in the tunica media and tunica adventitia [10,11]. Possible mechanisms involved in the increased risk of cardiovascular disease in patients with IBD include increased levels of inflammatory cytokines and oxidative stress, altered platelet function, hypercoagulability, endothelial dysfunction, and changes in gut microbiota [12]. Moreover, microbial translocation, defined as the migration of bacteria or their products from the gut to the extraintestinal space and eventually to the systemic circulation, might be promoted by increased intestinal permeability induced by disruption of intestinal epithelial barrier function, intestinal bacterial overgrowth, and changes in the composition of bacterial microbes in the gut, all conditions that could promote and perpetuate systemic inflammation [13,14].

Overall, IBD affects more than 6.8 million patients worldwide, and several meta-analyses, including up to 27 studies, showed an independent association between IBD and atherosclerotic cardiovascular disease (ASCVD) [15,16]. Chronic inflammation and endothelial dysfunction are the two most important factors of atherogenesis [17,18]. Several mechanisms maintain chronic inflammation. A disturbed intestinal barrier in IBD allows the products of luminal microorganisms (lipopolysaccharides and other endotoxins) to enter the bloodstream. Lipopolysaccharides induce the expression of proinflammatory cytokines and affect the oxidation of low-density cholesterol and the activation of macrophages, contributing to endothelial dysfunction, foam cell formation, and, consequently, atherosclerosis. Metabolism of lipids by gut microbiota can also affect atherosclerosis [19,20]. Intestinal microbiota contributes to atherosclerosis by increasing the trimethylamine N-oxide level and inducing Toll-like receptor expression 2 and 4 [17,18].

In addition to structural and functional vascular alterations induced by chronic systemic inflammation, dyslipidemia, and accelerated development of atherosclerosis contribute to arterial thromboembolism [21–31]. Patients with ulcerative colitis have altered lipid profiles. Although the exact mechanism behind this is unknown, it is thought to be due to chronic inflammation and/or malabsorption [32]. CRP, TNF-α, vascular endothelial growth factor, and IL-6 participate in atherogenesis development and the pathogenesis of inflammatory bowel diseases. Their elevated serum levels in patients with ulcerative colitis contribute to the accelerated process of atherogenesis [21]. The overlap of the pathogenetic mechanisms of ulcerative colitis and atherosclerosis is also reflected in the elevated value of calprotectin, an acute reactant phase of inflammation. Calprotectin binds to Toll-like receptor 4 (TLR4), which mediates inflammation and atherosclerosis [25].

Disturbed platelet function is recognized in the pathogenesis of clinical complications of atherosclerosis. Aggregation (Ag) and activation of platelets play a crucial role in myocardial infarction, unstable angina pectoris, and stroke [33]. Moreover, elevated proinflammatory cytokines in patients with IBD, such as TNF-α and IL-1, can induce changes in endothelial cells, monocytes, macrophages, and platelets, such as upregulation of tissue factor, which binds plasma factor VIIa, resulting in procoagulant activity [34–36]. In addition, in patients with IBD, decreased levels of protein C and protein S, increased plasma levels of PAI-1, and reduced plasma levels of thrombin-activatable fibrinolysis inhibitor (TAFI) were found, indicating the imbalance of fibrinolysis in IBD [35,37].

In patients with IBD, absorption of nutrients, including folate and vitamin B12, is impaired [38–45]. Literature data also confirm a reduced concentration of vitamin B6 and elevated homocysteine in these patients [46]. It is known that a high level of homocysteine is a risk factor for thrombosis [47–49]. Folic acid and vitamin B12 play an essential role in the metabolic reactions of homocysteine [50,51]. The demethylation of methionine produces homocysteine, and the lack of vitamin B complex is the leading cause of hyperhomocysteinemia in patients with IBD [46]. Among the B complex vitamins, pyridoxine deficiency is a significant risk factor for hyperhomocysteinemia in IBD [52].

Therefore, the main goal of this research was to examine the relationship between biochemical, haemostatic and immune parameters of atherosclerosis and ulcerative colitis patients and its relationship to platelet aggregation.

2. Material and Methods

2.1. Patients and Settings

A clinical, observational, cross-sectional study was performed at the Djordje Joanović General Hospital, Zrenjanin, University Clinical Center Kragujevac, Center for Gastroenterohepatology and the Faculty of Medical Sciences, University of Kragujevac. All research procedures were made to the Principle of Good Clinical Practice, and ethical approvals were obtained from relevant ethics committees.

A total of 120 patients were included in the trial. The patients were divided into four groups. The first group had 25 patients who had ulcerative colitis and atherosclerosis. The second group included 39 patients with ulcerative colitis without atherosclerosis. The third group consisted of 31 patients suffering from atherosclerosis without ulcerative colitis, and the fourth group consisted of 25 subjects as healthy control, without ulcerative colitis and atherosclerosis.

2.2. Inclusion and Exclusion Criteria

The presence of the following inclusion and exclusion criteria had to be met to participate in the study (depending on the assigned group).

1. Inclusion criteria for experimental groups (ulcerative colitis and atherosclerosis, ulcerative colitis only and atherosclerosis only groups).

(a) A diagnosis of ulcerative colitis based on the endoscopic examination of the colon and the pathohistological findings of the biopsies taken during the endoscopic examination of the colon, and following the criteria of the Third European Evidence-Based Consensus on Diagnosis and Management of Ulcerative Colitis from 2017 [53], and/or

(b) an established diagnosis of atherosclerosis based on laboratory, clinical, and ultrasound parameters measured on carotid blood vessels.

2. Inclusion criteria for the control group include

(a) normal findings on the endoscopic examination of the colon and negative laboratory and ultrasound parameters of atherosclerosis.

3. Signed voluntary consent to participate in the study (for all groups).

The exclusion criteria were the following.

(a) Respondents under 18, pregnant women, nursing mothers and persons with limited legal responsibility and reduced cognitive abilities;

(b) respondents who took vitamin supplements in the previous 6 months;

(c) subjects with other conditions or diseases that can cause vitamin deficiency (daily alcohol intake above 35 g, strict vegetarians, history of cancer, previous gastrectomy);

(d) respondents who take or have taken in the previous six months medications that could affect the status of vitamin B and homocysteine (proton pump inhibitors, oral contraceptives, metformin, phenytoin, theophylline);

(e) subjects with chronic and malignant diseases and/or therapy that may affect the investigated parameters including antilipidemic, antiaggregation, immunosuppressive, immunomodulatory, and corticosteroid therapy; and

(f) infection and infectious syndromes two months before and during research.

2.3. Biochemical Parameters and Platelet Aggregability

The complete blood count, biochemical analyses, and stool specimen analysis were determined in the Central Biochemical Laboratory of the University Clinical Center Kragujevac and the General Hospital Djordje Joanović laboratory Zrenjanin by using enzymatic methods on a Roche Cobas 6000 (c501module) analyzer (Roche Diagnostics, Basel Switzerland) and colourimetric assay by using commercially available kits, respectively. Serum concentrations of homocysteine were determined with high-performance liquid chromatography.

Heparinized whole blood samples were used to assess platelet aggregability by using the impedance aggregometry method with a multiplate analyzer (Dynabyte, Munchen, Germany). Omega-3 PUFA's antiplatelet impact was evaluated in two different ways. The first method involved taking precise measurements of platelet aggregability following the addition of agonists such as adenosine phosphate (ADP test) and arachidonate (ASPI test), with higher results indicating increased residual platelet aggregation and decreased antiplatelet effect of supplementation. When a patient did not take a glycoprotein IIb/IIIa antagonist, basal platelet aggregability was measured by using the thrombin receptor-activating protein (TRAP) test, which was used to evaluate the impact of inhibitors of glycoprotein IIb/IIIa receptors on the platelet aggregability.

2.4. Diagnosis of Atherosclerosis

The Acuson 128XP ultrasonography (Siemens, Germany) with 5 MHz or 7 MHz linear-array transducers were used for carotid duplex ultrasound and color Doppler flow imaging by a single skilled sonographer. Subjects were examined in supine positions with their necks extended and their heads turned 45 degrees to the left or right. The first proximal centimetre of the internal carotid arteries in three separate projections (anterior, lateral, and posterior), as well as the last distal centimetre of the right and left common carotid artery and the bifurcation, were all scanned by using ultrasound technology. Measurement of the increased intima-media thickness was performed as a valid marker of atherosclerosis.

The atherogenic index of plasma was calculated as the logarithm of triglycerides (TGL)/high-density lipoprotein (HDL) ratio, the atherogenic index was calculated as low-density lipoprotein (LDL)/high-density lipoprotein ratio, and the coronary risk index was calculated as total cholesterol/HDL ratio [54,55].

2.5. Measurement of Cytokines in the Serum

The separated serum of patients participating in the research was frozen at $-20\ ^\circ C$ until analysis. The concentration of cytokines involved in the pathogenesis of ulcerative colitis and atherosclerosis (TNF-α, IL-6) was measured by the ELISA method according to the established protocol of the manufacturer (R&D Systems, Minneapolis, MN, USA).

2.6. Statistical Analysis

Numeric variables are shown as mean $\pm$ standard deviation (SD) or median (IQR). The data distribution was examined using the Shapiro–Wilk test or Kolmogorov–Smirnov test. A statistically significant difference between the four groups was determined by a Kruskal–Wallis or one-way analysis of variance (ANOVA) test, depending on the normality of the distribution of the examined parameter. Post hoc (Mann–Whitney U or Tukey Test) tests were conducted to determine which specific groups statistically significant difference occurred. During the post hoc tests, Bonferroni's alpha value was corrected (0.05/6 = 0.008).

The ROC curve method was used, and the statistical analysis reliability level was determined by determining the sensitivity and specificity of the test. Statistics were deemed to be significant at values of $p < 0.05$. The statistical analysis was conducted by using SPSS version 20.0.

3. Results

A total of 120 patients were included in this study, 68 (56.7%) men and 52 (43.3%) women. The average age of the patients with ulcerative colitis and atherosclerosis was 68.76 ± 8.90 years, while the average age of the patients with ulcerative colitis was only 38.08 ± 9.84 years. The average age of the patients with atherosclerosis only was 62.10 ± 9.89 years, and the average age of the healthy controls was 39.52 ± 9.88 years old.

When compared to healthy controls, patients with ulcerative colitis and atherosclerosis, patients with ulcerative colitis without atherosclerosis and patients with atherosclerosis without ulcerative colitis had higher levels of SE, CRP, Ag PLT ADP, Ag PLT ASPI, Ag PLT TRAP, leukocytes, platelets, faecal calprotectin, TNF-α, and IL6 (Table 1). No significant difference was found between any groups regarding the parameters of vitamin B6, folic acid levels, coronary risk, atherogenic, and atherogenic index of plasma and TIBC values.

Table 1. The difference in patient parameters between the four study groups.

Variable	Ulcerative Colitis and Atherosclerosis (Median (IQR))	Ulcerative Colitis Only (Median (IQR))	Atherosclerosis Only (Median (IQR))	Healthy Controls (Median (IQR))	p Value
SE	30 (37.50)	13 (26.00)	12 (13.25)	2.5 (3.25)	0.001
CRP	49.0 (97.35)	23.8 (95.00)	3.7 (2.50)	1.0 (0.75)	0.000
B 12	245 (218.5)	350 (258.0)	456 (179.5)	417 (148.0)	0.000
B 6	15.00 (16.0)	16.00 (12.7)	15.00 (7.0)	16.35 (12.48)	0.500
Folic acid	12.0 (19.45)	7.5 (7.7)	9.0 (8.7)	7.65 (5.62)	0.246
LDL	1.87 (2.43)	1.89 (1.92)	2.45 (1.56)	2.33 (0.55)	0.052
HDL	1.56 (1.56)	1.33 (0.88)	1.87 (1.73)	3.09 (1.27)	0.000
Chol	4.10 (2.05)	4.20 (1.78)	5.55 (1.82)	5.08 (1.05)	0.003
TGL	1.22 (0.79)	1.10 (0.76)	2.33 (1.91)	0.95 (0.53)	0.000
Remnant cholesterol	0.60 (0.68)	0.44 (0.34)	0.90 (0.70)	0.44 (0.28)	0.000
Coronary risk index	0.79 (1.96)	0.72 (0.62)	0.58 (0.62)	0.60 (0.58)	0.477
Atherogenic index	1.27 (3.64)	2.17 (1.90)	2.29 (1.88)	1.81 (1.26)	0.241
Atherogenic index of plasma	2.52 (4.44)	3.17 (2.20)	3.46 (2.13)	2.29 (1.25)	0.135
Fe	8.50 (6.35)	10.00 (8.70)	13.10 (5.60)	17.50 (8.00)	0.000
Ferritin	74.00 (95.5)	122.00 (274.0)	236.00 (95.0)	79.40 (64.7)	0.000
Transferrin saturation	17.35 (14.65)	20.00 (17.40)	30.26 (12.02)	32.00 (14.50)	0.000
Ag PLT ADP	1212.00 (307)	1199.00 (762)	675.00 (342)	727.50 (294)	0.000
Ag PLT ASPI	1654.00 (519)	1387.00 (771)	988.00 (333)	1227.00 (267)	0.000
Ag PLT TRAP	1654.00 (412)	1320.00 (691)	1121.00 (334)	1198.00 (273)	0.000
TIBC	52.00 (13)	56.00 (21)	49.00 (13)	/	0.395
Le	9.45 (7.1)	8.65 (6.6)	4.87 (1.3)	5.70 (2.0)	0.000
PLT	404 (181)	386 (199)	298 (188)	230 (85)	0.000
FCP	987.60 (1331)	439.00 (1266)	13.40 (11)	/	0.000
TNF-α	379.67 (176.67)	395.00 (256.50)	391.67 (80.00)	0.00 (1.75)	0.000
IL-6	511.86 (122.86)	581.36 (491.43)	563.29 (114.29)	0.00 (0.00)	0.000
Non-HDL	3.52 (2.80)	2.68 (2.17)	4.10 (2.29)	3.86 (1.20)	0.013
Homocysteine	11.02 (5.15)	10.28 (3.90)	9.24 (3.40)	10.00 (4.00)	0.107
UIBC	35.56 (15)	40.62 (17)	42.84 (11)	/	0.051
Systolic BP	162 (20)	133 (0)	157 (25)	123 (12)	0.000
Diastolic BP	91 (5)	82 (5)	90 (5)	72 (15)	0.021

Acronyms: SE, erythrocyte sedimentation rate; CRP, C-reactive protein; B12, vitamin B12; B6, vitamin B6, LDL, low-density lipoprotein cholesterol; HDL, high-density lipoprotein cholesterol; Chol, Cholesterol; TGL, triglycerides; Fe, iron; Ag, aggregation; PLT, platelets; ADP, adenosine diphosphate; ASPI, arachidonic acid; TRAP, thrombin receptor activating peptide; TIBC, total iron-binding capacity; Le, leukocytes; FCP, fecal calprotectin; TNF-α, tumor necrosis factor α; IL-6, interleukin 6; UIBC, unsaturated iron-binding capacity; BP, blood pressure; IQR, interquartile range.

A significant difference in the values of erythrocyte sedimentation rate ($p = 0.008$), Ag PLT ASPI value ($p = 0.004$), and Ag PLT TRAP value ($p = 0.001$) was observed between patients with ulcerative colitis and atherosclerosis and patients with ulcerative colitis, with higher levels in patients with both ulcerative colitis and atherosclerosis.

Patients with ulcerative colitis and atherosclerosis had higher levels of erythrocyte sedimentation rate ($p = 0.000$), CRP ($p = 0.000$), Ag PLT ADP ($p = 0.000$), Ag PLT ASPI ($p = 0.000$), Ag PLT TRAP ($p = 0.000$), leukocyte ($p = 0.000$), platelet count ($p = 0.001$), and fecal calprotectin values ($p = 0.000$) when compared to the patients with atherosclerosis only. Values of vitamin B12 ($p = 0.000$), triglycerides ($p = 0.000$), ferritin ($p = 0.001$), and transferrin ($p = 0.000$) were significantly higher in patients with atherosclerosis only.

Significantly higher levels of erythrocyte sedimentation rate ($p = 0.000$), CRP ($p = 0.000$), HDL ($p = 0.000$), transferrin saturation ($p = 0.000$), Ag PLT ADP ($p = 0.000$), Ag PLT ASPI ($p = 0.000$), Ag PLT TRAP ($p = 0.000$), leukocyte ($p = 0.000$), platelet count ($p = 0.000$), IL-6 ($p = 0.000$) and TNF-α values ($p = 0.000$) were observed in patients with ulcerative colitis and atherosclerosis when compared to healthy controls. In comparison, higher levels of vitamin B12 ($p = 0.002$) and serum iron values ($p = 0.000$) were observed in healthy patients.

When patients with ulcerative colitis only and atherosclerosis only were compared, values of CRP ($p = 0.000$), transferrin saturation ($p = 0.000$), Ag PLT ADP ($p = 0.000$), leukocyte ($p = 0.001$) and fecal calprotectin ($p = 0.000$) were significantly higher in patients with ulcerative colitis only. Patients with atherosclerosis only had higher levels of vitamin B12 ($p = 0.004$), HDL ($p = 0.004$), cholesterol ($p = 0.001$), triglyceride ($p = 0.000$), remnant cholesterol ($p = 0.000$), and serum iron values ($p = 0.001$).

Patients with ulcerative colitis only had higher levels of erythrocyte sedimentation rate ($p = 0.000$), CRP ($p = 0.000$), triglyceride ($p = 0.000$), Ag PLT ADP ($p = 0.000$), leukocyte ($p = 0.001$), fecal calprotectin ($p = 0.000$), IL-6 ($p = 0.000$), and TNF-α values ($p = 0.000$) than healthy controls. Higher levels of vitamin B12 ($p = 0.004$), HDL ($p = 0.004$), cholesterol ($p = 0.001$), serum iron ($p = 0.001$), and transferrin saturation ($p = 0.000$) were observed in healthy controls.

Significantly higher values of erythrocyte sedimentation rate ($p = 0.001$), CRP ($p = 0.000$), LDL ($p = 0.002$), triglyceride ($p = 0.000$), remnant cholesterol ($p = 0.001$), ferritin ($p = 0.000$), Ag PLT ASPI ($p = 0.001$), IL-6 ($p = 0.000$), and TNF-α values ($p = 0.000$) were observed in patients with atherosclerosis only when compared to healthy controls.

A one-way ANOVA test was used to analyze the variables shown in Table 2. The groups were compared to determine between which groups there was a statistically significant difference in the observed variables.

Table 2. The difference in non-HDL, homocysteine, and UIBC between the four study groups.

Variable	Ulcerative Colitis and Atherosclerosis (Mean ± SD)	Ulcerative Colitis Only (Mean ± SD)	Atherosclerosis Only (Mean ± SD)	Healthy Controls (Mean ± SD)	p-Value
non-HDL	3.52 ± 2.039	2.68 ± 1.439	4.10 ± 1.589	3.86 ± 0.729	0.013
Homocysteine	11.02 ± 2.985	10.28 ± 2.398	9.24 ± 2.724	10.00 ± 2.872	0.107
UIBC	35.56 ± 12.322	40.62 ± 12.639	42.84 ± 7.546	/	0.051

Acronyms: HDL, high-density lipoprotein cholesterol; UIBC, unsaturated iron-binding capacity; SD, standard deviation.

No statistically significant difference in serum homocysteine values was shown between the examined groups. After the ANOVA test showed a significant difference between the four groups in values of non-HDL and UIBC (Table 2), the post-hoc Tukey test revealed that significantly higher levels of non-HDL in patients with atherosclerosis only, when compared to patients with ulcerative colitis only ($p = 0.013$). Levels of UIBC were significantly lower in patients with ulcerative colitis and atherosclerosis when compared to the patients with atherosclerosis only ($p = 0.044$) (Table 2).

The receiver operating characteristic (ROC) curve analysis showed that Ag PLT TRAP has the highest sensitivity and specificity in assessing the risk of developing atherosclerosis (area under the curve (AUC)) = 0.753, sensitivity 85.3%, specificity 70.8%) (Figure 1A–F).

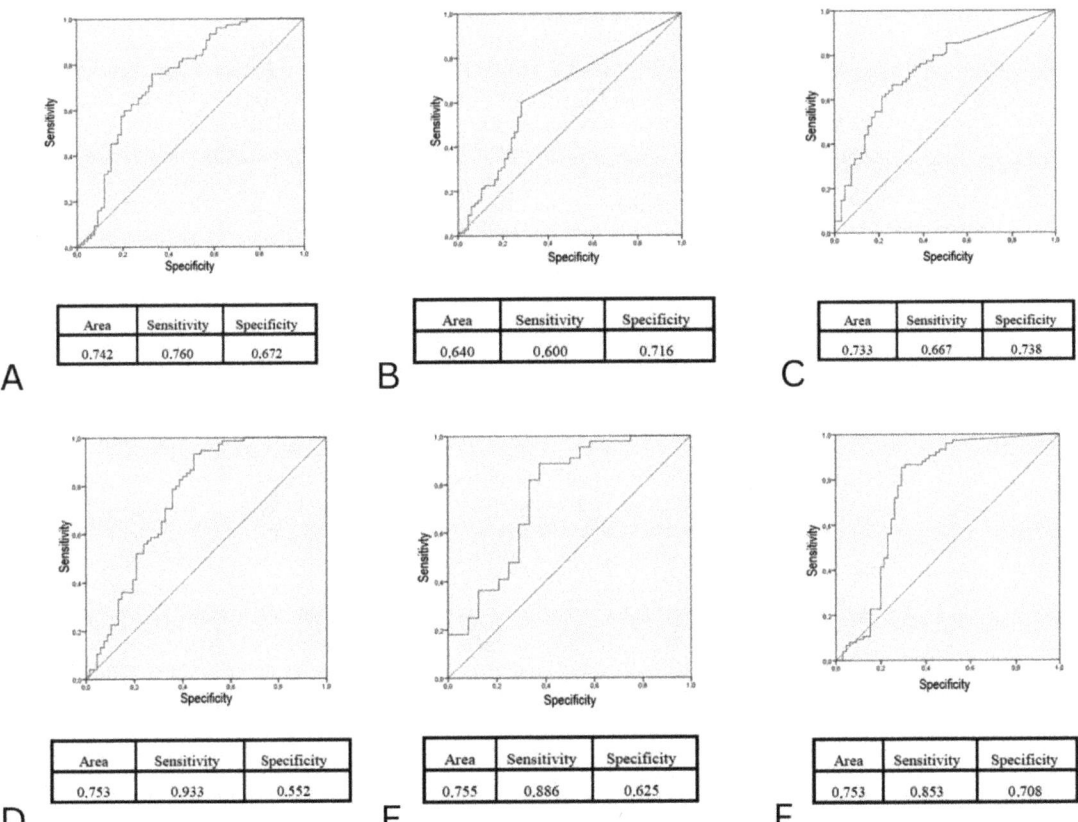

Figure 1. (A) ROC curve showing the relationship between sensitivity and specificity of CRP in patients with ulcerative colitis and its influence on the development of atherosclerosis (AUC = 0.742, sensitivity 76.0%, specificity 67.2%). (B) ROC curve showing the relationship between sensitivity and specificity of IL-6 in patients with ulcerative colitis and its influence on the development of atherosclerosis (AUC = 0.640, sensitivity 60.0%, specificity 71.6%). (C) ROC curve showing the relationship between sensitivity and specificity of TNF-α in patients with ulcerative colitis and its influence on the development of atherosclerosis. (AUC = 0.733, sensitivity 66.7%, specificity 73.8%). (D) ROC curve showing the relationship between sensitivity and specificity of Ag PLT ADP in patients with ulcerative colitis and its influence on the development of atherosclerosis (AUC = 0.753, sensitivity 93.3%, specificity 55.2%). (E) ROC curve showing the relationship between sensitivity and specificity of Ag PLT ASPI in patients with ulcerative colitis and its influence on the development of atherosclerosis (AUC = 0.755, sensitivity 88.6%, specificity 62.5%). (F) ROC curve showing the relationship between sensitivity and specificity of Ag PLT TRAP in patients with ulcerative colitis and its influence on the development of atherosclerosis (AUC = 0.753, sensitivity 85.3%, specificity 70.8%).

4. Discussion

The connection of atherosclerotic parameters as predictors of cardiovascular risk in patients with ulcerative colitis is explained by inflammation, which represents the pathophysiological basis of both conditions. Inflammation plays a strong role in the pathogenesis of the atherosclerotic cardiovascular disease (ASCVD). Although many serological markers of inflammation exist today, no marker alone seems to predict or identify disease activity in ulcerative colitis [56].

Our study shows higher levels of SE, CRP, Ag PLT ASPI, Ag PLT TRAP, Ag PLT ADP, Le, PLT, FCP, TNF-α, and IL-6 in patients with ulcerative colitis, when compared to the healthy controls, as well as lower levels of vitamins B12, B6, serum Fe, and transferrin saturation.

Several large studies have confirmed an increased risk of ASCVD, especially myocardial infarction, in those patients with elevated CRP and hs-CRP values [56,57]. On the other hand, different CRP levels correlate with the clinical and endoscopic activity of ulcerative colitis [58,59]. Determining these serum markers in daily clinical practice could assess the activity and dynamics of ulcerative colitis disease and the risk of ASCVD. In our study, the highest CRP values were in patients with ulcerative colitis and patients with ulcerative colitis and atherosclerosis, which was expected because CRP is a positive reactant of acute inflammation. A significant difference was also registered between patients with ulcerative colitis and patients with atherosclerosis compared to healthy patients, confirming that CRP is a good marker of chronic inflammation.

Vitamin B12 deficiency occurs in 5%, and folic acid deficiency is reported in 30–40% of ulcerative colitis patients [60]. Vitamin B12 and folate deficiency can contribute to hyperhomocysteinemia, a risk factor for thrombosis [42–44,47–49]. Literature data confirm that patients with IBD are at a higher risk of hyperhomocysteinemia [50,51]. Vitamin B deficiency, specifically vitamin B6, is a significant risk factor for hyperhomocysteinemia in patients with IBD [46,52]. Our research revealed no deficiency of vitamins B12, B6, folic acid, or hyperhomocysteinemia in any of the studied groups.

Numerous studies have analyzed lipid profiles in patients with ulcerative colitis, and results show significantly lower lipid concentrations in the blood than those without IBD. Despite these results, it was shown that early signs of ASCVD are still detected in patients with ulcerative colitis, including increased carotid artery thickness, elevated levels of homocysteine, and hs-CRP [56]. In our study, lower levels of total cholesterol and LDL were recorded in patients with ulcerative colitis and those with ulcerative colitis and atherosclerosis, similar to the study's results. Some studies favour triglycerides and remnant cholesterol as significant risk factors for atherosclerosis and ASCVD [61–64]. In our study, despite the lower triglyceride levels registered in patients with ulcerative colitis, the levels of triglycerides were higher in patients with ulcerative colitis and atherosclerosis. Additionally, patients with ulcerative colitis and atherosclerosis had higher remnant cholesterol and triglyceride values when compared to patients with ulcerative colitis.

Analyzing the atherosclerosis index, which was obtained by calculating based on the quotient of lipid values in the examined groups, we noticed that the atherogenic index and coronary risk index were the highest in patients with atherosclerosis, which was expected and then in patients with ulcerative colitis. The coronary risk index was the highest in patients with ulcerative colitis and the lowest in patients with atherosclerosis. Although different average values of the atherosclerosis index were registered, no statistically significant difference was recorded when comparing the groups.

Iron deficiency is registered in 60–80% of patients with IBD. Hypoferremia is the cause of microcytic anemia, which can also overlap with anemia due to chronic illness in these patients. In conditions in which biochemical and clinical signs of inflammation are absent in the patient, iron deficiency should be suspected when the serum ferritin level is lower than 30 µg/L [65,66]. Our research recorded no serum ferritin level lower than 30 µg/L. Higher serum ferritin values in patients with atherosclerosis and patients with ulcerative colitis than those with ulcerative colitis and atherosclerosis can be explained by low-grade chronic inflammation. In patients with ulcerative colitis and atherosclerosis, it can be observed that the ferritin is lower, and consequent microcytic anemia is in agreement with other literature data.

Leukocytosis, as a consequence of inflammation, is common in patients with atherosclerosis and those with ulcerative colitis [67,68]. In our research, leukocytosis was not recorded. However, leukocyte values were higher in patients with ulcerative colitis and atherosclerosis and patients with ulcerative colitis than in the other two groups, which was expected due to chronic inflammation.

Ulcerative colitis is also associated with thrombocytosis. The high platelet count is likely due to increased thrombopoiesis, which is induced by higher plasma levels of thrombopoietin and IL-6 [69–71] or is caused by iron deficiency [72]. Some studies describe a correlation between high platelet counts and atherosclerosis [73–75]. In our research, higher values of platelets were registered in patients with ulcerative colitis and atherosclerosis and patients with ulcerative colitis, which coincides with the results of the mentioned studies.

In addition to the value of platelets in patients with ulcerative colitis and atherosclerosis patients, perhaps even more important is the aggregation of platelets. The highest values of platelet aggregation—Ag PLT ADP, Ag PLT ASPI, and Ag PLT TRAP—were registered in patients with ulcerative colitis and atherosclerosis, and a statistically significant difference was registered in Ag PLT ASPI, Ag PLT ADP, and Ag PLT TRAP. The results are expected and potentially indicate a greater tendency for thrombosis in patients with ulcerative colitis and atherosclerosis as a result of increased platelet aggregation.

Fecal calprotectin in patients with ulcerative colitis has great clinical significance in monitoring disease activity [76,77]. Our research obtained results consistent with other research and clinical presentation. Namely, elevated values of fecal calprotectin were registered in patients with ulcerative colitis (with or without atherosclerosis), while in patients with atherosclerosis only, the value of fecal calprotectin was normal. In healthy control, the value of fecal calprotectin was not determined.

Our research included determining cytokine values with a significant and proven role in atherosclerosis and ulcerative colitis pathogenesis. Our results showed increased values of TNF-α and IL6 in patients with ulcerative colitis and atherosclerosis, ulcerative colitis only, and atherosclerosis only, considering that chronic inflammation is present in the aforementioned investigated groups [78–81].

The studied groups' average blood pressure (BP) values were also analyzed. The highest blood pressure values were recorded in patients with atherosclerosis (with or without ulcerative colitis). An elevated blood pressure value was not recorded in patients with ulcerative colitis and healthy controls. The obtained results were expected and simply can be interpreted by the presence of atherosclerosis, which is also the most crucial pathophysiological mechanism underlying hypertension.

According to our results, Ag PLT TRAP showed the highest sensitivity and specificity between all analysed serum markers, which allows discrimination of subjects with ulcerative colitis with the highest risk of developing atherosclerosis.

The limitations of this study are the small number of patients included in the research and, therefore, limited analysis. Regardless, this research provides insight into the possible mechanisms of the connection between ulcerative colitis and atherosclerosis, one of the most common cardiovascular manifestations. Moreover, in this study, there was no follow-up of patients that would provide temporal insight into the relationship between markers of inflammation, platelet aggregability, and outcomes in patients with ulcerative colitis and atherosclerosis.

This study provides insights into possible mechanisms of the connection between ulcerative colitis and atherosclerosis as one of the most common manifestations, as well as the role of inflammation and platelet aggregation. In our study, the levels of inflammatory markers were markedly elevated in patients with both ulcerative colitis and atherosclerosis when compared to patients with ulcerative colitis only, confirming the hypothesis that inflammation is a crucial mechanism of accelerated atherosclerosis in patients with ulcerative colitis. Further studies are needed to examine all possible mechanisms and associations.

Author Contributions: Conceptualization, S.I.L. and N.D.Z. (Natasa D. Zdravkovic); methodology, S.I.L.; software, N.D.Z. (Nebojsa D. Zdravkovic); validation, I.L.P., T.M.M. and R.H.M.; formal analysis, S.I.L. and Ž.D.T.; investigation, S.I.L. and N.D.Z. (Natasa D. Zdravkovic); resources, S.I.L.; data curation, S.M.S.; writing—original draft preparation, S.I.L. and B.M.D.; writing—review & editing, Ž.D.T., S.M.S., V.M.G., and N.D.Z. (Natasa D. Zdravkovic); visualization, V.M.G.; supervision, N.D.Z. (Natasa D. Zdravkovic); project administration, S.I.L.; funding acquisition, S.I.L. All authors have read and agreed to the published version of the manuscript.

Funding: This research received no external funding.

Institutional Review Board Statement: The study was conducted according to the guidelines of the Declaration of Helsinki, and approved by the Institutional Review Board (or Ethics Committee) of University Clinical Center Kragujevac (protocol code 01-7012, 02.07.2015.).

Informed Consent Statement: Informed consent was obtained from all subjects involved in the study.

Data Availability Statement: The data presented in this study are available on request from the corresponding author.

Conflicts of Interest: S.M.S. received lecture honorary, travel grants and/or fellowship grant from Abbot, Astra Zeneca, Bayer, Boehringer Ingelheim, Medtronic, and Novartis. All other authors declare no conflict of interest.

References

1. Fakhoury, M.; Al-Salami, H.; Negrulj, R.; Mooranian, A. Inflammatory Bowel Disease: Clinical Aspects and Treatments. *J. Inflamm. Res.* **2014**, *7*, 113. [CrossRef] [PubMed]
2. Venkateswaran, N.; Weismiller, S.; Clarke, K. Indeterminate Colitis—Update on Treatment Options. *J. Inflamm. Res.* **2021**, *14*, 6383–6395. [CrossRef] [PubMed]
3. Feuerstein, J.D.; Moss, A.C.; Farraye, F.A. Ulcerative Colitis. *Mayo Clin. Proc.* **2019**, *94*, 1357–1373. [CrossRef]
4. Maaser, C.; Sturm, A.; Vavricka, S.R.; Kucharzik, T.; Fiorino, G.; Annese, V.; Calabrese, E.; Baumgart, D.C.; Bettenworth, D.; Borralho Nunes, P.; et al. ECCO-ESGAR Guideline for Diagnostic Assessment in IBD Part 1: Initial Diagnosis, Monitoring of Known IBD, Detection of Complications. *J. Crohn's Colitis* **2019**, *13*, 144–164K. [CrossRef] [PubMed]
5. Sairenji, T.; Collins, K.L.; Evans, D.V. An Update on Inflammatory Bowel Disease. *Prim. Care Clin. Off. Pract.* **2017**, *44*, 673–692. [CrossRef]
6. Gajendran, M.; Loganathan, P.; Jimenez, G.; Catinella, A.P.; Ng, N.; Umapathy, C.; Ziade, N.; Hashash, J.G. A Comprehensive Review and Update on Ulcerative Colitis. *Dis. A Mon.* **2019**, *65*, 100851. [CrossRef]
7. Nóbrega, V.G.; Silva, I.N.D.N.; Brito, B.S.; Silva, J.; Silva, M.C.M.D.; Santana, G.O. The Onset of Clinical Manifestations in Inflammatory Bowel Disease Patients. *Arq. De Gastroenterol.* **2018**, *55*, 290–295. [CrossRef]
8. Olpin, J.D.; Sjoberg, B.P.; Stilwill, S.E.; Jensen, L.E.; Rezvani, M.; Shaaban, A.M. Beyond the Bowel: Extraintestinal Manifestations of Inflammatory Bowel Disease. *RadioGraphics* **2017**, *37*, 1135–1160. [CrossRef] [PubMed]
9. Karmiris, K.; Avgerinos, A.; Tavernaraki, A.; Zeglinas, C.; Karatzas, P.; Koukouratos, T.; Oikonomou, K.A.; Kostas, A.; Zampeli, E.; Papadopoulos, V.; et al. Prevalence and Characteristics of Extra-Intestinal Manifestations in a Large Cohort of Greek Patients with Inflammatory Bowel Disease. *J. Crohn's Colitis* **2016**, *10*, 429–436. [CrossRef]
10. Faxon, D.P.; Fuster, V.; Libby, P.; Beckman, J.A.; Hiatt, W.R.; Thompson, R.W.; Topper, J.N.; Annex, B.H.; Rundback, J.H.; Fabunmi, R.P.; et al. Atherosclerotic Vascular Disease Conference. *Circulation* **2004**, *109*, 2617–2625. [CrossRef]
11. Libby, P.; Ridker, P.M.; Hansson, G.K. Progress and Challenges in Translating the Biology of Atherosclerosis. *Nature* **2011**, *473*, 317–325. [CrossRef] [PubMed]
12. Wu, H.; Hu, T.; Hao, H.; Hill, M.A.; Xu, C.; Liu, Z. Inflammatory Bowel Disease and Cardiovascular Diseases: A Concise Review. *Eur. Heart J. Open* **2022**, *2*, oeab029. [CrossRef]
13. Oliva, A.; Aversano, L.; De Angelis, M.; Mascellino, M.T.; Miele, M.C.; Morelli, S.; Battaglia, R.; Iera, J.; Bruno, G.; Corazziari, E.S.; et al. Persistent Systemic Microbial Translocation, Inflammation, and Intestinal Damage during Clostridioides Difficile Infection. *Open Forum Infect. Dis.* **2019**, *7*, ofz507. [CrossRef]
14. Oliva, A.; Miele, M.C.; Di Timoteo, F.; De Angelis, M.; Mauro, V.; Aronica, R.; Al Ismail, D.; Ceccarelli, G.; Pinacchio, C.; d'Ettorre, G.; et al. Persistent Systemic Microbial Translocation and Intestinal Damage during Coronavirus Disease-19. *Front. Immunol.* **2021**, *12*, 708149. [CrossRef] [PubMed]
15. Alatab, S.; Sepanlou, S.G.; Ikuta, K.; Vahedi, H.; Bisignano, C.; Safiri, S.; Sadeghi, A.; Nixon, M.R.; Abdoli, A.; Abolhassani, H.; et al. The Global, Regional, and National Burden of Inflammatory Bowel Disease in 195 Countries and Territories, 1990–2017: A Systematic Analysis for the Global Burden of Disease Study 2017. *Lancet Gastroenterol. Hepatol.* **2020**, *5*, 17–30. [CrossRef] [PubMed]
16. Sun, H.-H.; Tian, F. Inflammatory Bowel Disease and Cardiovascular Disease Incidence and Mortality: A Meta-Analysis. *Eur. J. Prev. Cardiol.* **2018**, *25*, 1623–1631. [CrossRef]

17. Shen, X.; Li, L.; Sun, Z.; Zang, G.; Zhang, L.; Shao, C.; Wang, Z. Gut Microbiota and Atherosclerosis—Focusing on the Plaque Stability. *Front. Cardiovasc. Med.* **2021**, *8*, 668532. [CrossRef]
18. van den Munckhof, I.C.L.; Kurilshikov, A.; ter Horst, R.; Riksen, N.P.; Joosten, L.A.B.; Zhernakova, A.; Fu, J.; Keating, S.T.; Netea, M.G.; de Graaf, J.; et al. Role of Gut Microbiota in Chronic Low-Grade Inflammation as Potential Driver for Atherosclerotic Cardiovascular Disease: A Systematic Review of Human Studies. *Obes. Rev.* **2018**, *19*, 1719–1734. [CrossRef]
19. Vourakis, M.; Mayer, G.; Rousseau, G. The Role of Gut Microbiota on Cholesterol Metabolism in Atherosclerosis. *Int. J. Mol. Sci.* **2021**, *22*, 8074. [CrossRef] [PubMed]
20. Duttaroy, A.K. Role of Gut Microbiota and Their Metabolites on Atherosclerosis, Hypertension and Human Blood Platelet Function: A Review. *Nutrients* **2021**, *13*, 144. [CrossRef] [PubMed]
21. Reiss, A.B.; Siegart, N.M.; De Leon, J. Interleukin-6 in atherosclerosis: Atherogenic or atheroprotective. *Clin. Lipidol.* **2017**, *12*, 14–23. [CrossRef]
22. Yarur, A.J.; Deshpande, A.R.; Pechman, D.M.; Tamariz, L.; Abreu, M.T.; Sussman, D.A. Inflammatory Bowel Disease Is Associated with an Increased Incidence of Cardiovascular Events. *Am. J. Gastroenterol.* **2011**, *106*, 741–747. [CrossRef] [PubMed]
23. Manichanh, C.; Borruel, N.; Casellas, F.; Guarner, F. The Gut Microbiota in IBD. *Nat. Rev. Gastroenterol. Hepatol.* **2012**, *9*, 599–608. [CrossRef] [PubMed]
24. Tang, W.H.W.; Li, D.Y.; Hazen, S.L. Dietary Metabolism, the Gut Microbiome, and Heart Failure. *Nat. Rev. Cardiol.* **2018**, *16*, 137–154. [CrossRef] [PubMed]
25. Kruzliak, P.; Novák, J.; Novák, M.; Fodor, G.J. Role of Calprotectin in Cardiometabolic Diseases. *Cytokine Growth Factor Rev.* **2014**, *25*, 67–75. [CrossRef]
26. Tan, V.P.; Chung, A.; Yan, B.P.; Gibson, P.R. Venous and Arterial Disease in Inflammatory Bowel Disease. *J. Gastroenterol. Hepatol.* **2013**, *28*, 1095–1113. [CrossRef] [PubMed]
27. Zezos, P. Inflammatory Bowel Disease and Thromboembolism. *World J. Gastroenterol.* **2014**, *20*, 13863. [CrossRef] [PubMed]
28. Harper, J.W.; Zisman, T.L. Interaction of Obesity and Inflammatory Bowel Disease. *World J. Gastroenterol.* **2016**, *22*, 7868–7881. [CrossRef]
29. Kamperidis, N.; Kamperidis, V.; Zegkos, T.; Kostourou, I.; Nikolaidou, O.; Arebi, N.; Karvounis, H. Atherosclerosis and Inflammatory Bowel Disease—Shared Pathogenesis and Implications for Treatment. *Angiology* **2020**, *72*, 303–314. [CrossRef] [PubMed]
30. Zanoli, L.; Rastelli, S.; Granata, A.; Inserra, G.; Empana, J.-P.; Boutouyrie, P.; Laurent, S.; Castellino, P. Arterial Stiffness in Inflammatory Bowel Disease: A Systematic Review and Meta-Analysis. *J. Hypertens.* **2016**, *34*, 822–829. [CrossRef]
31. Scaldaferri, F. Haemostatic System in Inflammatory Bowel Diseases: New Players in Gut Inflammation. *World J. Gastroenterol.* **2011**, *17*, 594. [CrossRef]
32. Rungoe, C.; Nyboe Andersen, N.; Jess, T. Inflammatory Bowel Disease and Risk of Coronary Heart Disease. *Trends Cardiovasc. Med.* **2015**, *25*, 699–704. [CrossRef]
33. Wang, L.; Tang, C. Targeting Platelet in Atherosclerosis Plaque Formation: Current Knowledge and Future Perspectives. *Int. J. Mol. Sci.* **2020**, *21*, 9760. [CrossRef] [PubMed]
34. Kirchhofer, D.; Tschopp, T.B.; Hadváry, P.; Baumgartner, H.R. Endothelial Cells Stimulated with Tumor Necrosis Factor-Alpha Express Varying Amounts of Tissue Factor Resulting in Inhomogenous Fibrin Deposition in a Native Blood Flow System. Effects of Thrombin Inhibitors. *J. Clin. Investig.* **1994**, *93*, 2073–2083. [CrossRef] [PubMed]
35. Stadnicki, A.; Stadnicka, I. Venous and Arterial Thromboembolism in Patients with Inflammatory Bowel Diseases. *World J. Gastroenterol.* **2021**, *27*, 6757–6774. [CrossRef] [PubMed]
36. Butenas, S.; Orfeo, T.; Mann, K.G. Tissue Factor in Coagulation: Which? Where? When? *Arterioscler. Thromb. Vasc. Biol.* **2009**, *29*, 1989–1996. [CrossRef] [PubMed]
37. Koutroubakis, I.E.; Sfiridaki, A.; Tsiolakidou, G.; Coucoutsi, C.; Theodoropoulou, A.; Kouroumalis, E.A. Plasma Thrombin-Activatable Fibrinolysis Inhibitor and Plasminogen Activator Inhibitor-1 Levels in Inflammatory Bowel Disease. *Eur. J. Gastroenterol. Hepatol.* **2008**, *20*, 912–916. [CrossRef] [PubMed]
38. Leddin, D.; Tamim, H.; Levy, A.R. Is Folate Involved in the Pathogenesis of Inflammatory Bowel Disease? *Med. Hypotheses* **2013**, *81*, 940–941. [CrossRef]
39. Weisshof, R.; Chermesh, I. Micronutrient Deficiencies in Inflammatory Bowel Disease. *Curr. Opin. Clin. Nutr. Metab. Care* **2015**, *18*, 576–581. [CrossRef]
40. Massironi, S.; Rossi, R.E.; Cavalcoli, F.A.; Della Valle, S.; Fraquelli, M.; Conte, D. Nutritional Deficiencies in Inflammatory Bowel Disease: Therapeutic Approaches. *Clin. Nutr.* **2013**, *32*, 904–910. [CrossRef]
41. Battat, R.; Kopylov, U.; Byer, J.; Sewitch, M.J.; Rahme, E.; Nedjar, H.; Zelikovic, E.; Dionne, S.; Bessissow, T.; Afif, W.; et al. Vitamin B12 Deficiency in Inflammatory Bowel Disease. *Eur. J. Gastroenterol. Hepatol.* **2017**, *29*, 1361–1367. [CrossRef] [PubMed]
42. Owczarek, D. Diet and Nutritional Factors in Inflammatory Bowel Diseases. *World J. Gastroenterol.* **2016**, *22*, 895. [CrossRef]
43. Ratajczak, A.E.; Szymczak-Tomczak, A.; Rychter, A.M.; Zawada, A.; Dobrowolska, A.; Krela-Kaźmierczak, I. Does Folic Acid Protect Patients with Inflammatory Bowel Disease from Complications? *Nutrients* **2021**, *13*, 4036. [CrossRef]
44. Pan, Y.; Liu, Y.; Guo, H.; Jabir, M.S.; Liu, X.; Cui, W.; Li, D. Associations between Folate and Vitamin B12 Levels and Inflammatory Bowel Disease: A Meta-Analysis. *Nutrients* **2017**, *9*, 382. [CrossRef] [PubMed]

45. Jayawardena, D.; Dudeja, P.K. Micronutrient Deficiency in Inflammatory Bowel Diseases: Cause or Effect? *Cell. Mol. Gastroenterol. Hepatol.* **2020**, *9*, 707–708. [CrossRef]
46. Erzin, Y.; Uzun, H.; Celik, A.F.; Aydin, S.; Dirican, A.; Uzunismail, H. Hyperhomocysteinemia in Inflammatory Bowel Disease Patients without Past Intestinal Resections: Correlations with Cobalamin, Pyridoxine, Folate Concentrations, Acute Phase Reactants, Disease Activity, and Prior Thromboembolic Complications. *J. Clin. Gastroenterol.* **2008**, *42*, 481–486. [CrossRef]
47. Vasilopoulos, S.; Saiean, K.; Emmons, J.; Berger, W.L.; Abu-Hajir, M.; Seetharam, B.; Binion, D.G. Terminal Ileum Resection Is Associated with Higher Plasma Homocysteine Levels in Crohn's Disease. *J. Clin. Gastroenterol.* **2001**, *33*, 132–136. [CrossRef] [PubMed]
48. Chowers, Y.; Sela, B.A.; Holland, R.; Fidder, H.; Simoni, F.B.; Bar-Meir, S. Increased Levels of Homocysteine in Patients with Crohn's Disease Are Related to Folate Levels. *Am. J. Gastroenterol.* **2000**, *95*, 3498–3502. [CrossRef]
49. Oussalah, A.; Guéant, J.-L.; Peyrin-Biroulet, L. Meta-Analysis: Hyperhomocysteinaemia in Inflammatory Bowel Diseases. *Aliment. Pharmacol. Ther.* **2011**, *34*, 1173–1184. [CrossRef]
50. Stipanuk, M.H. SULFUR AMINO ACID METABOLISM: Pathways for Production and Removal of Homocysteine and Cysteine. *Annu. Rev. Nutr.* **2004**, *24*, 539–577. [CrossRef]
51. Hwang, C.; Ross, V.; Mahadevan, U. Micronutrient Deficiencies in Inflammatory Bowel Disease: From a to Zinc. *Inflamm. Bowel Dis.* **2012**, *18*, 1961–1981. [CrossRef] [PubMed]
52. Vagianos, K.; Bector, S.; McConnell, J.; Bernstein, C.N. Nutrition Assessment of Patients with Inflammatory Bowel Disease. *JPEN. J. Parenter. Enter. Nutr.* **2007**, *31*, 311–319. [CrossRef] [PubMed]
53. Magro, F.; Gionchetti, P.; Eliakim, R.; Ardizzone, S.; Armuzzi, A.; Barreiro-de Acosta, M.; Burisch, J.; Gecse, K.B.; Hart, A.L.; Hindryckx, P.; et al. Third European Evidence-Based Consensus on Diagnosis and Management of Ulcerative Colitis. Part 1: Definitions, Diagnosis, Extra-Intestinal Manifestations, Pregnancy, Cancer Surveillance, Surgery, and Ileo-Anal Pouch Disorders. *J. Crohn's Colitis* **2017**, *11*, 649–670. [CrossRef]
54. Kim, S.H.; Cho, Y.K.; Kim, Y.-J.; Jung, C.H.; Lee, W.J.; Park, J.-Y.; Huh, J.H.; Kang, J.G.; Lee, S.J.; Ihm, S.-H. Association of the Atherogenic Index of Plasma with Cardiovascular Risk beyond the Traditional Risk Factors: A Nationwide Population-Based Cohort Study. *Cardiovasc. Diabetol.* **2022**, *21*, 81. [CrossRef] [PubMed]
55. Kazemi, T.; Hajihosseini, M.; Moossavi, M.; Hemmati, M.; Ziaee, M. Cardiovascular Risk Factors and Atherogenic Indices in an Iranian Population: Birjand East of Iran. *Clin. Med. Insights Cardiol.* **2018**, *12*, 117954681875928. [CrossRef] [PubMed]
56. Bigeh, A.; Sanchez, A.; Maestas, C.; Gulati, M. Inflammatory Bowel Disease and the Risk for Cardiovascular Disease: Does All Inflammation Lead to Heart Disease? *Trends Cardiovasc. Med.* **2019**, *30*, 463–469. [CrossRef] [PubMed]
57. Grundy, S.M.; Stone, N.J.; Bailey, A.L.; Beam, C.; Birtcher, K.K.; Blumenthal, R.S.; Braun, L.T.; de Ferranti, S.; Faiella-Tommasino, J.; Forman, D.E.; et al. 2018 AHA/ACC/AACVPR/AAPA/ABC/ACPM/ADA/AGS/APhA/ASPC/NLA/PCNA Guideline on the Management of Blood Cholesterol. *Circulation* **2018**, *139*, e1082–e1143. [CrossRef]
58. Croft, A.; Lord, A.; Radford-Smith, G. Markers of Systemic Inflammation in Acute Attacks of Ulcerative Colitis: What Level of C-Reactive Protein Constitutes Severe Colitis? *J. Crohn's Colitis* **2022**, *16*, 1089–1096. [CrossRef] [PubMed]
59. Bakkaloglu, O.K.; Eskazan, T.; Celik, S.; Kurt, E.A.; Hatemi, I.; Erzin, Y.; Celik, A.F. Can We Predict Mucosal Remission in Ulcerative Colitis More Precisely with a Redefined Cutoff Level of C-Reactive Protein? *Color. Dis. Off. J. Assoc. Coloproctology Great Br. Irel.* **2022**, *24*, 77–84. [CrossRef] [PubMed]
60. Guagnozzi, D.; Lucendo, A.J. Anemia in Inflammatory Bowel Disease: A Neglected Issue with Relevant Effects. *World J. Gastroenterol. WJG* **2014**, *20*, 3542–3551. [CrossRef]
61. Castañer, O.; Pintó, X.; Subirana, I.; Amor, A.J.; Ros, E.; Hernáez, Á.; Martínez-González, M.Á.; Corella, D.; Salas-Salvadó, J.; Estruch, R.; et al. Remnant Cholesterol, Not LDL Cholesterol, Is Associated with Incident Cardiovascular Disease. *J. Am. Coll. Cardiol.* **2020**, *76*, 2712–2724. [CrossRef] [PubMed]
62. Nordestgaard, B.G. Triglyceride-Rich Lipoproteins and Atherosclerotic Cardiovascular Disease. *Circ. Res.* **2016**, *118*, 547–563. [CrossRef] [PubMed]
63. Sandesara, P.B.; Virani, S.S.; Fazio, S.; Shapiro, M.D. The Forgotten Lipids: Triglycerides, Remnant Cholesterol, and Atherosclerotic Cardiovascular Disease Risk. *Endocr. Rev.* **2018**, *40*, 537–557. [CrossRef] [PubMed]
64. Jepsen, A.-M.K.; Langsted, A.; Varbo, A.; Bang, L.E.; Kamstrup, P.R.; Nordestgaard, B.G. Increased Remnant Cholesterol Explains Part of Residual Risk of All-Cause Mortality in 5414 Patients with Ischemic Heart Disease. *Clin. Chem.* **2016**, *62*, 593–604. [CrossRef] [PubMed]
65. Stein, J.; Dignass, A.U. Management of Iron Deficiency Anemia in Inflammatory Bowel Disease—A Practical Approach. *Ann. Gastroenterol.* **2013**, *26*, 104–113. [PubMed]
66. Dignass, A.U.; Gasche, C.; Bettenworth, D.; Birgegård, G.; Danese, S.; Gisbert, J.P.; Gomollon, F.; Iqbal, T.; Katsanos, K.; Koutroubakis, I.; et al. European Consensus on the Diagnosis and Management of Iron Deficiency and Anaemia in Inflammatory Bowel Diseases. *J. Crohn's Colitis* **2015**, *9*, 211–222. [CrossRef]
67. Cioffi, M. Laboratory Markers in Ulcerative Colitis: Current Insights and Future Advances. *World J. Gastrointest. Pathophysiol.* **2015**, *6*, 13. [CrossRef] [PubMed]
68. Madjid, M.; Awan, I.; Willerson, J.T.; Casscells, S.W. Leukocyte Count and Coronary Heart Disease. *J. Am. Coll. Cardiol.* **2004**, *44*, 1945–1956. [CrossRef]

69. Chen, Z.; Lu, Y.; Wu, J.; Zhang, H. Clinical Significance of Blood Platelets and Mean Platelet Volume in Patients with Ulcerative Colitis. *J. Int. Med. Res.* **2021**, *49*, 3000605211009715. [CrossRef]
70. Giannotta, M.; Tapete, G.; Emmi, G.; Silvestri, E.; Milla, M. Thrombosis in Inflammatory Bowel Diseases: What's the Link? *Thromb. J.* **2015**, *13*, 14. [CrossRef]
71. Heits, F.; Stahl, M.; Ludwig, D.; Stange, E.F.; Jelkmann, W. Elevated Serum Thrombopoietin and Interleukin-6 Concentrations in Thrombocytosis Associated with Inflammatory Bowel Disease. *J. Interferon Cytokine Res.* **1999**, *19*, 757–760. [CrossRef]
72. Evstatiev, R.; Bukaty, A.; Jimenez, K.; Kulnigg-Dabsch, S.; Surman, L.; Schmid, W.; Eferl, R.; Lippert, K.; Scheiber-Mojdehkar, B.; Michael Kvasnicka, H.; et al. Iron Deficiency Alters Megakaryopoiesis and Platelet Phenotype Independent of Thrombopoietin. *Am. J. Hematol.* **2014**, *89*, 524–529. [CrossRef]
73. Bath, P.M.; Missouris, C.G.; Buckenham, T.; MacGregor, G.A. Increased Platelet Volume and Platelet Mass in Patients with Atherosclerotic Renal Artery Stenosis. *Clin. Sci.* **1994**, *87*, 253–257. [CrossRef]
74. Liu, K.; Xu, J.; Tao, L.; Yang, K.; Sun, Y.; Guo, X. Platelet Counts Are Associated with Arterial Stiffness in Chinese Han Population: A Longitudinal Study. *BMC Cardiovasc. Disord.* **2020**, *20*, 353. [CrossRef]
75. Lee, M.K.S.; Kraakman, M.J.; Dragoljevic, D.; Hanssen, N.M.J.; Flynn, M.C.; Al-Sharea, A.; Sreejit, G.; Bertuzzo-Veiga, C.; Cooney, O.D.; Baig, F.; et al. Apoptotic Ablation of Platelets Reduces Atherosclerosis in Mice with Diabetes. *Arterioscler. Thromb. Vasc. Biol.* **2021**, *41*, 1167–1178. [CrossRef] [PubMed]
76. Khaki-Khatibi, F.; Qujeq, D.; Kashifard, M.; Moein, S.; Maniati, M.; Vaghari-Tabari, M. Calprotectin in Inflammatory Bowel Disease. *Clin. Chim. Acta* **2020**, *510*, 556–565. [CrossRef]
77. Xiang, J.-Y.; Ouyang, Q.; Li, G.-D.; Xiao, N.-P. Clinical Value of Fecal Calprotectin in Determining Disease Activity of Ulcerative Colitis. *World J. Gastroenterol.* **2008**, *14*, 53. [CrossRef]
78. Ridker, P.M.; Everett, B.M.; Thuren, T.; MacFadyen, J.G.; Chang, W.H.; Ballantyne, C.; Fonseca, F.; Nicolau, J.; Koenig, W.; Anker, S.D.; et al. Antiinflammatory Therapy with Canakinumab for Atherosclerotic Disease. *N. Engl. J. Med.* **2017**, *377*, 1119–1131. [CrossRef] [PubMed]
79. Kirii, H.; Niwa, T.; Yamada, Y.; Wada, H.; Saito, K.; Iwakura, Y.; Asano, M.; Moriwaki, H.; Seishima, M. Lack of Interleukin-1β Decreases the Severity of Atherosclerosis in ApoE-Deficient Mice. *Arterioscler. Thromb. Vasc. Biol.* **2003**, *23*, 656–660. [CrossRef]
80. Shimokawa, H.; Ito, A.; Fukumoto, Y.; Kadokami, T.; Nakaike, R.; Sakata, M.; Takayanagi, T.; Egashira, K.; Takeshita, A. Chronic Treatment with Interleukin-1 Beta Induces Coronary Intimal Lesions and Vasospastic Responses in Pigs in Vivo. The Role of Platelet-Derived Growth Factor. *J. Clin. Investig.* **1996**, *97*, 769–776. [CrossRef] [PubMed]
81. Duewell, P.; Kono, H.; Rayner, K.J.; Sirois, C.M.; Vladimer, G.; Bauernfeind, F.G.; Abela, G.S.; Franchi, L.; Nuñez, G.; Schnurr, M.; et al. NLRP3 Inflamasomes Are Required for Atherogenesis and Activated by Cholesterol Crystals That Form Early in Disease. *Nature* **2010**, *464*, 1357–1361. [CrossRef] [PubMed]

Disclaimer/Publisher's Note: The statements, opinions and data contained in all publications are solely those of the individual author(s) and contributor(s) and not of MDPI and/or the editor(s). MDPI and/or the editor(s) disclaim responsibility for any injury to people or property resulting from any ideas, methods, instructions or products referred to in the content.

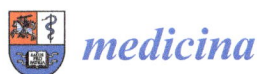

Article

Evaluation of Artificial Intelligence-Calculated Hepatorenal Index for Diagnosing Mild and Moderate Hepatic Steatosis in Non-Alcoholic Fatty Liver Disease

Zita Zsombor [1], Aladár D. Rónaszéki [1], Barbara Csongrády [1], Róbert Stollmayer [1], Bettina K. Budai [1], Anikó Folhoffer [2], Ildikó Kalina [1], Gabriella Győri [1], Viktor Bérczi [1], Pál Maurovich-Horvat [1], Krisztina Hagymási [3,†] and Pál Novák Kaposi [1,*,†]

1. Medical Imaging Center, Department of Radiology, Faculty of Medicine, Semmelweis University, Korányi S. u. 2/A., 1083 Budapest, Hungary
2. Department of Internal Medicine and Oncology, Faculty of Medicine, Semmelweis University, Korányi S. u. 2/A., 1083 Budapest, Hungary
3. Department of Surgery, Transplantation and Gastroenterology, Faculty of Medicine, Semmelweis University, Üllői út 78., 1082 Budapest, Hungary
* Correspondence: kaposi.pal@med.semmelweis-univ.hu
† These authors contributed equally to this work.

Abstract: *Background and Objectives*: This study aims to evaluate artificial intelligence-calculated hepatorenal index (AI-HRI) as a diagnostic method for hepatic steatosis. *Materials and Methods*: We prospectively enrolled 102 patients with clinically suspected non-alcoholic fatty liver disease (NAFLD). All patients had a quantitative ultrasound (QUS), including AI-HRI, ultrasound attenuation coefficient (AC,) and ultrasound backscatter-distribution coefficient (SC) measurements. The ultrasonographic fatty liver indicator (US-FLI) score was also calculated. The magnetic resonance imaging fat fraction (MRI-PDFF) was the reference to classify patients into four grades of steatosis: none < 5%, mild 5–10%, moderate 10–20%, and severe ≥ 20%. We compared AI-HRI between steatosis grades and calculated Spearman's correlation (r_s) between the methods. We determined the agreement between AI-HRI by two examiners using the intraclass correlation coefficient (ICC) of 68 cases. We performed a receiver operating characteristics (ROC) analysis to estimate the area under the curve (AUC) for AI-HRI. *Results*: The mean AI-HRI was 2.27 (standard deviation, ±0.96) in the patient cohort. The AI-HRI was significantly different between groups without (1.480 ± 0.607, $p < 0.003$) and with mild steatosis (2.155 ± 0.776), as well as between mild and moderate steatosis (2.777 ± 0.923, $p < 0.018$). AI-HRI showed moderate correlation with AC ($r_s = 0.597$), SC ($r_s = 0.473$), US-FLI ($r_s = 0.5$), and MRI-PDFF ($r_s = 0.528$). The agreement in AI-HRI was good between the two examiners (ICC = 0.635, 95% confidence interval (CI) = 0.411–0.774, $p < 0.001$). The AI-HRI could detect mild steatosis (AUC = 0.758, 95% CI = 0.621–0.894) with fair and moderate/severe steatosis (AUC = 0.803, 95% CI = 0.721–0.885) with good accuracy. However, the performance of AI-HRI was not significantly different ($p < 0.578$) between the two diagnostic tasks. *Conclusions*: AI-HRI is an easy-to-use, reproducible, and accurate QUS method for diagnosing mild and moderate hepatic steatosis.

Keywords: ultrasound; liver; artificial intelligence; non-alcoholic fatty liver disease; hepatorenal index

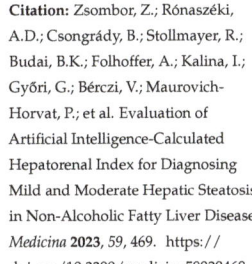

Citation: Zsombor, Z.; Rónaszéki, A.D.; Csongrády, B.; Stollmayer, R.; Budai, B.K.; Folhoffer, A.; Kalina, I.; Győri, G.; Bérczi, V.; Maurovich-Horvat, P.; et al. Evaluation of Artificial Intelligence-Calculated Hepatorenal Index for Diagnosing Mild and Moderate Hepatic Steatosis in Non-Alcoholic Fatty Liver Disease. *Medicina* **2023**, *59*, 469. https://doi.org/10.3390/medicina59030469

Academic Editors: Ludovico Abenavoli and Marcello Candelli

Received: 17 January 2023
Revised: 12 February 2023
Accepted: 23 February 2023
Published: 27 February 2023

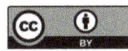

Copyright: © 2023 by the authors. Licensee MDPI, Basel, Switzerland. This article is an open access article distributed under the terms and conditions of the Creative Commons Attribution (CC BY) license (https://creativecommons.org/licenses/by/4.0/).

1. Introduction

Non-alcoholic fatty liver disease (NAFLD) is the most common cause of chronic liver disease in Western countries, and it has a 25% prevalence worldwide [1]. There is a strong association with type 2 diabetes; NAFLD is a frequent indication for liver transplantation and a significant cause of cardiovascular morbidity. Fat accumulation in ≥5% of the hepatocytes detected either by histology, or magnetic resonance imaging (MRI) is a prerequisite to the NAFLD diagnosis. To facilitate early diagnosis and prevent complications from NAFLD, current European practice guidelines recommend screening individuals with increased metabolic risk using non-invasive methods. Moreover, according to the guidelines, hepatic steatosis should be identified with imaging methods, preferably ultrasound (US), because it is more widely available and cheaper than the gold standard, MRI [2].

Although liver biopsy is considered the most accurate method to diagnose hepatic steatosis, it has multiple drawbacks, including sampling only a small portion of the parenchyma, non-negligible risk of complications, and limited accessibility. Therefore, clinical practice has shifted towards non-invasive imaging techniques to detect fatty liver, as these are more readily available, put less burden on the patient, and can be used to assess focal variations in fat content [3]. Grayscale US is an efficient method to diagnose hepatic steatosis based on well-established morphological signs such as increased liver reflectivity, distal attenuation of US signal, blurring of hepatic vessels and gallbladder wall, or focal sparing at typical locations. The disadvantages of grayscale US are its relatively weak sensitivity for lower grades (<20%) of steatosis, the difficulties with scanning morbidly obese patients with body mass index (BMI) > 40 kg/m^2, and considerable dependence on the observer's experience [4]. Computed tomography (CT) is an alternative imaging technique that could quantify hepatic steatosis with good accuracy; however, it exposes patients to a significant amount of ionizing radiation [5]. MRI is the most sensitive imaging method, which can reliably detect even low-grade, between 5% and 10%, steatosis. MRI-PDFF has become a universally accepted reference technique as it can stage steatosis with accuracy comparable to liver biopsy; also, the entire liver can be evaluated with a single scan [6]. However, MRI-PDFF's high cost and limited availability do not allow screening of large patient populations.

Semi-quantitative scores such as the ultrasonographic fatty liver indicator (US-FLI) can improve the reproducibility of US diagnosis, and identify patients who have non-alcoholic steatohepatitis (NASH) [7]. Another semi-quantitative metric is the hepatorenal index (HRI), which is the ratio between the brightness of the liver and the right renal cortex on grayscale US. HRI is less operator-dependent, and it has been shown to have a good detection rate of mild and even better detection of moderate and severe steatosis [8–10]. Meanwhile, the calculation of HRI can be time-consuming, and selecting a region of interest (ROI) can be subjective, weakening the measurement's reproducibility. Recently, artificial intelligence-calculated HRI (AI-HRI) measurement has become available, where pixels of the liver and renal cortex are delineated by a deep convolutional neural network (DCNN), and positioning of the ROIs, and calculation of the HRI are fully-automated [11]. Furthermore, multiple quantitative ultrasound (QUS) parameters, which allow for simultaneous assessment of liver fibrosis, inflammation, and steatosis in chronic liver diseases, can be measured on advanced systems [12–14]. The performance of some of the QUS metrics, such as the ultrasound attenuation coefficient (AC) and ultrasound backscatter-distribution coefficient (SC), has been very good in the classification of all steatosis grades according to multiple studies [15,16].

In the present study, we have used AI-HRI to diagnose hepatic steatosis in NAFLD patients and evaluated its interobserver reproducibility and diagnostic accuracy using MRI-PDFF as the reference method. According to our knowledge, this is the first study that has directly compared AI-HRI with other US parameters for classifying steatosis grades.

2. Materials and Methods

2.1. Patients

This single-center prospective cohort study was approved by the regional and institutional committee of science and research ethics of our university and written informed consent was obtained from all participants according to the World Medical Association Declaration of Helsinki, revised in Edinburgh in 2000. We prospectively enrolled 271 participants who were examined for suspected liver steatosis in our institution between July 2020 and November 2022. The eligibility criteria to participate in the study included the following: 18 years or older, referral to an imaging study to rule out clinically suspected hepatic steatosis, completed artificial intelligence augmented HRI and MRI-PDFF measurements of liver fat content, clinical findings consistent with NAFLD based on the diagnostic criteria of the European Clinical Practice guidelines [2]. The participants' demographic data, including the history of alcohol consumption, were collected from a personal survey, and the medical history and laboratory tests were collected from electronic medical reports. We excluded participants who reported daily alcohol consumption in excess of 20 g (2 drinks) for females or 30 g (3 drinks) for males in the last two years, patients with a history of chronic liver disease due to an etiology other than NAFLD, including chronic viral hepatitis, autoimmune hepatitis, PBC, PSC, long term use of hepatotoxic drugs, as well as patients whose liver iron content was above the normal range (≥ 2 mg/g) or had a positive genetic test for hereditary hemochromatosis. Patients with acute liver failure (ALF), acute on chronic liver failure (ACLF), decompensated liver cirrhosis (DLC: hepatic encephalopathy, moderate ascites, esophageal bleeding), or extrahepatic biliary obstruction were excluded (Figure 1).

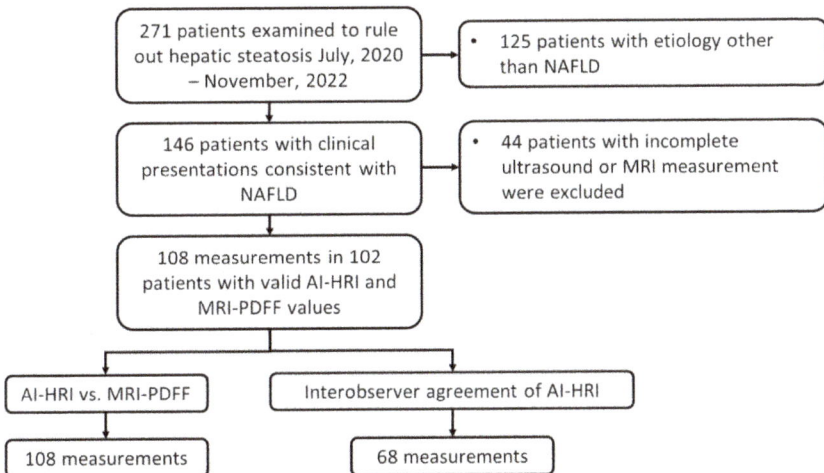

Figure 1. The flowchart demonstrates patient selection and study design. We prospectively enrolled 102 participants with suspected non-alcoholic fatty liver disease (NAFLD) in our study. Two hundred and seventy-one patients were referred to either an ultrasound or an MRI scan at our department to rule out hepatic steatosis; out of these, in 146 patients who did not show signs of acute liver failure, clinical findings were consistent with NAFLD. Forty-four patients who did not have a complete artificial intelligence-calculated hepatorenal index (AI-HRI) and magnetic resonance imaging proton density fat fraction (MRI-PDFF) measurements were excluded from the study. We evaluated the diagnostic accuracy of AI-HRI by comparing it to MRI-PDFF as a reference using 108 independent measurements of 102 patients. The interobserver agreement of AI-HRI was assessed in 68 cases, where measurements by two different examiners were available.

The final patient cohort included 102 subjects (50 females and 52 males) who fulfilled the eligibility criteria, did not meet any exclusion criteria, and had 108 valid ultrasonography and MRI measurements of hepatic steatosis. There were six patients who were followed for chronic liver disease and had US and MRI scans during the study period at two different time points with a 6-month interval. The participants' mean age ($\pm$standard deviation, SD) was 55 ± 13 years. Among the participants, 23 (23/102, 23%) had type 2 diabetes mellitus (T2DM), and 31 (31/102, 30%) were severely overweight with a BMI ≥ 30 kg/m^2. Demographic information and results of laboratory tests in the patient cohort are summarized in Table 1.

Table 1. Demographic variables and laboratory tests in the NAFLD patient cohort.

Patient Number:	102
Females/males:	50/52
* Age (years):	55 ± 13
* BMI:	28.95 ± 4.63
T2DM:	23/102 (22.5%)
* Platelet($\times 10^9$/L):	245.17 ± 67.35
* Albumin (g/L):	43.82 ± 3.66
* AST (IU/L):	37.38 ± 26.57
* ALT (IU/L):	48.80 ± 39.84
* ALP (IU/L):	86.93 ± 48.62
* Total bilirubin (μmol/L):	13.89 ± 7.60
* Sodium (mmol/L):	139.89 ± 2.24
* Creatinine (μmol/L):	78.10 ± 21.35
*$ APRI:	0.41 ± 0.28
*$ Fibrosis-4 Index:	1.38 ± 0.85
*$ NAFLD Fibrosis Score:	1.57 ± 1.65
** HSI:	37.83 ± 6.21

* Values are reported as mean ± standard deviation; $ Clinical and laboratory test indices were calculated using the MDCalc website (www.mdcalc.org (accessed on 2 December 2022)); ** hepatic steatosis index = 8 × (ALT/AST ratio) + BMI (+2, if female; +2, if diabetes mellitus) [17]; BMI: body mass index, T2DM: type 2 diabetes mellitus, AST: aspartate aminotransferase, ALT: alanine aminotransferase, ALP: alkaline phosphatase, APRI: AST to platelet ratio index, HSI: hepatic steatosis index.

2.2. Ultrasound Scanning and AI-HRI Measurements

Patients were asked to fast for at least four hours before the ultrasound scan. We used a Samsung RS85 Prestige ultrasound system (Samsung Medison Co. Ltd., Hongcheon, Republic of Korea) equipped with a CA 1-7S convex probe to scan all participants. The ultrasound scans were performed by an expert radiologist with more than ten years of experience in abdominal ultrasound. The AI-HRI model used in this study has been trained and validated by Cha et al. on pre-transplantation liver US scans as has been reported previously [11]. For AI-HRI measurements, a right intercostal or subcostal view was obtained in supine patients and showing the longitudinal cross-section of the right kidney and the right liver lobe. Then, the EzHRI™ application was selected, which automatically detected the outlines of the renal cortex and the liver parenchyma based on a DCNN image segmentation, and placed two identical-size circular ROIs in the liver and the renal cortex at the same depth from the skin surface avoiding large vessels and high-intensity areas of the medulla. The HRI was calculated from the ratio of average pixel intensity values between the two ROIs (Figure 1). The average time to complete a single measurement was less than ten seconds. The AI-HRI value in each case was the median of repeated measurements on five different images. In the few instances, <5% of the measurements, when the algorithm incorrectly placed an ROI, i.e., in an area concealed by rib shadows, the ROI was repositioned manually. The image acquisition parameters, including gain, dynamic range, and focal depth were selected by the examiner to obtain the best available image quality. If the average pixel intensity value was below ten units in any ROI, the gain was increased to avoid large variations in the intensity ratios. A second examiner, a radiology trainee with more than four years of experience in abdominal ultrasound also measured the AI-HRI in 68 patients on the same day. Both examiners were blinded from each other's and the patients' prior results.

2.3. Measurement of AC, SC, and Semi-Quantitative Scoring of Hepatic Steatosis on US Images

Together with AI-HRI, during the same scan, we also measured two additional QUS parameters, the AC and the SC, as alternative biomarkers of hepatic steatosis. The detailed protocols of the AC and SC measurements have been published previously [14]. Briefly, the right lobe of the liver was visualized from an intercostal window, and from the QUS application of the scanner, either tissue attenuation imaging (TAI™) or tissue scatter distribution imaging (TSI^{TM}) mode was selected. Then, the examiner placed a color-coded ROI in the liver parenchyma and recorded the mean AC in dB/cm/MHz units or the mean SC in arbitrary units. AC measurements with an R-squared (R^2) value > 0.6 were considered unreliable and discarded. Finally, we calculated the median of valid AC and SC measurements and used them in consecutive analyses.

We also took images of the liver in standard views and used them to calculate the ultrasonographic fatty liver indicator (US-FLI) score [7]. The US-FLI is a semi-quantitative scoring system for grading hepatic steatosis based on B-mode images. The US-FLI is a sum of scores given on multiple different features. A trainee and expert radiologist performed the scoring individually, and the final score reflected the consensus between the examiners. The most important feature was the liver/kidney contrast, which could be absent (score 0), mild/moderate (score 1), or severe (score 2). Other features included the posterior attenuation of the beam, vessel blurring, difficult visualization of the gallbladder wall, difficult visualization of the diaphragm, and areas of focal sparing; each of these was scored as either absent (score 0) or present (score 1). We calculated the US-FLI score for 107 US examinations of 103 participants based on archived images retrieved from our PACS system. The US-FLI score of the patients ranged from 0 to 8; a score ≥ 2 was needed for the diagnosis of steatosis, while a score ≥ 4 was indicative of non-alcoholic steatohepatitis (NASH).

2.4. Measurement of the MRI-PDFF

The MRQuantif examination protocol and software (https://imagemed.univ-rennes1.fr/en/mrquantif (accessed on 16 September 2022) were used to measure the MRI-PDFF in the participants' livers [18]. During the MRI scan, two-dimensional (2D) axial images of the liver at the level of the porta hepatis were acquired with a multi-echo gradient echo sequence, which included twelve echoes with gradually spaced echo times (TE) starting from 1.2 msec with 1.2 msec increments. Other scanning parameters included a repetition time (TR) of 120 msec, a flip angle (FA) of 20 degrees, a pixel bandwidth (Bw) of 2712 Hz, a field-of-view of 400 × 350 mm, a reconstruction matrix of 128 × 116 pixels, and an interslice gap of 10 mm. Each slab was scanned during a single breath-hold of 18 s or less. All participants were scanned with the same Philips Ingenia^{TM} 1.5 T MRI scanner (Philips Healthcare, Amsterdam, the Netherlands) using the Q-Body coil. The software calculated the R2* and the MRI-PDFF using a magnitude-based exponential decay model integrating the variation of the signal linked to the six main fat peaks determined by Hamilton et al. [19]. For visual reference, we performed a complex-based estimation of MRI-PDFF and reconstructed color-coded fat fraction maps in a selection of cases using Matlab (The Mathworks, Natick, MA, USA) code (https://github.com/welcheb/FattyRiot (accessed on 30 September 2020) of Berglund et al. [20] (Figure 2). The MRI scans were completed within a month after the ultrasound scans and evaluated blinded from US results. Similar to previous publications, we classified patients into four severity grades (none: <5%, mild: 5–10%, moderate: 10–20%, severe: $\geq$20%) based on the amount of hepatic steatosis measured with MRI-PDFF [4,14,16,21].

2.5. Statistical Analysis

We used the Shapiro–Wilk test to confirm normal distribution of continuous demographic, biochemical, and imaging variables. The analysis of variance (ANOVA) and post-hoc Tukey's honestly significant difference (HSD) tests were applied to compare continuous variables with normal distributions (i.e., AC and SC) between multiple groups. We used the Kruskal–Wallis rank sum test and, post hoc, the pairwise Wilcoxon rank sum test to compare not normally distributed variables (i.e., AI-HRI and US-FLI). We adjusted p-values with the Benjamini–Hochberg method to control the false discovery rate (FDR) in multiple comparisons. The Spearman's rank correlation coefficient (r_s) was calculated to assess the strength of the relationship between different image-based biomarkers of hepatic steatosis and between the AI-HRI measurements of the two examiners. We constructed a Bland–Altman plot to evaluate the interobserver agreement between the AI-HRI values measured by two examiners and calculated the intraclass correlation coefficient (ICC) using a two-way mixed effect model.

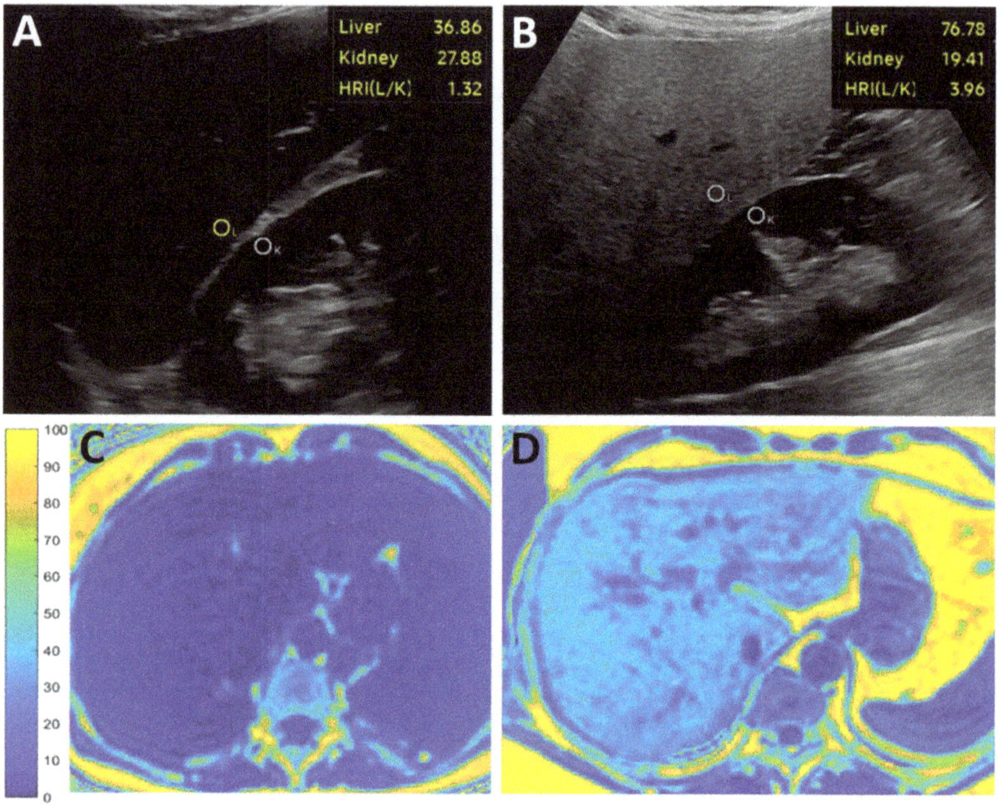

Figure 2. Representative images show measurements of the artificial intelligence-calculated hepatorenal index (HRI) and magnetic resonance imaging fat fraction (MRI-PDFF). The examiner took a longitudinal brightness mode image of the right liver lobe and the right kidney. The HRI was calculated from the pixel intensity ratio of two circular regions of interest (ROI) automatically placed in the liver (L) and the kidney cortex (K) by the software after segmentation of the ultrasound image with a deep convolutional neural network. (**A**) The brightness of a non-steatotic liver was similar to the kidney's cortex resulting in a low HRI. (**B**) The brightness of a severely steatotic liver was much higher than the kidney's cortex, causing an elevated HRI in a patient diagnosed with NAFLD. The MRI-PDFF maps reconstructed with a complex method were used as a reference. (**C**) In the first cases, the blue color of a non-steatotic liver corresponded to <5% MRI-PDFF on the scale ranging from 0–100%. (**D**) Meanwhile, severe steatosis ($\geq$20% MRI-PDFF) was indicated by the turquoise color of the liver in the second case.

We built multiple univariable regression models to identify significant associations between clinical variables and AI-HRI. The age, gender, weight, height, BMI, liver-to-skin distance, type 2 diabetes, blood glucose, hematocrit, platelet count, international normalized ratio (INR), serum albumin, aspartate aminotransferase (AST), alanine aminotransferase (ALT), alkaline phosphatase (ALP), γ-glutamil transferase (GGT), total bilirubin, blood urea nitrogen (BUN), serum creatinine were tested as independent variables against AI-HRI as the dependent variable. Clinical factors achieving significance in the univariable analysis were also evaluated in a multivariable model. The adjusted R-squared (R^2) metric was used to assess the strength of the associations.

We performed receiver operating characteristic (ROC) curve analyses to assess the performance of the different diagnostic methods of hepatic steatosis with MRI-PDFF used as the reference method. We also calculated multiple performance metrics, including area under the ROC curve (AUC), sensitivity (sens.), specificity (spec.), negative predictive value (NPV), positive predictive value (PPV), and accuracy (acc.). The thresholds of AI-HRI, which could accurately differentiate between consecutive steatosis grades, were also calculated. The Delong test was used to compare the AUC values between different hepatic steatosis metrics. A ROC curve power analysis was also completed using the formula described by Obuchowski et al. to estimate the smallest sample size that allows for accurate discrimination between categories with a type I error rate < 0.05 and a type II error rate < 0.2 [22].

Continuous variables were reported in a mean and standard deviation (SD) format, and categorical variables as numbers and percentages. The r_s, ICC, and AUC values were reported as median and 95% confidence intervals (CI). We applied a $p < 0.05$ threshold to declare statistical significance in all comparisons. We performed all statistical analysis with the RStudio 2022.07.2 software package (https://rstudio.com (accessed on 2 December 2022).

3. Results

3.1. Comparison of AI-HRI and Other QUS Parameters between Different Grades of Steatosis

We measured multiple QUS parameters, AI-HRI, AC, and SC, and calculated the semi-quantitative US-FLI score to determine the severity of steatosis in 108 independent measurements in 102 NAFLD patients. The study cohort consisted of 30 cases (30/108, 27.7%) without steatosis (<5% MRI-PDFF), 24 cases (24/108, 22.2%) of mild (from 5% $\leq$ to <10% MRI-PDFF), 37 cases (37/108, 34.3%) of moderate (from 10% $\leq$ to <20% MRI-PDFF) and 17 cases (17/108, 15.7%) of severe ($\geq$20% MRI-PDFF) steatosis. The AI-HRI ranged from 0.45 to 5.90, with a mean of 2.27 $\pm$ 0.96 for all participants. The AI-HRI was significantly higher in mild steatosis (2.155 $\pm$ 0.776) compared to the normal liver (1.480 $\pm$ 0.607, $p < 0.003$) and was elevated in moderate steatosis (2.777 $\pm$ 0.923, $p < 0.018$) compared to mild steatosis. However, the AI-HRI values were not significantly different between moderate and severe steatosis (2.711 $\pm$ 0.822, $p < 0.787$) (Figure 3). The US-FLI score was not significantly higher in mild steatosis (0.900 $\pm$ 1.398) compared to the normal liver (1.542 $\pm$ 1.318, $p < 0.074$), but it showed significant increase both in moderate (4.000 $\pm$ 1.509, $p < 0.001$) and in severe (5.941 $\pm$ 0.966, $p < 0.001$) steatosis compared to lower grades. The AC values showed significant gradual increase through all consecutive steatosis grades. Meanwhile, SC was significantly different only between normal liver (91.75 $\pm$ 11.03) and mild (101.37 $\pm$ 7.15, $p < 0.001$) steatosis (Table 2). No adverse events occurred during the patient scans.

3.2. Evaluation of AI-HRI for Detection of Different Grades of Hepatic Steatosis

We performed a ROC curve analysis with AI-HRI, AC, SC, and US-FLI to evaluate the performance of these methods in differentiating normal liver (<5% MRI-PDFF) from mild ($\geq$5% MRI-PDFF) steatosis. The MRI-PDFF was used as the reference method to determine steatosis grades. AI-HRI was able to classify patients into normal and mild steatosis groups with fair accuracy (AUC = 0.758, 95% CI = 0.621–0.894) (Figure 4). We also calculated the spec., sens., PPV, NPV, and acc. metrics for thresholds enabled the most accurate classification (Table 3). The AC (AUC = 0.829, 95% CI = 0.713–0.945, $p < 0.281$) performed relatively better, while SC (AUC = 0.772, 95% CI = 0.645–0.898, $p < 0.851$) similar, and US-FLI (AUC = 0.639, 95% CI = 0.497–0.781, $p < 0.175$) relatively worse than AI-HRI in the same classification task. Due to the low correct prediction rate, the ROC analysis performed with US-FLI had limited statistical power (true positives = 43.6%). The probability of type II error was <20% in all other ROC analyses with the current sample size.

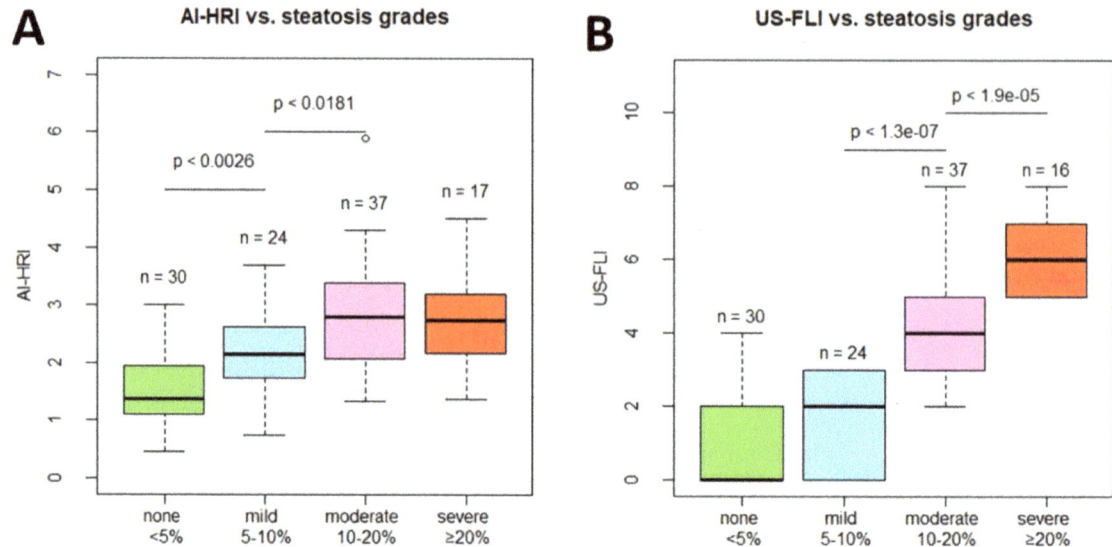

Figure 3. Box plots show the distribution of (**A**) artificial intelligence-calculated hepatorenal index (AI-HRI) values and (**B**) ultrasonographic fatty liver indicator (US-FLI) scores in increasing grades of hepatic steatosis. Magnetic resonance imaging proton density fat fraction (MRI-PDFF) was used as the reference method. We compared AI-HRI and US-FLI between different steatosis grades with the pairwise Wilcoxon rank sum test and labeled significant differences with the p-value.

Table 2. Values measured with QUS methods in increasing grades of hepatic steatosis.

* Steatosis Grade:	None	Mild	Moderate	Severe
AI-HRI	1.480 ± 0.607	2.155 ± 0.776	2.777 ± 0.923	2.711 ± 0.822
** p-value<	NA	0.003	0.018	0.787
*** AC (dB/cm/Mhz)	0.674 ± 0.084	0.797 ± 0.089	0.895 ± 0.097	1.004 ± 0.139
** p-value<	NA	0.001	0.002	0.003
*** SC	91.75 ± 11.03	101.37 ± 7.15	105.98 ± 5.40	106.17 ± 4.81
** p-value<	NA	0.001	0.115	1.00
*** US-FLI	0.900 ± 1.398	1.542 ± 1.318	4.000 ± 1.509	5.941 ± 0.966
** p-value<	NA	0.074	0.001	0.001

* Classification is based on MRI-PDFF as the reference method (none: <5%, mild: 5–10%, moderate: 10–20%, severe: ≥20%), ** Compared to lower grade(s) of steatosis, *** Mean ± standard deviation, AI-HRI: artificial intelligence-calculated hepatorenal index, AC: ultrasound attenuation coefficient, MRI-PDFF: magnetic resonance imaging proton density fat fraction, SC: ultrasound backscatter-distribution coefficient, US-FLI: ultrasonographic fatty liver indicator.

We also evaluated the same US methods for the classification of absent and mild (<10% MRI-PDFF) versus moderate and severe (≥10% MRI-PDFF) steatosis. The AI-HRI could differentiate between advanced and mild or absent steatosis (AUC = 0.803, 0.721–0.885) with good accuracy. The SC (AUC = 0.805, 95% CI = 0.720–0.890, p < 0.997), performed very similarly to AI-HRI in the second classification. Meanwhile, both AC (AUC = 0.895, 0.835–0.955, p < 0.031) and US-FLI (AUC = 0.937, 95% CI = 0.898–0.975, p < 0.002) significantly outperformed AI-HRI in diagnostic accuracy for advanced steatosis. The performance of AI-HRI was not significantly different (p < 0.578) between the classification problems. The power for the detection of moderate/severe steatosis was above 90% in the case of all tested diagnostic methods.

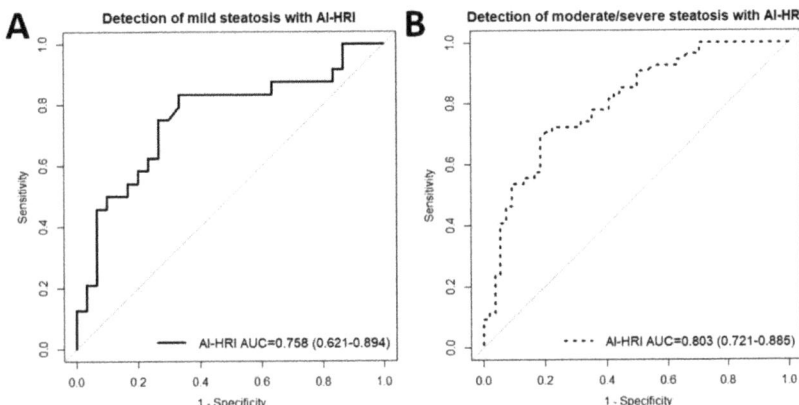

Figure 4. (**A**) The plot shows receiver operating characteristics (ROC) curve analyses with artificial intelligence-calculated hepatorenal index (AI-HRI) for the classification of normal liver and mild steatosis. The accuracy of AI-HRI was fair based on the area under the curve (AUC) value of 0.758. The 95% confidence intervals of the AUC are listed inside the brackets. (**B**) The plot shows that AI-HRI could detect moderate/severe steatosis with an AUC of 0.803, indicating good classification accuracy. The magnetic resonance imaging fat fraction (MRI-PDFF) was used as the reference method in both classifications.

Table 3. Performance metrics from ROC analyses with QUS parameters.

Method	Thresh.	Spec.	Sens.	PPV	NPV	Acc.
* For differentiation between normal liver (<5%) and mild (≥5%) steatosis						
	1.23	0.367	0.875	0.525	0.786	0.593
AI-HRI (AUC = 0.85)	** 1.53	0.667	0.833	0.667	0.833	0.741
	1.85	0.733	0.750	0.692	0.786	0.741
	0.74	0.828	0.750	0.783	0.800	0.792
AC (AUC = 0.922)	** 0.77	0.897	0.708	0.850	0.788	0.811
	0.79	0.931	0.583	0.875	0.730	0.774
	90.47	0.414	0.958	0.575	0.923	0.660
SC (AUC = 0.860)	** 93.93	0.552	0.875	0.618	0.842	0.698
	94.87	0.586	0.792	0.613	0.773	0.679
US-FLI (AUC = 0.85)	*** 2	0.733	0.583	0.636	0.688	0.667
* For differentiation between absent/mild (<10%) and moderate/severe (≥10%) steatosis						
	2.21	0.778	0.722	0.765	0.737	0.750
AI-HRI (AUC = 0.803)	** 2.25	0.796	0.704	0.776	0.729	0.750
	2.29	0.815	0.685	0.787	0.721	0.750
	0.81	0.792	0.840	0.792	0.840	0.816
AC (AUC = 0.895)	** 0.83	0.849	0.800	0.833	0.818	0.825
	0.85	0.868	0.760	0.844	0.793	0.816
	98.37	0.547	0.940	0.662	0.906	0.738
SC (AUC = 0.805)	** 100.22	0.623	0.920	0.697	0.892	0.767
	101.35	0.642	0.860	0.694	0.829	0.748
US-FLI (AUC = 0.937)	*** 4	0.944	0.667	0.923	0.739	0.806

* The magnetic resonance imaging fat fraction (MRI-PDFF) was used as the reference method. ** Labels the best thresholds with the highest diagnostic accuracy. *** Diagnostic thresholds of US-FLI for non-alcoholic fatty liver disease (NAFLD) and non-alcoholic steatohepatitis (NASH) were defined by Ballestri et al. [7]. Acc: accuracy, AI-HRI: artificial intelligence-calculated hepatorenal index, AC: ultrasound attenuation coefficient, AUC: area under the ROC curve, NPV: negative predictive value, PPV: positive predictive value, SC: ultrasound backscatter-distribution coefficient, Sens.: sensitivity, Spec.: specificity, Thresh.: threshold, US-FLI: ultrasonographic fatty liver indicator.

3.3. Correlation of AI-HRI with Other Methods

We found moderate but significant positive correlation between AI-HRI and MRI-PDFF (r_s = 0.528, 95% CI = 0.377–0.651, p < 0.001), as well as between AI-HRI and US-FLI measurements (r_s = 0.498, 95% CI = 0.329–0.635, p < 0.001) (Figure 5). The US-FLI values showed very strong significant correlation with MRI-PDFF (r_s = 0.804, 95% CI = 0.706–0.863, p < 0.001) and a strong correlation with AC (r_s = 0.690, 95% CI = 0.565–0.782, p < 0.001). The correlation was also strong between AC and MRI-PDFF (r_s = 0.775, 95% CI = 0.660–0.849, p < 0.001), but only moderate, although significant, between AC and AI-HRI (r_s = 0.597, 95% CI = 0.464–0.700, p < 0.001). SC showed strong correlation with MRI-PDFF (r_s = 0.6, 95% CI = 0.442–0.724, p < 0.001) but only moderate with AI-HRI (r_s = 0.473, 95% CI = 0.296–0.621, p < 0.001).

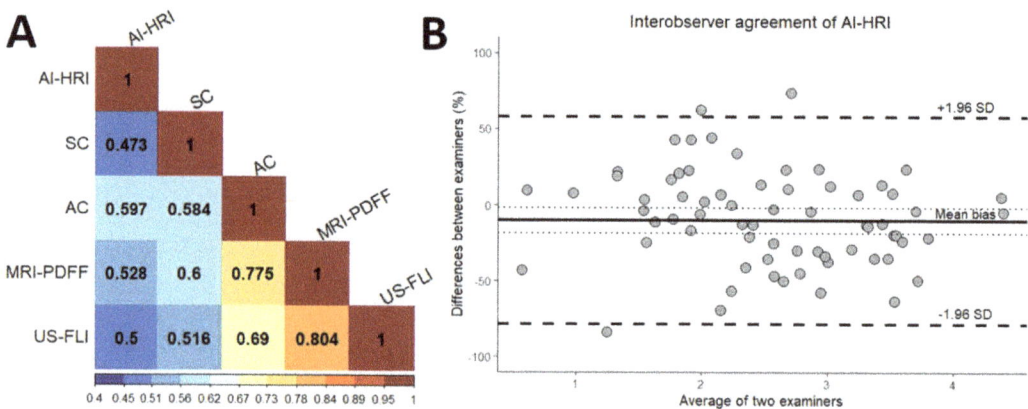

Figure 5. (**A**) The correlation matrix between imaging methods is displayed on a colored heat map. The amount of steatosis was determined with quantitative ultrasound (QUS) metrics, including artificial intelligence-calculated hepatorenal index (AI-HRI) and ultrasound attenuation coefficient (AC), ultrasound backscatter-distribution coefficient (SC), and semi-quantitative ultrasonographic fatty liver indicator (US-FLI); while magnetic resonance imaging fat fraction (MRI-PDFF) was the reference method. The Spearman's rank correlation coefficients were calculated from pairwise comparisons. (**B**) The Bland–Altman plot shows interobserver agreement between AI-HRI measured by two examiners. The mean of the bias is labeled with a solid, and the upper and lower limits of agreement are with dashed lines.

In the univariable regression analysis, four independent variables, including age (R^2 = 0.044, p < 0.0395), BUN (R^2 = 0.103, p < 0.004), height (R^2 = 0.042, p < 0.0368), and INR (R^2 = 0.057, p < 0.0333) showed very weak but significant association with AI-HRI. In the multivariable model, none of these factors was a significant predictor of AI-HRI.

3.4. Interobserver Agreement of AI-HRI Measurements

There was a moderate but significant correlation between AI-HRI measurements performed by the two examiners (r_s = 0.572, 95% CI = 0.340–0.728, p < 0.001). The ICC was 0.635 (95% CI = 0.411–0.774, p < 0.001), which indicated good interobserver agreement. The Bland–Altman analysis revealed −10.29% average bias between the examiners, while the limits of agreement (LOA) were at 57.70% and −78.28% (Figure 5).

4. Discussion

In the present study, we have demonstrated that AI-HRI is a reliable method for the diagnosis and classification of hepatic steatosis in NAFLD. In previous studies, which evaluated HRI, the liver and kidney ROIs were manually selected, which caused significant differences between the diagnostic protocols [8–10,23,24].

In previous studies evaluating non-invasive biomarkers of steatosis, 5%, 10%, and 20% MRI-PDFF were used as optimal thresholds for diagnosing mild, moderate, and severe hepatic steatosis, respectively, as these cutoff values closely approximate the classification into S1, S2, and S3 histology grades [6,16,21,25]. We think that for the unambiguous comparability of our results with other non-invasive diagnostic techniques, it was important to use the same classification for steatosis severity as in previous studies.

The accuracy of manually labeled HRI in the detection of mild steatosis showed considerable variability between different studies, with AUC values ranging between 0.68 and 0.92 [8–10]. The performance of AI-HRI was within the above range; however, its AUC of 0.76 was superior to some recently published results obtained with high-end ultrasound systems, which measured HRI manually [8]. The best diagnostic threshold for the detection of mild steatosis was 1.53, which is almost identical to the threshold at 1.54 reported for manual HRI in a study that compared US metrics with magnetic resonance spectroscopy proton density fat fraction (MRS-PDFF). Using nearly identical thresholds, the sensitivity was higher (83% vs. 50%), and the specificity was lower (67% vs. 92%) with AI-HRI than with HRI. In another study comparing HRI with histology grades, the cutoff value for mild steatosis was 1.46, which had only 43% sensitivity and 91% specificity. These data suggest that AI-HRI may outperform conventional HRI in detecting low-grade hepatic steatosis as it has greater sensitivity at similar thresholds. Thus, AI-HRI could be an efficient tool for screening patients with suspected NAFLD.

The AI-HRI performed slightly better in diagnosing at least moderate steatosis, although its AUC of 0.81 was not significantly different from the AUC calculated for mild steatosis. The accuracy of AI-HRI was also better compared to manually labeled HRI, which had an AUC of 0.71 and 0.74 for the detections of moderate and severe S2 and S3 histology grade steatosis, respectively [8]. The sensitivity of AI-HRI was again better (70% vs. 47–52%), and its specificity is lower (80% vs. 85–94%) compared to HRI. Meanwhile, the diagnostic threshold for AI-HRI was considerably higher (2.25 vs. 1.48 and 1.79). However, the direct comparison between the two studies is difficult as they used different reference methods, and the exact relationship between MRI-PDFF and steatosis grade detected with histology is still undetermined [6].

The range of AI-HRI (0.45–5.90) was comparable to the conventional HRI (0.77–4.2) as reported previously [9]. The mean AI-HRI (2.27) in the study cohort was higher than the mean HRI (1.4–1.56) in previous studies. This can be mainly attributed to the lower percentage of patients without significant steatosis (27.7%) in our study cohort compared to patient populations in previous studies where the percentage of negative cases (47.8–69.2%) was much higher [8–10]. We also found significant differences between AI-HRI measured in normal liver, mild steatosis, and mild and moderate steatosis, indicating robust diagnostic performance.

The agreement between AI-HRI measured by two examiners (ICC = 0.64) was good, and it was in the range of the interobserver agreement reported for manually labeled HRI (ICC = 0.58–0.68) [11]. The correlation between the two observers' measurements was weaker with AI-HRI than with conventional HRI (r_s =0.57 vs. Pearson's r =0.70). Meanwhile, the mean interobserver bias of −10% and the LOA of −78% and 58% in a Bland–Altman analysis were all higher compared to the bias of 2% and LOA of −47% and 51% reported for HRI [10]. The disagreement between the results can be partly explained by the differences in the study protocol. In our investigation, the mean of five repeated measurements was recorded by both examiners as the AI-HRI. In contrast, in the other study, HRI measurements were preselected, and only the three closest values with a difference of less than 0.2 were used to calculate the mean HRI, which could reduce interobserver variability. In addition, our study cohort included relatively higher numbers of obese patients, the mean BMI was 29 kg/m^2 vs. 23 kg/m^2, which could also influence the reproducibility.

Our study is the first to directly compare AI-HRI with other QUS methods for diagnosing hepatic steatosis. The AC was the most accurate in diagnosing all steatosis grades, with excellent and good prediction rates for moderate (AUC = 0.90) and mild steatosis (AUC = 0.83), respectively. A potential drawback of AC is the relatively small difference between diagnostic thresholds for mild (AC = 0.77) and moderate steatosis (AC = 0.83), which can cause miss diagnosis if the interobserver variation is large, especially in difficult-to-scan patients. The SC's performance was very similar to AI-HRI in the classification of steatosis. Meanwhile, US-FLI, which relies on semi-quantitative scoring of US signs on grayscale images, had a low detection rate for mild steatosis (AUC = 0.64, and sens. = 58%) but high for moderate to severe steatosis (AUC = 0.94, and sens. = 67%). These findings are in line with reports, which indicated that the sensitivity of grayscale US is poor for detecting mild steatosis and excellent for high-grade steatosis [26,27]. We also agree with Petzold et al. that AI-HRI should be evaluated together with grayscale US signs, as these can identify patients with high-grade steatosis with greater accuracy [8]. However, our study has also clearly demonstrated that AI-HRI is better for detecting low-grade steatosis than grayscale US.

This study has several limitations. First, we did not use histology grading as a reference for steatosis as NAFLD patients, especially those with low-grade steatosis, are seldom biopsied; and recent studies have shown that MRI-PDFF can classify all grades of steatosis with extremely high accuracy and reliability [6,28]. There has been a large amount of evidence published in multiple papers that MRI-PDFF is a quantitative noninvasive biomarker that objectively estimates liver fat content providing values over the entire range of biologically relevant liver fat content and, thus, it can be used as a surrogate marker for liver biopsy in clinical studies [3]. Moreover, liver biopsy is not routinely recommended by current European guidelines for diagnosing NAFLD [2]. Therefore, we think that using MRI-PDFF as a reference standard of AI-HRI in our study is rational. Second, a single ultrasound scanner was used for all patient examinations, and the manufacturer trained the DCNN algorithm, which generated the AI-HRI measurements. Other AI software may have very different diagnostic capabilities. Meanwhile, Cha et al. have already evaluated the precision of the same DCNN algorithm and concluded that it achieved similar performance to radiologists for calculating HRI in normal livers and mild steatosis [11]. Third, this is a single-center prospective study conducted in a relatively small patient cohort of 102 subjects. Thus, our result cannot be generalized, and further studies in larger patient groups and preferably in a multi-center setting are required to demonstrate the advantages of AI-HRI in routine clinical practice. Meanwhile, the sample size of 108 independent paired US and MRI-PDFF measurements analyzed in our study is well comparable to other single-center studies investigating the diagnostic performance of the non-invasive diagnostic techniques of steatosis, such as the reports by Caussy et al. on controlled attenuation parameter (CAP), and Jeon et al. on AC, and SC conducted in cohorts of 119 and 120 NAFLD patients, respectively [16,21].

5. Conclusions

New, AI-based image analysis techniques can transform US diagnostics by automating the collection of quantitative biomarkers. The AI-HRI is an algorithm developed for automated measurement of HRI on grayscale US. The most significant advantages of AI-HRI are the much shorter measurement time, the reduced workload of the examiners as there is no need for external image processing, the straightforward interpretation of the results, and the uniformity of the diagnostic protocol across all institutions using the same software. The results of our investigation have shown that AI-HRI could detect mild and moderate steatosis with good diagnostic accuracy. AI-HRI has shown great potential as a fast and objective screening tool for detecting hepatic steatosis as it had 83.3% NPV at the 1.53 suggested cutoff value, much higher compared to the 68.8% NPV of the grayscale US signs. The reproducibility of AI-HRI was similar to conventional HRI measurement. Therefore, AI-HRI may be efficiently used to screen large populations for NAFLD and follow up on disease severity.

Author Contributions: Z.Z.—conceptualization, formal analysis, investigation, data curation, writing original draft, project administration; A.D.R.—conceptualization, methodology, investigation, writing original draft; B.C.—investigation, data curation; R.S.—data curation, software; B.K.B.—investigation, data curation; A.F.—validation, manuscript reviewing and editing; I.K.—resources, supervision; G.G.—investigation, resources, supervision; V.B.—supervision, manuscript reviewing and editing; P.M.-H.—resources, supervision; K.H.—conceptualization, methodology, investigation, validation, manuscript reviewing and editing, supervision; P.N.K.—conceptualization, methodology, formal analysis, investigation, writing original draft, supervision. All authors have read and agreed to the published version of the manuscript.

Funding: This research received no external funding.

Institutional Review Board Statement: The study was approved by Semmelweis University's Regional and Institutional Science and Research Ethics Committee (Protocol number: SE RKEB 140/2020, 16 July 2020) and conducted in accordance with ethical standards specified in the Declaration of Helsinki.

Informed Consent Statement: All patients gave informed written consent to participate in the study.

Data Availability Statement: Not applicable.

Acknowledgments: We would like to acknowledge Lilla Petovsky for her help in the MRI examination.

Conflicts of Interest: P.N.K. is a consultant and speaker for Samsung Medison Ltd. All other authors declare no conflict of interest.

References

1. Huang, D.Q.; El-Serag, H.B.; Loomba, R. Global epidemiology of NAFLD-related HCC: Trends, predictions, risk factors and prevention. *Nat. Rev. Gastroenterol. Hepatol.* **2020**, *18*, 223–238. [CrossRef] [PubMed]
2. European Association for the Study of the Liver (EASL); European Association for the Study of Diabetes (EASD); European Association for the Study of Obesity (EASO). EASL-EASD-EASO Clinical Practice Guidelines for the management of non-alcoholic fatty liver disease. *J. Hepatol.* **2016**, *64*, 1388–1402. [CrossRef] [PubMed]
3. Ferraioli, G.; Kumar, V.; Ozturk, A.; Nam, K.; de Korte, C.L.; Barr, R.G. US Attenuation for Liver Fat Quantification: An AIUM-RSNA QIBA Pulse-Echo Quantitative Ultrasound Initiative. *Radiology* **2022**, *302*, 495–506. [CrossRef] [PubMed]
4. Dasarathy, S.; Dasarathy, J.; Khiyami, A.; Joseph, R.; Lopez, R.; McCullough, A.J. Validity of real time ultrasound in the diagnosis of hepatic steatosis: A prospective study. *J. Hepatol.* **2009**, *51*, 1061–1067. [CrossRef] [PubMed]
5. Pickhardt, P.J.; Blake, G.M.; Graffy, P.M.; Sandfort, V.; Elton, D.C.; Perez, A.A.; Summers, R.M. Liver Steatosis Categorization on Contrast-Enhanced CT Using a Fully Automated Deep Learning Volumetric Segmentation Tool: Evaluation in 1204 Healthy Adults Using Unenhanced CT as a Reference Standard. *Am. J. Roentgenol.* **2021**, *217*, 359–367. [CrossRef]
6. Gu, J.; Liu, S.; Du, S.; Zhang, Q.; Xiao, J.; Dong, Q.; Xin, Y. Diagnostic value of MRI-PDFF for hepatic steatosis in patients with non-alcoholic fatty liver disease: A meta-analysis. *Eur. Radiol.* **2019**, *29*, 3564–3573. [CrossRef] [PubMed]
7. Ballestri, S.; Lonardo, A.; Romagnoli, D.; Carulli, L.; Losi, L.; Day, C.P.; Loria, P. Ultrasonographic fatty liver indicator, a novel score which rules out NASH and is correlated with metabolic parameters in NAFLD. *Liver Int.* **2012**, *32*, 1242–1252. [CrossRef]
8. Petzold, G.; Lasser, J.; Rühl, J.; Bremer, S.C.B.; Knoop, R.F.; Ellenrieder, V.; Kunsch, S.; Neesse, A. Diagnostic accuracy of B-Mode ultrasound and Hepatorenal Index for graduation of hepatic steatosis in patients with chronic liver disease. *PLoS ONE* **2020**, *15*, e0231044. [CrossRef]
9. Marshall, R.H.; Eissa, M.; Bluth, E.I.; Gulotta, P.M.; Davis, N.K. Hepatorenal Index as an Accurate, Simple, and Effective Tool in Screening for Steatosis. *Am. J. Roentgenol.* **2012**, *199*, 997–1002. [CrossRef]
10. Van Tran, B.; Ujita, K.; Taketomi-Takahashi, A.; Hirasawa, H.; Suto, T.; Tsushima, Y. Reliability of ultrasound hepatorenal index and magnetic resonance imaging proton density fat fraction techniques in the diagnosis of hepatic steatosis, with magnetic resonance spectroscopy as the reference standard. *PLoS ONE* **2021**, *16*, e0255768. [CrossRef]
11. Cha, D.I.; Kang, T.W.; Min, J.H.; Joo, I.; Sinn, D.H.; Ha, S.Y.; Kim, K.; Lee, G.; Yi, J. Deep learning-based automated quantification of the hepatorenal index for evaluation of fatty liver by ultrasonography. *Ultrasonography* **2021**, *40*, 565–574. [CrossRef] [PubMed]
12. Kaposi, P.N.; Unger, Z.; Fejér, B.; Kucsa, A.; Tóth, A.; Folhoffer, A.; Szalay, F.; Bérczi, V. Interobserver agreement and diagnostic accuracy of shearwave elastography for the staging of hepatitis C virus-associated liver fibrosis. *J. Clin. Ultrasound* **2019**, *48*, 67–74. [CrossRef] [PubMed]
13. Folhoffer, A.; Rónaszéki, A.; Budai, B.; Borsos, P.; Orbán, V.; Győri, G.; Szalay, F.; Kaposi, P. Follow-Up of Liver Stiffness with Shear Wave Elastography in Chronic Hepatitis C Patients in Sustained Virological Response Augments Clinical Risk Assessment. *Processes* **2021**, *9*, 753. [CrossRef]
14. Rónaszéki, A.D.; Budai, B.K.; Csongrády, B.; Stollmayer, R.; Hagymási, K.M.; Werling, K.M.; Fodor, T.; Folhoffer, A.M.; Kalina, I.M.; Győri, G.; et al. Tissue attenuation imaging and tissue scatter imaging for quantitative ultrasound evaluation of hepatic steatosis. *Medicine* **2022**, *101*, e29708. [CrossRef]

15. Park, J.; Lee, J.M.; Lee, G.; Jeon, S.K.; Joo, I. Quantitative Evaluation of Hepatic Steatosis Using Advanced Imaging Techniques: Focusing on New Quantitative Ultrasound Techniques. *Korean J. Radiol.* **2022**, *23*, 13–29. [CrossRef]
16. Jeon, S.K.; Lee, J.M.; Joo, I.; Park, S.-J. Quantitative Ultrasound Radiofrequency Data Analysis for the Assessment of Hepatic Steatosis in Nonalcoholic Fatty Liver Disease Using Magnetic Resonance Imaging Proton Density Fat Fraction as the Reference Standard. *Korean J. Radiol.* **2021**, *22*, 1077–1086. [CrossRef]
17. Lee, J.-H.; Kim, D.; Kim, H.J.; Lee, C.-H.; Yang, J.I.; Kim, W.; Kim, Y.J.; Yoon, J.-H.; Cho, S.-H.; Sung, M.-W.; et al. Hepatic steatosis index: A simple screening tool reflecting nonalcoholic fatty liver disease. *Dig. Liver Dis.* **2010**, *42*, 503–508. [CrossRef]
18. Henninger, B.; Alustiza, J.; Garbowski, M.; Gandon, Y. Practical guide to quantification of hepatic iron with MRI. *Eur. Radiol.* **2019**, *30*, 383–393. [CrossRef]
19. Hamilton, G.; Yokoo, T.; Bydder, M.; Cruite, I.; Schroeder, M.E.; Sirlin, C.B.; Middleton, M.S. In vivo characterization of the liver fat ^{1}H MR spectrum. *NMR Biomed.* **2010**, *24*, 784–790. [CrossRef]
20. Berglund, J.; Skorpil, M. Multi-scale graph-cut algorithm for efficient water-fat separation. *Magn. Reson. Med.* **2016**, *78*, 941–949. [CrossRef]
21. Caussy, C.; Alquiraish, M.H.; Nguyen, P.; Hernandez, C.; Cepin, S.; Fortney, L.E.; Ajmera, V.; Bettencourt, R.; Collier, S.; Hooker, J.; et al. Optimal threshold of controlled attenuation parameter with MRI-PDFF as the gold standard for the detection of hepatic steatosis. *Hepatology* **2017**, *67*, 1348–1359. [CrossRef] [PubMed]
22. Obuchowski, N.A.; Lieber, M.L.; Wians, F.H. ROC Curves in Clinical Chemistry: Uses, Misuses, and Possible Solutions. *Clin. Chem.* **2004**, *50*, 1118–1125. [CrossRef] [PubMed]
23. Kwon, H.-J.; Kim, K.W.; Jung, J.-H.; Choi, S.H.; Jeong, W.K.; Kim, B.; Song, G.-W.; Lee, S.-G. Noninvasive quantitative estimation of hepatic steatosis by ultrasound: A comparison of the hepato-renal index and ultrasound attenuation index. *Med. Ultrason.* **2016**, *18*, 431–437. [CrossRef]
24. Johnson, S.; Fort, D.; Shortt, K.; Therapondos, G.; Galliano, G.; Nguyen, T.; Bluth, E. Ultrasound Stratification of Hepatic Steatosis Using Hepatorenal Index. *Diagnostics* **2021**, *11*, 1443. [CrossRef] [PubMed]
25. Kramer, H.; Pickhardt, P.J.; Kliewer, M.A.; Hernando, D.; Chen, G.-H.; Zagzebski, J.A.; Reeder, S.B. Accuracy of Liver Fat Quantification with Advanced CT, MRI, and Ultrasound Techniques: Prospective Comparison with MR Spectroscopy. *Am. J. Roentgenol.* **2017**, *208*, 92–100. [CrossRef] [PubMed]
26. Lee, D.H. Imaging evaluation of non-alcoholic fatty liver disease: Focused on quantification. *Clin. Mol. Hepatol.* **2017**, *23*, 290–301. [CrossRef] [PubMed]
27. Palmentieri, B.; Sio, I.D.; LA Mura, V.; Masarone, M.; Vecchione, R.; Bruno, S.; Torella, R.; Persico, M. The role of bright liver echo pattern on ultrasound B-mode examination in the diagnosis of liver steatosis. *Dig. Liver Dis.* **2006**, *38*, 485–489. [CrossRef]
28. Lee, S.S.; Park, S.H.; Kim, H.J.; Kim, S.Y.; Kim, M.-Y.; Kim, D.Y.; Suh, D.J.; Kim, K.M.; Bae, M.H.; Lee, J.Y.; et al. Non-invasive assessment of hepatic steatosis: Prospective comparison of the accuracy of imaging examinations. *J. Hepatol.* **2010**, *52*, 579–585. [CrossRef]

Disclaimer/Publisher's Note: The statements, opinions and data contained in all publications are solely those of the individual author(s) and contributor(s) and not of MDPI and/or the editor(s). MDPI and/or the editor(s) disclaim responsibility for any injury to people or property resulting from any ideas, methods, instructions or products referred to in the content.

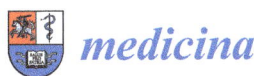 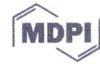

Article

Development and Validation of a Difficulty Scoring System for Laparoscopic Liver Resection to Treat Hepatolithiasis

Yeongsoo Jo *, Jai Young Cho *, Ho-Seong Han, Yoo-Seok Yoon, Hae Won Lee, Jun Suh Lee, Boram Lee, Eunhye Lee, Yeshong Park, MeeYoung Kang and Junghyun Lee

Department of Surgery, Seoul National University Bundang Hospital, Seoul National University College of Medicine, Seongnam-si 13590, Republic of Korea
* Correspondence: dudtn87411@gmail.com (Y.J.); jychogs@gmail.com (J.Y.C.)

Abstract: *Background and Objectives*: A difficulty scoring system was previously developed to assess the difficulty of laparoscopic liver resection (LLR) for liver tumors; however, we need another system for hepatolithiasis. Therefore, we developed a novel difficulty scoring system (nDSS) and validated its use for predicting postoperative outcomes. *Materials and Methods*: This was a retrospective study. We used clinical data of 123 patients who underwent LLR for hepatolithiasis between 2003 and 2021. We analyzed the data to determine which indices were associated with operation time or estimated blood loss (EBL) to measure the surgical difficulty. We validated the nDSS in terms of its ability to predict postoperative outcomes, namely red blood cell (RBC) transfusion, postoperative hospital stay (POHS), and major complications defined as grade ≥IIIa according to the Clavien–Dindo classification (CDC). *Results*: The nDSS included five significant indices (range: 5–17; median: 8). The RBC transfusion rate ($p < 0.001$), POHS ($p = 0.002$), and major complication rate ($p = 0.002$) increased with increasing nDSS score. We compared the two groups of patients divided by the median nDSS (low: 5–7; high: 8–17). The operation time (210.7 vs. 240.7 min; $p < 0.001$), EBL (281.9 vs. 702.6 mL; $p < 0.001$), RBC transfusion rate (5.3% vs. 37.9%; $p < 0.001$), POHS (8.0 vs. 13.3 days; $p = 0.001$), and major complication rate (8.8% vs. 25.8%; $p = 0.014$) were greater in the high group. *Conclusions*: The nDSS can predict the surgical difficulty and outcomes of LLR for hepatolithiasis and may help select candidates for the procedure and surgical approach.

Keywords: difficulty scoring system; laparoscopic liver resection; hepatolithiasis

Citation: Jo, Y.; Cho, J.Y.; Han, H.-S.; Yoon, Y.-S.; Lee, H.W.; Lee, J.S.; Lee, B.; Lee, E.; Park, Y.; Kang, M.; et al. Development and Validation of a Difficulty Scoring System for Laparoscopic Liver Resection to Treat Hepatolithiasis. *Medicina* **2022**, *58*, 1847. https://doi.org/10.3390/medicina58121847

Academic Editors: Ludovico Abenavoli and Marcello Candelli

Received: 26 November 2022
Accepted: 13 December 2022
Published: 15 December 2022

Publisher's Note: MDPI stays neutral with regard to jurisdictional claims in published maps and institutional affiliations.

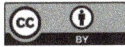

Copyright: © 2022 by the authors. Licensee MDPI, Basel, Switzerland. This article is an open access article distributed under the terms and conditions of the Creative Commons Attribution (CC BY) license (https:// creativecommons.org/licenses/by/ 4.0/).

1. Introduction

The difficulty of surgical techniques is somewhat subjective and can be influenced by patient characteristics, disease severity, surgical equipment, type of surgery, and the surgeon's experience [1]. Many scoring systems for surgical procedures have been proposed, including difficulty scores for laparoscopic cholecystectomy [2] and spinal anesthesia [3], the complexity of endotracheal intubation [4], and for predicting the complications of ophthalmological surgery [5]. Such systems can reveal a road map for young surgeons who are learning surgical techniques, via a step-by-step training regime [6] and can help surgeons provide patients with better information about the predicted risk of the procedure [7]. Scoring systems can also be used to make unbiased comparisons of cases of various difficulties among surgeons [8].

Laparoscopic liver resection (LLR) has shown impressive developments in the field of liver surgery in the last few decades [9,10]. In an effort to measure operative difficulty and generate a roadmap for surgeons advancing from simple to highly technical LLR, a difficulty scoring system (DSS) was developed to assess the difficulty of LLR for liver tumors [11]. The resulting DSS was determined based on the extent of liver resection, tumor location, tumor size, proximity to major vessels, hand-assisted laparoscopic surgery (HALS) or hybrid surgery, and liver function [12,13].

For hepatolithiasis, also known as intrahepatic duct (IHD) stones, hepatectomy is a safe and definitive treatment to treat diseased IHD. However, unlike liver tumors, non-anatomical resection is not recommended because of the IHD's distribution, which can be easily distorted by stones or combined atrophy of liver parenchyma. Some indices used in the published DSS cannot be applied to LLR for hepatolithiasis, particularly proximity to major vessels and tumor size. Furthermore, HALS or hybrid surgery has not been performed for hepatolithiasis in recent years. Therefore, we developed a novel DSS for LLR to treat hepatolithiasis [14].

2. Materials and Methods

2.1. Study Design

This was a single-center retrospective study. We reviewed the clinical data for 138 patients who underwent LLR for hepatolithiasis between June 2003 and April 2021 at Seoul National University Bundang Hospital, Seongnam, South Korea. We excluded 15 patients who either underwent combined surgery at the same time ($n = 8$) or were diagnosed with malignant tumors postoperatively ($n = 7$); therefore, their surgical records and data were not appropriate to calculate the novel difficulty scoring system (nDSS) for LLR. We had nine patients who were converted to open approach, but six of them were confirmed with malignant disease and the others underwent combined surgery. These factors already corresponded to the exclusion criteria of this study, so we did not analyze open conversion cases. Accordingly, we analyzed data for 123 patients. To estimate the surgical difficulty, we calculated scores using indices that were significantly associated with operation time and estimated blood loss (EBL), which are generally thought to be the key markers for the difficulty of LLR. We validated the nDSS in terms of its ability to predict postoperative outcomes, namely red blood cell (RBC) transfusion, postoperative hospital stay (POHS), and major complications defined as grade $\geq$IIIa according to the Clavien–Dindo classification (CDC). We also divided the patients into two groups according to their nDSS (low, 5–7; high, $\geq$8) and evaluated the short-term outcomes to simplify the surgical decisions. This study was approved by the hospital's Institutional Review Board (B-2208-773-105).

2.2. Surgical Techniques

The LLR techniques used at our institution are described in a previous report [15]. If remnant duct stones were suspected, intraoperative bile duct exploration was performed [16]. After dividing the liver parenchyma, the duct of the section or hemiliver was isolated. If the surgeon presumed that stones were close to the resection plane, the duct was divided with endo scissors. The stones near the open duct were extracted and the duct was closed using intracorporeal sutures. To detect any remnant stones, further exploration was performed via intraoperative choledochoscopy through the open duct before closing the duct [17]. Similarly, if common bile duct stones were suspected, the surgeon performed intraoperative common bile duct exploration in the same way. In this study, the operations were performed by five different surgeons and all of them had sufficient experiences of LLR, at least 30 cases each.

2.3. Definitions

Hepatolithiasis could be associated with IHD stricture, which can be observed by magnetic resonance cholangiopancreatography (MRCP; Figure 1A,B). The proximity to the bifurcation was defined as the distance between the distal end of the stricture and the confluence of the IHD affected by the stricture. We used this definition because, when planning anatomical liver resection, it is very important to draw the resection plane distal to the IHD confluence to avoid bile duct injury. If the distance is <1 cm, it might be more difficult to perform LLR properly without causing bile duct injury. Figure 1 shows two examples of MRCP depicting the proximity to the bifurcation. As an example, in a patient who was undergoing left hemihepatectomy, we drew the imaginary resection line just on the confluence of the left hepatic duct and common hepatic duct, and measured the distance between the imaginary resection line and the distal end of the left hepatic duct stricture (Figure 1A). Similarly, in a patient who was undergoing right hemihepatectomy, we measured the distance between the imaginary resection line and the distal end of the right hepatic duct stricture (Figure 1B). We reviewed all MRCP images from each patient and measured the distance in this way.

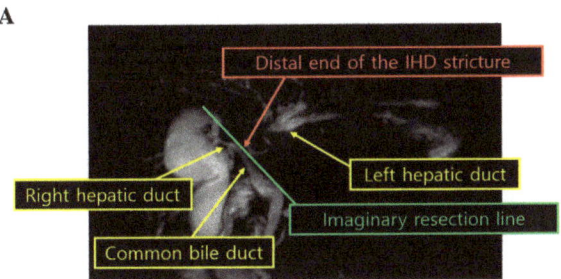

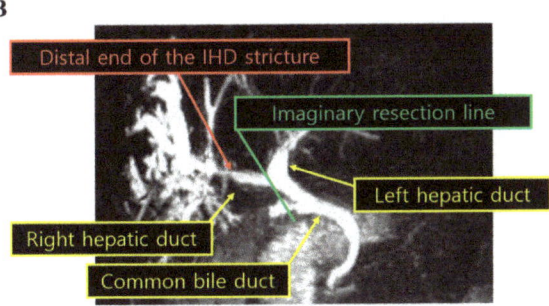

Figure 1. Preoperative magnetic resonance cholangiopancreatography. The proximity to the bifurcation was defined as the distance between the distal end of the stricture and the confluence of the IHD affected by the stricture. The straight line represents imaginary resection line, and we measured the distance between the imaginary resection line and the distal end of the stricture in representative patients undergoing left hemihepatectomy ((**A**); distance < 1 cm) and right hemihepatectomy ((**B**); distance ≥ 1 cm). IHD intrahepatic duct.

2.4. Statistics

All data were analyzed using SPSS version 20.0 for Windows (SPSS, Chicago, IL, USA). Continuous variables were compared using Student's *t* test. Categorical variables were compared using the χ2 test or Fisher's exact test. We also performed univariate and multivariable logistic regression analyses. In multivariate logistic regression analysis, we selected all significant variables from univariate logistic regression analysis. In all tests, a *p* value of ≤0.05 was regarded as significant.

3. Results
3.1. Patient Characteristics

We analyzed data for 46 males (37.4%) and 77 females (62.6%) (Table 1). Their mean age was 60 years and the mean BMI was 23.7 kg/m^2. Twenty-nine patients (23.6%) had a history of upper abdominal surgery, including hepatobiliary and pancreatic surgery or gastroduodenal surgery, and some of them underwent multiple procedures. The prior procedures were cholecystectomy in most of these patients (*n* = 22), extrahepatic bile duct surgery (*n* = 9), pancreaticoduodenectomy (*n* = 3), hepatectomy (*n* = 2), and gastrectomy (*n* = 1). The LLR was classified into two types: left lateral sectionectomy (*n* = 43; 35.0%) and major hepatectomy (*n* = 80; 65.0%). The resection side was also classified into two groups: left (n = 106; 86.2%) and right (n = 17; 13.8%). Atrophy of the liver parenchyma was observed in 64 patients (52.0%). Fifty-one patients (41.5%) underwent IHD exploration, as described in the Methods (Surgical techniques). The hepatolithiasis was in close proximity to the bifurcation in 63 patients (51.2%). Among the patients who were corresponded to the inclusion criteria, nobody underwent biliary reconstructions with Roux-en-Y hepaticojejunostomy.

Table 1. Preoperative characteristics.

Characteristics (n = 123)	Value
Age, years (mean)	59.98 ± 9.25
Sex, n (%)	
Male	46 (37.4%)
Female	77 (62.6%)
BMI, kg/m^2 (mean)	23.67 ± 3.01
History of upper abdominal surgery, n (%)	29 (23.6%)
Resection type, n (%)	
Left lateral sectionectomy	43 (35.0%)
Major hepatectomy	80 (65.0%)
Resection side, n (%)	
Left hemiliver	106 (86.2%)
Right hemiliver	17 (13.8%)
Liver parenchyma atrophy, n (%)	64 (52.0%)
Bile duct exploration, n (%)	51 (41.5%)
IHD stricture <1 mm from the bifurcation, n (%)	63 (51.2%)

BMI body mass index, IHD intrahepatic duct.

3.2. Surgical Outcomes

The median operation time was 260 min and the median EBL was 300 mL. In total, 28 patients (22.8%) received RBC transfusion and the median POHS was 8 days. Eleven patients (8.9%) had remnant stones. Twenty-two patients (17.9%) experienced severe postoperative complications with CDC grade of ≥IIIa (Table 2). To determine which factors were associated with the surgical difficulty, we performed a logistic regression analysis using operation time longer than the median (260 min) as the dependent variable. In the multivariable analysis, four variables were significantly associated with this outcome: resection type (odds ratio [OR]: 3.984; 95% confidence interval [CI]: 1.596–9.947; p = 0.003), resection side (OR: 4.173; 95% CI: 1.018–17.104; p = 0.047), intraoperative bile duct exploration (OR: 3.891; 95% CI: 1.678–9.021; p = 0.002), and proximity to the bifurcation (OR: 2.683; 95% CI: 1.1487–6.269; p = 0.023) (Table 3). We also performed logistic regression using EBL greater than the median (300 mL) as the dependent variable. In the multivariable analysis, three variables were significantly associated with this outcome: resection side (OR: 16.209; 95% CI: 2.007–130.901; p = 0.009), intraoperative bile duct exploration (OR: 2.812; 95% CI: 1.225–6.455; p = 0.015), and history of upper abdominal surgery (OR: 3.976; 95% CI: 1.408–11.231; p = 0.009) (Table 3).

Table 2. Surgical outcomes.

Variable	Value
Operation time (min)	Mean: 280.46 ± 141.63; median: 260
EBL (mL)	Mean: 507.64 ± 590.43; median: 300
RBC transfusion, n (%)	28 (22.8%)
RBC transfusion (mL)	Mean: 302.44 ± 784.01
POHS (days)	Mean: 10.85 ± 9.70, median: 8
Remnant stone, n (%)	11 (8.9%)
Recurrent stone, n (%)	6 (4.9%)

Table 2. Cont.

Variable	Value
CDC grade ≥IIIa, n (%)	22 (17.9%)
Fluid collection, n (%)	10 (8.1%)
Biliary fistula, n (%)	6 (4.9%)
Pleural effusion, n (%)	2 (1.6%)
Biliary stricture, n (%)	1 (0.8%)
Septic shock, n (%)	1 (0.8%)
Pseudoaneurysm rupture, n (%)	1 (0.8%)
Wound complication, n (%)	1 (0.8%)

EBL estimated blood loss, RBC red blood cell, POHS postoperative hospital stay, CDC Clavien–Dindo classification.

Table 3. Logistic regression analysis for operation time ≥ 260 min and estimated blood loss ≥ 300 mL as the dependent variables.

	Operation Time ≥ 260 min						Estimated Blood Loss ≥ 300 mL					
		Univariate			Multivariable			Univariate			Multivariable	
Variables	OR	95% CI	p Value	OR	95% CI	p Value	OR	95% CI	p Value	OR	95% CI	p Value
Age [1]	0.979	0.394–2.435	0.964	-	-	-	1.123	0.461–2.735	0.798	-	-	-
Sex [2]	0.760	0.313–1.848	0.545	-	-	-	0.628	20.259–1.520	0.302	-	-	-
BMI [3]	1.771	0.701–4.474	0.227	-	-	-	1.582	0.628–3.985	0.331	-	-	-
Resection type [4]	4.479	1.702–11.785	0.002	3.984	1.596–9.947	0.003	1.759	0.740–4.183	0.201	-	-	-
Resection side [5]	4.267	1.018–17.886	0.047	4.173	1.018–17.104	0.047	13.172	1.562–111.047	0.018	16.209	2.007–130.901	0.009
Liver parenchyma atrophy [6]	0.744	0.312–1.770	0.504	-	-	-	0.622	0.267–1.452	0.272	-	-	-
Bile duct exploration [7]	4.172	1.761–9.883	0.001	3.891	1.678–9.021	0.002	2.712	1.164–6.318	0.021	2.812	1.225–6.455	0.015
Proximity to the bifurcation [8]	2.744	1.136–6.624	0.025	2.683	1.148–6.269	0.023	1.425	0.624–3.255	0.400	-	-	-
History of UAS [9]	1.708	0.728–4.004	0.218	-	-	-	3.096	1.155–8.301	0.025	3.976	1.408–11.231	0.009

[1] <65 vs. ≥65 years; [2] male vs. female; [3] <25 vs. ≥25 kg/m^2; [4] LLS vs. major; [5] left vs. right; [6] no vs. yes; [7] no vs. yes; [8] ≥1 cm vs. <1 cm; [9] no vs. yes. p values in bold are statistically significant at ≤0.05. OR odds ratio, CI confidence interval, BMI body mass index, LLS left lateral sectionectomy, UAS upper abdominal surgery.

3.3. Development of the nDSS and Associations between nDSS and Short-Term Outcomes

Five variables, including those that overlapped both multivariable regression models, were included in the nDSS: resection type, resection side, intraoperative bile duct exploration, proximity to the bifurcation, and history of upper abdominal surgery. When a patient had some factors, we assigned points to each factor according to their odds ratios. We multiplied the odds ratios from the results of multivariable analyses based on operation time and EBL, and extracted the square root of them, and rounded off to the nearest whole number; for example, when it comes to resection side and if it is the right side, the point is 8 ($\approx \sqrt{4.173 \times 16.209}$). If the factor had a significance on only one dependent variable, the odds ratio from the other side was considered as 1; for example, when it comes to proximity to the bifurcation and if IHD stricture is <1 cm from the bifurcation, the point is 2 ($\approx \sqrt{2.683 \times 1}$). If a patient did not have some specific factors, we assigned 1 point to each factor. In conclusion, each factor had their own points (resection type, 2; resection side, 8; intraoperative bile duct exploration, 3; proximity to the bifurcation, 2; history of upper abdominal surgery, 2), which are summed to provide the nDSS with a possible range of 5 to 17 points. However, in contrast to common perception, liver parenchyma atrophy was not a significant variable in either model, and this was excluded from the nDSS.

Scatter plots for operation time and EBL versus nDSS are shown in Figure 2. Both graphs showed that operation time and EBL tended to increase with greater nDSS. To evaluate the use of nDSS for predicting short-term outcomes, we performed univariate logistic regression analyses for five variables each, and three variables showed significance with increasing nDSS: RBC transfusion rate (OR: 1.383; 95% CI: 1.186–1.614; $p < 0.001$), POHS ≥ 8 days (OR: 1.307; 65% CI: 1.107–1.544; $p = 0.002$), and CDC grade ≥IIIa (OR: 1.267; 95% CI: 1.092–1.470; $p = 0.002$) (Table 4). Remnant stones (OR: 0.928; 95% CI: 0.722–1.194; $p = 0.564$) and recurrent stones (OR: 0.948; 95% CI: 0.686–1.310; $p = 0.746$) were not significantly associated with nDSS.

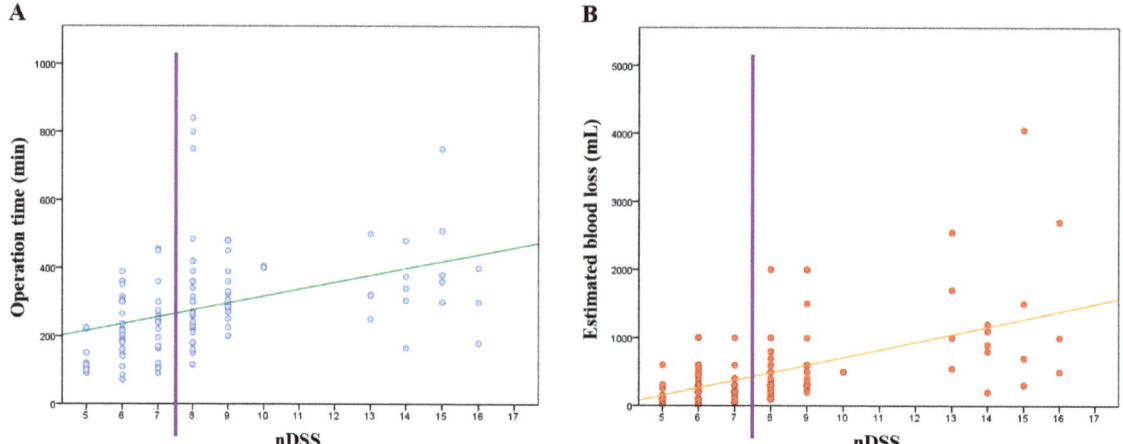

Figure 2. Scatter plots for nDSS versus operation time (**A**) and EBL (**B**). The vertical line splits the patients into two groups, low and high groups, and the oblique lines represent the correlations between the variables. nDSS modified difficulty scoring system.

Table 4. Surgical outcomes based on the novel difficulty scoring system.

Variable	OR	95% CI	p Value
RBC transfusion	1.383	1.186–1.614	**<0.001**
POHS ≥ 8 days	1.307	1.107–1.544	**0.002**
CDC grade ≥ IIIa	1.267	1.092–1.470	**0.002**
Remnant stone	0.928	0.722–1.194	0.564
Recurrent stone	0.948	0.686–1.310	0.746

p values in bold are statistically significant at ≤0.05. OR odds ratio, CI confidence interval, EBL estimated blood loss, RBC red blood cell, POHS postoperative hospital stay, CDC Clavien–Dindo classification.

To understand whether the nDSS can be useful for treatment decisions, including surgical approach and patient selection, we divided the patients into two groups based on the median nDSS and compared the surgical outcomes between the two groups. The low group comprised patients with a score of 5–7 points and the high group comprised patients with a score of 8–17 points. As shown in Table 5, the low group had significantly better short-term outcomes than the high group for operation time ≥260 min (28.1% vs. 72.7%; OR: 6.833; $p < 0.001$), EBL ≥ 300 mL (42.1% vs. 77.3%; OR: 4.675; $p < 0.001$), RBC transfusion rate (5.3% vs. 37.9%; OR: 10.976; $p < 0.001$), POHS ≥ 8 days (35.1% vs. 66.7%; OR 3.700; $p = 0.001$), and CDC grade ≥IIIa (8.8% vs. 25.8%; OR: 3.608; $p = 0.014$), but no differences were found for remnant or recurrent stones.

Table 5. Surgical outcomes in patients divided into high and low nDSS scores.

Variable	nDSS 5–7	nDSS ≥ 8	OR	p Value
Operation time, min (mean)	210.67	240.74	-	**<0.001**
Operation time ≥ 260 min, n (%)	16 (28.1%)	48 (72.7%)	6.833	**<0.001**
EBL, mL (mean)	281.93	702.58	-	**<0.001**
EBL ≥ 300 mL, n (%)	24 (42.1%)	51 (77.3%)	4.675	**<0.001**
RBC transfusion, n (%)	3 (5.3%)	25 (37.9%)	10.976	**<0.001**
POHS, days (mean)	8.00	13.32	-	**0.001**
POHS ≥ 8 days, n (%)	20 (35.1%)	44 (66.7%)	3.700	**0.001**
CDC grade ≥ IIIa, n (%)	5 (8.8%)	17 (25.8%)	3.608	**0.014**
Remnant stone, n (%)	4 (7.0%)	7 (10.6%)	1.572	0.543
Recurrent stone, n (%)	2 (3.5%)	4 (6.1%)	1.774	0.685

p values in bold are statistically significant at ≤0.05. nDSS modified difficulty scoring system, OR odds ratio, EBL estimated blood loss, RBC red blood cell, POHS postoperative hospital stay, CDC Clavien–Dindo classification.

4. Discussion

Although there are many different treatment modalities for hepatolithiasis, hepatectomy seems to be one of the most effective options because it can reduce the risk of recurrence and cholangiocarcinoma [18–21]. With advances in laparoscopic techniques and accumulating clinical evidence for better short-term outcomes and comparable long-term outcomes [22–27], LLR is increasingly being used for treating hepatolithiasis [28,29]. However, LLR for hepatolithiasis may be more technically challenging than for tumors because inflammation of the liver associated with hepatolithiasis leads to perihepatic adhesion and anatomical distortion [30]. Furthermore, parenchymal transection is often difficult because of parenchymal fibrosis and deformation of the IHD due to atrophic changes [16]. These factors could extend the operation time and increase the risk of postoperative complications. Moreover, intraoperative choledochoscopic evaluation of the remaining biliary tract is often required, and further prolongs the operation time and increases the surgical difficulty [16,31].

Several studies have developed a surgical DSS for LLR [11–13,32,33]. However, very few studies have evaluated the difficulty of LLR for hepatolithiasis. Here, we found that the surgical difficulty varies among patients undergoing the same LLR procedure and that the nDSS can be applied to LLR for hepatolithiasis. The surgical difficulty increases with nDSS (Figure 2) and the surgical outcomes are worse at higher nDSS (Table 4). Therefore, surgeons can use this system to predict the surgical difficulty and outcomes, and share the information with anesthesiologists, intensivists, hospitalists, nurses, and any other medical team members involved in the treatment, for appropriate pre-, intra-, and postoperative arrangements, such as preparation of blood transfusion, anesthetic drugs, surgical equipment, and intensive care. Furthermore, if the patients can be divided into low or high scores, based on the median score of 8 points, it is simpler to inform the patients about the likelihood of longer hospital stay or greater risk of postoperative complications, and to facilitate decisions on the surgical approach. Furthermore, because the nDSS is an unbiased tool that measures surgical difficulty quantitatively, it can be used to compare cases and determine which factor(s) may affect the surgery and postoperative outcomes. Thus, we believe the nDSS can be used as a roadmap for using LLR to treat hepatolithiasis.

We had a few unexpected results. One of them was about history of upper abdominal surgery. We defined upper abdominal surgery as hepatobiliary and pancreatic surgery or gastroduodenal surgery. If the patient had undergone very extensive surgery, for example, pancreaticoduodenectomy or hepatectomy, the surgeon might have decided to perform open surgery worrying about surgical difficulty. Otherwise, if the patient had undergone minor surgery, such as laparoscopic cholecystectomy, it might not have been a serious matter to go with laparoscopic surgery. That might have been one of the reasons that history of upper abdominal surgery was not a significant factor when it comes to operation time. However, we could not find any acceptable reasons to explain why it had a significant effect on EBL.

Another unexpected result was about bile duct exploration: even though it is not always difficult for experienced surgeons, once the procedure is performed, it is quite reasonable that surgery takes longer than that without the procedure. However, we could not find any explainable reasons of the result for why it had a significant effect on EBL as well. Otherwise, when it comes to resection type, it did not show any significant effect on EBL in contrast with common knowledge. Hence, further studies are warranted on these issues.

Regardless of the usefulness of nDSS, this study has some limitations to discuss. First, this was a single-center retrospective study with a risk of selection bias and other disadvantages inherent to such studies. For example, patients with severe liver parenchyma atrophy would not have been considered as candidates for laparoscopic surgery. If liver parenchyma atrophy is very severe, it could be very difficult to determine whether there is malignant tumor or not just based on preoperative image findings. Due to this reason, when liver parenchyma atrophy was very severe, we performed open surgery in case of achieving appropriate resection margins, performing lymph node dissection or hepaticojejunostomy according to intraoperative findings. This might explain why liver parenchyma atrophy was not a significant factor for surgical difficulty in our study, and that is the same with the matter of the 'few unexpected results' that we discussed before. Second, the nDSS was not associated with the remnant stone and recurrent stone rate. Of course, if the stones were located in both hemilivers, we resected the atrophied or more severe side of the liver and observed the patient prior to further resection. Accordingly, some IHD stones were intentionally left in situ ($n = 4$; 36.4%); this could affect the short-term outcome of the remnant stone rate. Considering the goal of surgery, it is important to perform further studies to determine the curability of this strategy. Third, because not all operations were performed by the same surgeons, even though the surgeons used near-identical techniques and had sufficient experiences of LLR (at least ≥ 30 cases each), differences in their surgical skill levels might affect the surgical difficulty and outcomes. Furthermore, we cannot ignore the evolution of laparoscopic equipment and devices during the study period. Finally, although some patients had chronic liver disease or liver cirrhosis, which could affect the difficulty or outcomes, we did not incorporate this factor due to limited data, and future studies should investigate the impact of these diseases.

5. Conclusions

In conclusion, we found that the surgical difficulty varies among patients undergoing LLR for hepatolithiasis. We know that more difficult surgical procedures carry greater risk of worse postoperative outcomes. The nDSS developed here can predict the surgical difficulty and short-term outcomes of LLR for hepatolithiasis. Furthermore, we expect the nDSS will also be useful for selecting candidate patients and deciding between laparoscopic or open surgery.

Author Contributions: Conceptualization, Y.J. and J.Y.C.; methodology, Y.J. and J.Y.C.; software, Y.J. and J.Y.C.; formal analysis Y.J. and J.Y.C.; resources, all authors; data curation, all authors; writing—original draft preparation, Y.J. and J.Y.C.; writing—review and editing, Y.J. and J.Y.C.; project administration, Y.J. and J.Y.C. All authors have read and agreed to the published version of the manuscript.

Funding: This work was supported by grant no 02-2022-0029 from the SNUBH Research Fund.

Institutional Review Board Statement: The study was conducted according to the guidelines of the Declaration of Helsinki and approved by the Institutional Review Board of Seoul National University Bundang Hospital (B-2208-773-105).

Informed Consent Statement: Patient consent was waived due to this study being retrospective research and does not harm patients.

Data Availability Statement: Data will be made available by the authors upon reasonable request.

Conflicts of Interest: The authors declare no conflict of interest.

References

1. Kim, T.H.; Kim, S.Y.; Tang, A.; Lee, J.M. Comparison of international guidelines for noninvasive diagnosis of hepatocellular carcinoma: 2018 update. *Clin. Mol. Hepatol.* **2019**, *25*, 245–263. [CrossRef] [PubMed]
2. Vivek, M.A.; Augustine, A.J.; Rao, R. A comprehensive predictive scoring method for difcult laparoscopic cholecystectomy. *J. Minim. Access Surg.* **2014**, *10*, 62–67. [CrossRef]
3. Khoshrang, H.; Falahatkar, S.; Heidarzadeh, A.; Abad, M.; Herfeh, N.R.; Nabi, B.N. Predicting difculty score for spinal anesthesia in transurethral lithotripsy surgery. *Anesth. Pain Med.* **2014**, *4*, e16244. [CrossRef] [PubMed]
4. Adnet, F.; Borron, S.W.; Racine, S.X.; Clemessy, J.L.; Fournier, J.L.; Plaisance, P.; Lapandry, C. The intubation difficulty scale (IDS): Proposal and evaluation of a new score characterizing the complexity of endotracheal intubation. *Anesthesiology* **1997**, *87*, 1290–1297. [CrossRef] [PubMed]
5. Osborne, S.A.; Severn, P.; Bunce, C.V.; Fraser, S.G. The use of a pre-operative scoring system for the prediction of phacoemulsification case difficulty and the selection of appropriate cases to be performed by trainees. *BMC Ophthalmol.* **2006**, *6*, 38. [CrossRef]

6. Lee, M.K.; Gao, F.; Strasberg, S.M. Perceived complexity of various liver resections: Results of a survey of experts with development of a complexity score and classification. *J. Am. Coll. Surg.* **2015**, *220*, 64–69. [CrossRef]
7. Muangkaew, P.; Cho, J.Y.; Han, H.S.; Yoon, Y.S.; Choi, Y.; Jang, J.Y.; Choi, H.; Jang, J.S.; Kwon, S.U. Defining surgical difficulty according to the perceived complexity of liver resection: Validation of a complexity classification in patients with hepatocellular carcinoma. *Ann. Surg. Oncol.* **2016**, *23*, 2602–2609. [CrossRef]
8. Osborne, S.A.; Adams, W.E.; Bunce, C.V.; Fraser, S.G. Validation of two scoring systems for the prediction of posterior capsule rupture during phacoemulsification surgery. *Br. J. Ophthalmol.* **2006**, *90*, 333–336. [CrossRef]
9. Jia, C.; Li, H.; Wen, N.; Chen, J.; Wei, Y.; Li, B. Laparoscopic liver resection: A review of current indications and surgical techniques. *Hepatobiliary Surg. Nutr.* **2018**, *7*, 277–288. [CrossRef]
10. Wakabayashi, G. What has changed after the Morioka consensus conference 2014 on laparoscopic liver resection? *Hepatobiliary Surg. Nutr.* **2016**, *5*, 281–289. [CrossRef]
11. Tanaka, S.; Kawaguchi, Y.; Kubo, S.; Kanazawa, A.; Takeda, Y.; Hirokawa, F.; Nitta, H.; Nakajima, T.; Kaizu, T.; Kaibori, M.; et al. Validation of index-based IWATE criteria as an improved difficulty scoring system for laparoscopic liver resection. *Surgery* **2019**, *165*, 731–740. [CrossRef] [PubMed]
12. Ban, D.; Tanabe, M.; Ito, H.; Otsuka, Y.; Nitta, H.; Abe, Y.; Hasegawa, Y.; Katagiri, T.; Takagi, C.; Itano, O.; et al. A novel difficulty scoring system for laparoscopic liver resection. *J. Hepatobiliary Pancreat. Sci.* **2014**, *21*, 745–753. [CrossRef] [PubMed]
13. Im, C.; Cho, J.Y.; Han, H.S.; Yoon, Y.S.; Choi, Y.; Jang, J.Y.; Choi, H.; Jang, J.S.; Kwon, S.U. Validation of difficulty scoring system for laparoscopic liver resection in patients who underwent laparoscopic left lateral sectionectomy. *Surg. Endosc.* **2017**, *31*, 430–436. [CrossRef]
14. Han, H.S.; Cho, J.Y.; Yoon, Y.S. Techniques for performing laparoscopic liver resection in various hepatic locations. *J. Hepatobiliary Pancreat. Surg.* **2009**, *16*, 427–432. [CrossRef] [PubMed]
15. Yoon, Y.S.; Han, H.S.; Shin, S.H.; Cho, J.Y.; Min, S.K.; Lee, H.K. Laparoscopic treatment for intrahepatic duct stones in the era of laparoscopy: Laparoscopic intrahepatic duct exploration and laparoscopic hepatectomy. *Ann. Surg.* **2009**, *249*, 286–291. [CrossRef] [PubMed]
16. Lee, K.B. Histopathology of a benign bile duct lesion in the liver: Morphologic mimicker or precursor of intrahepatic cholangiocarcinoma. *Clin. Mol. Hepatol.* **2016**, *22*, 400–405. [CrossRef]
17. Jeong, C.Y.; Kim, K.J.; Hong, S.C.; Jeong, S.H.; Ju, Y.T.; Lee, Y.J.; Choi, S.K.; Ha, W.S.; Park, S.T.; Jung, E.J. Laparoscopic left hemihepatectomy for left intrahepatic duct stones. *J. Korean Surg. Soc.* **2012**, *83*, 149–154. [CrossRef]
18. Liu, X.; Miao, X.; Zhong, D.; Yao, H.; Wen, Y.; Dai, W.; Liu, G. Laparoscopic left hemihepatectomy for treatment of left intrahepatic duct stones. *Am. Surg.* **2014**, *80*, E350–E351. [CrossRef]
19. Tan, J.; Tan, Y.; Chen, F.; Zhu, Y.; Leng, J.; Dong, J. Endoscopic or laparoscopic approach for hepatolithiasis in the era of endoscopy in China. *Surg. Endosc.* **2015**, *29*, 154–162. [CrossRef]
20. Yang, T.; Lau, W.Y.; Lai, E.C.; Yang, L.Q.; Zhang, J.; Yang, G.S.; Lu, J.H.; Wu, M.C. Hepatectomy for bilateral primary hepatolithiasis: A cohort study. *Ann. Surg.* **2010**, *251*, 84–90. [CrossRef]
21. Suzuki, Y.; Mori, T.; Yokoyama, M.; Nakazato, T.; Abe, N.; Nakanuma, Y.; Tsubouchi, H.; Sugiyama, M. Hepatolithiasis: Analysis of Japanese nationwide surveys over a period of 40 years. *J. Hepatobiliary Pancreat. Sci.* **2014**, *21*, 617–622. [CrossRef] [PubMed]
22. Buell, J.F.; Cherqui, D.; Geller, D.A.; O'rourke, N.; Iannitti, D.; Dagher, I.; Koffron, A.J.; Thomas, M.; Gayet, B.; Han, H.S.; et al. The international position on laparoscopic liver surgery: The Louisville Statement, 2008. *Ann. Surg.* **2009**, *250*, 825–830. [CrossRef] [PubMed]
23. Han, H.S.; Shehta, A.; Ahn, S.; Yoon, Y.S.; Cho, J.Y.; Choi, Y. Laparoscopic versus open liver resection for hepatocellular carcinoma: Case-matched study with propensity score matching. *J. Hepatol.* **2015**, *63*, 643–650. [CrossRef] [PubMed]
24. Wakabayashi, G.; Cherqui, D.; Geller, D.A.; Buell, J.F.; Kaneko, H.; Han, H.S.; Asbun, H.; O'Rourke, N.; Tanabe, M.; Koffron, A.J.; et al. Recommendations for laparoscopic liver resection: A report from the second international consensus conference held in Morioka. *Ann. Surg.* **2015**, *261*, 619–629. [CrossRef] [PubMed]
25. Cherqui, D. Laparoscopic liver resection: A new paradigm in the management of hepatocellular carcinoma? *J. Hepatol.* **2015**, *63*, 540–542. [CrossRef]
26. Korean Liver Cancer Association (KLCA); National Cancer Center (NCC) Korea. 2022 KLCA-NCC Korea practice guidelines for the management of hepatocellular carcinoma. *Clin. Mol. Hepatol.* **2022**, *28*, 583–705. [CrossRef]
27. Kim, J.M.; Kim, D.G.; Kim, J.; Lee, K.; Lee, K.W.; Ryu, J.H.; Kim, B.W.; Choi, D.L.; You, Y.K.; Kim, D.S.; et al. Outcomes after liver transplantation in Korea: Incidence and risk factors from Korean transplantation registry. *Clin. Mol. Hepatol.* **2021**, *27*, 451–462. [CrossRef]
28. Cai, X.; Wang, Y.; Yu, H.; Liang, X.; Peng, S. Laparoscopic hepatectomy for hepatolithiasis: A feasibility and safety study in 29 patients. *Surg. Endosc.* **2007**, *21*, 1074–1078. [CrossRef]
29. Lai, E.C.; Ngai, T.C.; Yang, G.P.; Li, M.K. Laparoscopic approach of surgical treatment for primary hepatolithiasis: A cohort study. *Am. J. Surg.* **2010**, *199*, 716–721. [CrossRef]
30. Kim, Y.K.; Han, H.S.; Yoon, Y.S.; Cho, J.Y.; Lee, W. Laparoscopic approach for right-sided intrahepatic duct stones: A comparative study of laparoscopic versus open treatment. *World J. Surg.* **2015**, *39*, 1224–1230. [CrossRef]
31. Gough, V.; Stephens, N.; Ahmed, Z.; Nassar, A.H. Intrahepatic choledochoscopy during trans-cystic common bile duct exploration; technique, feasibility and value. *Surg. Endosc.* **2012**, *26*, 3190–3194. [CrossRef] [PubMed]

32. Kawaguchi, Y.; Fuks, D.; Kokudo, N.; Gayet, B. Difficulty of laparoscopic liver resection: Proposal for a new classification. *Ann. Surg.* **2018**, *267*, 13–17. [CrossRef] [PubMed]
33. Hasegawa, Y.; Wakabayashi, G.O.; Nitta, H.; Takahara, T.; Katagiri, H.; Umemura, A.; Makabe, K.; Sasaki, A. A novel model for prediction of pure laparoscopic liver resection surgical difficulty. *Surg. Endosc.* **2017**, *31*, 5356–5363. [CrossRef] [PubMed]

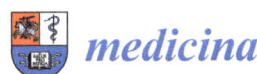

Article

Kawasaki Disease with Hepatobiliary Manifestations

Siti Aisyah Suhaini [1], Abdullah Harith Azidin [1], Chooi San Cheah [1], Wendy Lee Wei Li [1], Mohammad Shukri Khoo [2], Noor Akmal Shareela Ismail [3] and Adli Ali [1,*]

1 Department of Paediatric, Faculty of Medicine, Universiti Kebangsaan Malaysia, Jalan Yaacob Latif, Kuala Lumpur 56000, Malaysia
2 Department of Paediatric, Universiti Kebangsaan Malaysia Specialist Children's Hospital (HPKK), Jalan Yaacob Latif, Bandar Tun Razak, Cheras, Kuala Lumpur 56000, Malaysia
3 Department of Biochemistry, Faculty of Medicine, Universiti Kebangsaan Malaysia, Jalan Yaacob Latif, Kuala Lumpur 56000, Malaysia
* Correspondence: adli.ali@ppukm.ukm.edu.my; Tel.: +603-9174-8510

Abstract: *Background and Objectives:* Kawasaki Disease (KD) incidence has been on the rise globally throughout the years, particularly in the Asia Pacific region. KD can be diagnosed based on several clinical criteria. Due to its systemic inflammatory nature, multi-organ involvement has been observed, making the diagnosis of KD more challenging. Notably, several studies have reported KD patients presenting with hepatobiliary abnormalities. Nonetheless, comprehensive data regarding the hepatobiliary manifestations of KD are limited in Malaysia, justifying a more in-depth study of the disease in this country. Thus, in this article, we aim to discuss KD patients in Malaysia with hepatobiliary manifestations. *Materials and Methods:* A total of six KD patients with hepatobiliary findings who presented at Hospital Canselor Tuanku Muhriz (HCTM) from 2004 to 2021 were selected and included. Variables including the initial presenting signs and symptoms, clinical progress, laboratory investigations such as liver function test (LFT), and ultrasound findings of hepatobiliary system were reviewed and analyzed. *Results:* Out of these six KD patients, there were two patients complicated with hepatitis and one patient with gallbladder hydrops. Different clinical features including jaundice ($n = 3$) and hepatomegaly ($n = 4$) were also observed. All patients received both aspirin and intravenous immunoglobulin (IVIG) as their first-line treatment and all of them responded well to IVIG. The majority of them ($n = 5$) had a complete recovery and did not have any cardiovascular and hepatobiliary sequelae. *Conclusions:* Despite KD mostly being diagnosed with the classical clinical criteria, patients with atypical presentations should always alert physicians of KD as one of the possible differential diagnoses. This study discovered that hepatobiliary manifestations in KD patients were not uncommon. More awareness on the epidemiology, diagnosis, and management of KD patients with hepatobiliary manifestations are required to allow for the initiation of prompt treatment, thus preventing further complications.

Keywords: hepatobiliary manifestation; Kawasaki disease; gallbladder hydrops; hepatitis; hepatomegaly; hyperbilirubinemia; complications

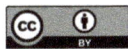

1. Introduction

Kawasaki disease (KD) is an acute systemic vasculitis that was first reported in 1961 [1]. Over the past few years, multiple papers have been published to provide a better insight of this disease. KD is characterized as an acute systemic vascular disease that mostly affects the small and medium vessels [2]. KD is self-limiting and happens commonly among children under 5 years old, following the diagnostic criteria in the American Heart Association (AHA) guidelines [3,4]. Most of the morbidity and mortality in KD patients stem from cardiac involvement with the development of arrhythmias or coronary artery aneurysms (CAA) [5]. However, in many patients, the clinical manifestations of KD are incomplete and atypical, which leads to delayed diagnosis and a worse prognosis for CAA.

In this study, we refer to atypical presentations of KD as clinical presentations that were not listed as the classical manifestations under the AHA guideline [4]. Various atypical presentations of KD occur at an early age including hepatobiliary manifestations. Some KD patients presented initially with hepatobiliary manifestations, such as jaundice, abdominal pain, nausea, vomiting, diarrhea, hepatosplenomegaly, gallbladder hydrops, laboratory, and radiological hepatobiliary abnormalities, thus masking the classical symptoms of KD, leading to misdiagnosis of hepatobiliary or gastrointestinal system diseases such as hepatitis or acute acalculous cholecystitis (ACC) [6–9]. Although hepatobiliary manifestations do not belong to the classical criteria of KD, there were approximately 15% to 45% of patients who presented with these atypical presentations [10]. In terms of complications, CAA is most commonly reported, but the inflammatory lesions of KD are not only limited to the coronary arteries but can also involve the abdominal arteries [11]. It has been suggested that hepatic dysfunction has a relation with KD systemic inflammation; however, its nature is still not clearly understood [12]. Thus, patients with atypical hepatobiliary manifestation should raise the index of suspicion of KD as one of the differential diagnoses. Since there is a scarcity of studies on KD in Malaysia, this study aims at discussing KD patients presenting with hepatobiliary manifestations at our center to further aid in the understanding of KD clinical presentations.

2. Material and Methods

2.1. Study Location and Period

The search for KD cases with hepatobiliary manifestation was conducted at Hospital Canselor Tuanku Muhriz (HCTM), a tertiary medical center and a teaching hospital under the administration of Universiti Kebangsaan Malaysia (UKM). The study was conducted from October 2021 to October 2022. Ethical approval was obtained from the institute itself (HCTM) prior to the commencement of this study (JEP-2021-868).

2.2. Research Design

The study was conducted as a retrospective cohort study. A total of 103 patients who attended HCTM with the diagnosis of KD from 2004 to 2021 were initially retrieved from the HCTM Case Mix system by using the International Classification of Diseases (ICD) code, ICD-10 (M30.3), for mucocutaneous lymph node syndrome, which is another name for KD. From this cohort, a total of 6 KD cases with hepatobiliary manifestations, such as jaundice, hepatomegaly, hepatitis, or gallbladder hydrops, were identified and included in this study. Variables including the initial presenting signs and symptoms, clinical progress, laboratory investigations such as liver function tests, and ultrasound findings of the hepatobiliary system were reviewed and analyzed.

2.3. Inclusion and Exclusion Criteria

All registered data of patients who were admitted to HCTM between 2004 and 2021 with the diagnosis of KD based on the health information system were retrieved. With this approach, there were two methodological limitations. The first limitation was the type I error, which happened when non-KD patients were coded as KD in the system. These patients did not meet the criteria to be diagnosed as complete or incomplete KD and were excluded from this study. The second limitation was the type II error, which happened when KD patients were not coded as KD in the system. These patients' data could not be traced and subsequently were not included in this study. From the total of 103 KD patients' data that were retrieved, those who had hepatobiliary manifestations, such as jaundice, hepatomegaly, hepatitis, or gallbladder hydrops, were identified and included in this study.

Meanwhile, the exclusion criteria of this study are (i) patient data with repeated names and reference numbers and (ii) patient data that could not be accessed at all due to loss of information or the patient's file. Repetitions of data were considered as a single entry. However, any incomplete dataset was accepted and reported as it is. After considering all the inclusion and exclusion criteria, the total of this study's subject is 6.

3. Results

3.1. Hepatitis

Out of the six KD patients, there were two patients diagnosed with hepatitis simultaneously with KD. Both patients presented with jaundice and abnormal liver function test. Patient 1 had incomplete KD, and serological investigation for hepatitis A immunoglobulin G (Ig G) tested positive, which led to the delayed diagnosis of KD. Meanwhile, Patient 2 had hepatomegaly with the typical presentations of KD, making an earlier diagnosis of KD complicated with hepatitis.

Patient 1, with underlying glucose-6-phosphate dehydrogenase (G6PD) deficiency, presented with fever and cough for 3 days. Acute gastroenteritis (AGE) was diagnosed by a general practitioner and symptomatic treatment was given. On the next day, rashes started to develop over the chest, trunk, and upper limbs. Jaundice was also noted. Upon admission on day 4 of illness, examination revealed bilateral cervical and inguinal lymphadenopathy, injected throat, cracked red lips, desquamation of scrotal area, and mild hepatomegaly. Laboratory investigations showed neutrophilic leukocytosis (white cell count 16.4×10^9 L; neutrophil 92%), direct hyperbilirubinemia (total serum bilirubin 142 µmol/L; direct bilirubin 111 µmol/L), and elevated alanine aminotransferase (ALT: 75 U/L). The patient was initially managed as viral hepatitis with concurrent G6PD hyperbilirubinemia. Serological investigations showed positive for Hepatitis A immunoglobulin G (IgG), indicating a previous history of infection. Kawasaki disease (KD) with atypical presentation was only diagnosed after the onset of edema and widespread rash over the extremities.

Patient 2 was initially treated for tonsilitis and received antibiotics. However, the fever (average recorded temperature of 39 °C) and left-sided neck pain persisted. Referral to our hospital for further evaluation was only done on the 7th day of fever with rashes over the back, neck, and cubital and popliteal fossa; bilateral non-purulent conjunctivitis; unilateral lymphadenopathy; and jaundice. Upon admission, the patient's liver was 3 cm palpable below the right subcostal margin, indicating the presence of hepatomegaly. Other systemic examinations were unremarkable. Laboratory studies revealed leukocytosis (white cell count 29.7×10^9/L), hemoglobin of 11.1 g/dL, normal platelet count (230×10^9/L) and raised C-reactive protein (CRP) (30 mg/dL). Serum alkaline phosphatase (ALP: 447 U/L) and serum ALT (82 U/L) were elevated. Diagnosis of typical KD with mild hepatitis was considered, and echocardiographic (ECHO) examination was performed revealing a normal cardiac finding.

In terms of management, both patients received intravenous immunoglobulin (IVIG) 2 g/kg with high-dose aspirin therapy followed by subsequent low-dose aspirin therapy. Both patients were subsequently on follow-ups at cardiology clinic and were later discharged with no complications.

3.2. Gallbladder Hydrops

There was one KD patient within our cohort with the finding of gallbladder hydrops. Patient 3 presented with fever for 8 days with the highest temperature of 39 °C associated with rigors and rashes. Rashes started to develop on day 4 of illness and initially appeared around the perioral region, then radiated to the ear, scalp, trunk, and limbs within a few hours. However, these rashes subsided on day 6 of illness. Upon admission, there were red lips and tongue, bilateral conjunctival injection, left axillary lymphadenopathy, and flaring of the bacille Calmette-Guérin scar (BCGitis), hence the diagnosis of complete KD. Examinations of other systems were unremarkable. Laboratory investigations showed leukocytosis (16.3×10^9 L, neutrophils 4.7×10^9) and hypoalbuminemia with normal ALT and ALP levels. Ultrasound of the abdomen was done, and gallbladder hydrops was confirmed, in which the gallbladder wall was distended without debris measured 4.9 cm in length (normal pediatric gallbladder measurement for 0–1-year-old, length of gallbladder range between 1.3 and 3.4 cm). The echocardiography result was normal. Treatment with IVIG of 2 g/kg over 12 h and oral aspirin of 30 mg/kg/day for 6 days was given. The patient was then continued with low-dose aspirin of 4 mg/kg/day for 6 weeks and subsequently discharged with no complications.

3.3. Hepatomegaly

Hepatomegaly is one of the hepatobiliary manifestations in KD. Four out of six patients in this study were found to have hepatomegaly findings. Two of the patients (Patient 1 and Patient 2) had concurrent hepatitis and we described the patients in Section 3.1. Under this subsection, we will focus on the two cases presented with hepatomegaly with normal LFT results.

The first patient, Patient 4, presented with 9 days of non-resolving low-grade fever (38 °C), which was temporarily relieved by tepid sponging. Maculopapular rashes developed on day 2 of illness and spread from both lower limbs towards the upper limbs, trunk, and face. Lips were dry; however, no classic KD mucosal lesions were noted. On systemic examination, other systems were normal, except the liver was 2 cm palpable (hepatomegaly). Blood investigations showed raised white cell count (47.2 × 10^9 with neutrophilia) and elevated CRP (20.78 mg/dL) with normal liver function test. The patient was tested to be rotavirus positive and was diagnosed with acute gastroenteritis (AGE). Ultrasound of the abdomen showed hepatomegaly with non-specific pericholecystic fluid. After 12 h of admission, pustular lesions developed and were noted to worsen especially around the thigh region, and the patient was started on intravenous antibiotics. On day 3 of admission, the patient was noted to have redness of both eyes and peeling of periungual region on his back eventually spreading to the abdomen and right upper limb. With this constellation of signs, the patient was eventually diagnosed with typical KD.

The second patient, Patient 5, presented with prolonged cough for 2 months and high-grade fever for 5 days associated with maculopapular rash that started on the trunk and abdomen, then later became generalized, while only sparing the face. There were also eye redness and reduced oral intake. On examination, there were generalized maculopapular rash, BCGitis, and hepatomegaly with the liver palpable 2 cm below the right subcostal margin. Otherwise, systemic examinations were normal. Laboratory investigations revealed high CRP (10.52 mg/dL). Incomplete KD was subsequently considered, and treatment was initiated.

In terms of management, both patients were treated well with IVIG at 2 g/kg over 12 h and high-dose oral aspirin. Echocardiography results of Patient 4 revealed right coronary artery ectasia of a 4 mm diameter, and the patient was prescribed low-dose aspirin (5 mg/kg/day) for 2 months. Meanwhile, Patient 5's echocardiography result was normal, and the patient was only given low-dose aspirin (5 mg/kg/day) for 6 weeks.

3.4. Cholestatic Jaundice

Our study found that cholestatic jaundice can also be one of the hepatobiliary manifestations of KD. Patient 6, with underlying G6PD deficiency, presented with 5 days history of fever associated with swollen lips and tongue, bilateral non-purulent conjunctivitis, and BCGitis with generalized macular rashes, as well as 1 day history of jaundice with passing of tea-colored urine. On examination, the patient appeared fretful and had jaundice with red and dry crack lips, generalized macular rash, and flaring of BCG scar. Cervical lymph nodes were palpable with the biggest measuring 1 cm × 1.5 cm. The throat was injected, and tonsils were enlarged. Systemic examinations were unremarkable.

Laboratory investigations revealed leukocytosis (white cell count 21.5 × 10^9/L) with neutrophilia. His CRP was elevated at 28.94 mg/dL. The total bilirubin was 142 μmol/L with the direct component of 112.8 μmol/L, indicating direct hyperbilirubinemia. The patient also had high levels of ALP (451 U/L), ALT (139 U/L), lactate dehydrogenase (LDH: 407 mmol/L), and Gamma-glutamyl transferase (GGT; 338 U/L). However, ultrasound abdomen revealed no evidence of gallbladder hydrops.

The patient was treated with IVIG 2 g/kg over 16 h. After completion of IVIG, the patient remained afebrile. Oral aspirin of 30 mg/kg/day was given for 6 days and later tapered down to 4 mg/kg/day for 6 weeks. Upon discharge, the patient was well with improving liver function and no other complications noted.

4. Discussion

The cohort of KD patients reported in this series highlights the importance of the high level of suspicion that is required for KD to be diagnosed accurately, especially if patients come in with the atypical hepatobiliary presentations (Table 1).

Table 1. Summary of the Clinical Hepatobiliary Presentation and Management of the KD patients.

	Patient 1	Patient 2	Patient 3	Patient 4	Patient 5	Patient 6
Age (months)	24	72	6	4	4	22
Duration of fever (days)	3	7	8	9	5	5
Highest temperature (°C)	40	39	39	38	39	39
Classical features of KD	Incomplete	Complete	Complete	Complete	Incomplete	Complete
Bilateral non-purulent conjunctivitis	-	+	+	+	+	+
Extremity changes	-	+	+	+	+	-
Maculopapular rash	+	+	+	+	+	+
Oral mucosal changes	+	-	+	-	-	+
Cervical lymphadenopathy	+	+	+	+	-	+
BCGitis	-	-	+	-	+	+
URTI symptoms	+	+	-	+	+	-
GIT symptoms	+	-	-	+	-	-
Jaundice	+	+	-	-	-	+
Hepatomegaly	+	+	-	+	+	-
Gallbladder hydrops	-	-	+	-	-	-
CRP (mg/dL)	12.30	30.00	7.14	20.78	10.52	28.94
ALT (U/L)	75	82	43	17	46	136
ALP (U/L)	264	447	143	99	232	497
GGT (U/L)	NA	NA	NA	NA	NA	338
Bilirubin (μmol/L)	142.0	96.1	3.9	6.0	6.2	149.9
Treatment	IVIG 2 g/kg over 12 h Aspirin 30 mg/kg/day for 2 weeks followed by 5 mg/kg/day for 3 months	IVIG 2 g/kg over 16 h Aspirin 30 mg/kg/day for 5 days followed by 5 mg/kg/day for 6 weeks	IVIG 2 g/kg over 12 h Aspirin 30 mg/kg/day for 6 days followed by 4 mg/kg/day for 6 weeks	IVIG 2 g/kg over 12 h Aspirin 30 mg/kg/day for 6 days followed by 5 mg/kg/day for 2 months	IVIG 2 g/kg over 12 h Aspirin 30 mg/kg/day for 3 days followed by 5 mg/kg/day for 6 weeks	IVIG 2 g/kg over 16 h Aspirin 30 mg/kg/day for 6 days followed by 4 mg/kg/day for 6 weeks.
Complications	No	No	No	CAA	No	No

+ Present; - Absent; NA Not available; CAA Coronary artery aneurysm.

The clinical manifestations of KD can be diverse. The diagnosis of KD can be difficult as not all the clinical features appear simultaneously. Hematological and biochemical investigations are not immensely helpful; however, these could exclude other diagnosis. Moreover, establishing the diagnosis of KD can be further complicated by the occurrence of other diseases, such as hepatitis and gallbladder hydrops, as seen in our cases. Our study reported six KD patients with hepatobiliary system manifestations, of which two had hepatitis, one had gallbladder hydrops, four had hepatomegaly, and three had jaundice, with one case manifested as cholestatic jaundice. All these patients presented with hepatobiliary manifestation simultaneously with the appearance of KD features, which further made the diagnosis of KD more challenging. In some cases, we reported a misdiagnosis in the first phase of the disease, causing delayed diagnosis of KD and late definitive treatment to be offered to the patients. This was similarly reported in previous study, where there was a delayed diagnosis of KD due to the initial misdiagnosis of viral hepatitis [13].

There were four KD patients noted to have hepatomegaly, which is an uncommon feature in KD. This was suggested by the possible involvement of portal area inflammation during acute phase of KD [14]. This clearly showed that hepatobiliary manifestations can affect the judgement of physicians to diagnose KD especially when patients had prominent hepatobiliary symptoms. Undeniably, hepatobiliary manifestations were widely reported as one of the clinical features of KD; however, they are not included in the classical clinical criteria [12,13,15].

We reported several KD patients with jaundice but without gallbladder hydrops, which was also observed by Taddio et.al [16]. This has been found to be a rarer occurrence, in which patients who presented with clinical jaundice had no sonographic evidence of gallbladder hydrops or mechanical obstruction [17–21]. In other studies, KD patients presented with obstructive jaundice were later found to develop gallbladder hydrops with symptoms mimicking acute abdomen [22]. One of the possible explanations behind this occurrence is lymphadenopathy causing compression effect of the hilum of the liver (porta hepatis) [7].

Apart from atypical clinical manifestations of KD, laboratory and radiological investigations demonstrating hepatobiliary abnormalities could also assist in the confirmation of the diagnosis. Three patients were reported to have abnormal LFT with either elevated ALT, ALP, or both. The pathogenesis of LFT derangement in KD is incompletely understood but is thought to be multifactorial [12]. Proposed etiologies include generalized inflammation, vasculitis, congestive cardiac failure secondary to myocarditis, non-steroidal anti-inflammatory antipyretics, toxin-mediated effects, or a combination of these conditions [12]. Liver dysfunction in KD patients is usually self-limiting, and the median recovery time ranges from 2 days to 99 days [23,24]. Although LFT is not the diagnostic tool of KD, it may indicate the severity of ongoing inflammation, thus serving as a prognostic marker for the development of IVIG resistance or coronary artery aneurysm (CAA) [12,15,25]. Having said that, patients can also present with normal LFT, as ALT was only elevated in less than 40% of KD patients and hyperbilirubinemia only occur in 10% of KD patients. Meanwhile, hypoalbuminemia was common among patients with severe and prolonged KD [4].

Based on our study, although hepatobiliary manifestation is not one of the criteria to diagnose KD, it is important to remember such unusual presentations do not exclude KD. Diagnosing KD in those who presented with atypical presentations of KD remains a challenge for physicians. Undeniably, one of the reasons for delayed diagnosis of KD is due to the atypical presentations [26]. Investigations, discussion with experts, and review of published guideline are mandatory to confirm or exclude the diagnosis of KD [27]. Delayed diagnosis causing delayed treatment will lead to increased risk for CAA to develop [28]. Therefore, a good and broad awareness of the various KD presentations is of utmost important to avoid delayed in the diagnosis, so that prompt treatment can be achieved.

Being known as an X-linked recessive genetic disorder, certain variants of G6PD deficiency including Class I, II, and III will cause potentially life-threatening hemolytic anemia with exposure of triggers, such as infection, drugs, and fava beans [29]. To date, the relationship between aspirin treatment and hemolytic anemia in KD patients with G6PD remains unknown due to limited studies [30]. Two of our KD patients within the studied cohort had underlying G6PD deficiency. However, both patients had direct hyperbilirubinemia during the acute phase of KD, indicating hepatocellular injury and negating the possibility of hemolytic anemia secondary to G6PD deficiency, which further suggests that aspirin treatment is not absolutely contraindicated in KD patients with underlying G6PD deficiency.

One of the major limitations of our study is the loss of patient's data since this is a retrospective analysis of KD patients in HCTM. Therefore, some of the information, such as laboratory investigation and duration of follow-up and subsequent treatment, was missing and could not be reported completely.

5. Conclusions

In this study, we discussed six KD patients who presented with hepatobiliary manifestations. Some of them initially had atypical presentations of KD, while others were misdiagnosed with other diseases before KD was considered. Therefore, abnormal results from laboratory investigations, such as LFT and imaging study including ultrasound of the hepatobiliary system, should always raise a suspicion of KD in patients who fulfilled only some of the classical clinical features of KD. KD with unusual presentations require for extreme alertness, rapid diagnosis, and prompt treatment to prevent progression to coronary artery lesions or potentially life-threatening disease with severe long-term consequences.

Author Contributions: All authors are equally responsible for the initial conceptualization, S.A.S., C.S.C., A.H.A., W.L.W.L., M.S.K., N.A.S.I. and A.A.; Writing—Original Draft Preparation, S.A.S., A.H.A., C.S.C. and W.L.W.L., Writing—Review and Editing, M.S.K., N.A.S.I. and A.A.; Supervision, M.S.K., N.A.S.I. and A.A. All authors have read and agreed to the published version of the manuscript.

Funding: The publication fee is sponsored by the Faculty of Medicine, Universiti Kebangsaan Malaysia.

Institutional Review Board Statement: This study is a part of a research study approved by the Universiti Kebangsaan Malaysia Ethics Review Board (JEP-2021-868), on 24 December 2021.

Informed Consent Statement: Not applicable.

Data Availability Statement: Not applicable.

Acknowledgments: We are thankful to the Faculty of Medicine, Universiti Kebangsaan Malaysia for supporting our publication.

Conflicts of Interest: The authors report no conflict of interest in this manuscript.

References

1. Kim, G.B. Reality of Kawasaki Disease Epidemiology. *Korean J. Pediatr.* **2019**, *62*, 292–296. [CrossRef]
2. de Graeff, N.; Groot, N.; Ozen, S.; Eleftheriou, D.; Avcin, T.; Bader-Meunier, B.; Dolezalova, P.; Feldman, B.M.; Kone-Paut, I.; Lahdenne, P.; et al. European Consensus-Based Recommendations for the Diagnosis and Treatment of Kawasaki Disease—The SHARE Initiative. *Rheumatology* **2019**, *58*, 672–682. [CrossRef] [PubMed]
3. Sánchez-Manubens, J.; Bou, R.; Anton, J. Diagnosis and Classification of Kawasaki Disease. *J. Autoimmun.* **2014**, *48–49*, 113–117. [CrossRef] [PubMed]
4. McCrindle, B.W.; Rowley, A.H.; Newburger, J.W.; Burns, J.C.; Bolger, A.F.; Gewitz, M.; Baker, A.L.; Jackson, M.A.; Takahashi, M.; Shah, P.B.; et al. Diagnosis, Treatment, and Long-Term Management of Kawasaki Disease: A Scientific Statement for Health Professionals from the American Heart Association. *Circulation* **2017**, *135*, e927–e999. [CrossRef]
5. Duarte, R.; Cisneros, S.; Fernandez, G.; Castellon, D.; Cattani, C.; Melo, C.A.; Apocada, A. Kawasaki Disease: A Review with Emphasis on Cardiovascular Complications. *Insights Imaging* **2010**, *1*, 223–231. [CrossRef] [PubMed]
6. Mammadov, G.; Liu, H.H.; Chen, W.X.; Fan, G.Z.; Li, R.X.; Liu, F.F.; Samadli, S.; Wang, J.J.; Wu, Y.F.; Luo, H.H.; et al. Hepatic Dysfunction Secondary to Kawasaki Disease: Characteristics, Etiology and Predictive Role in Coronary Artery Abnormalities. *Clin. Exp. Med.* **2020**, *20*, 21–30. [CrossRef] [PubMed]
7. Kuo, H.-C.; Yang, K.D.; Chang, W.-C.; Ger, L.-P.; Hsieh, K.-S. Kawasaki Disease: An Update on Diagnosis and Treatment. *Pediatr. Neonatol.* **2012**, *53*, 4–11. [CrossRef] [PubMed]
8. Colomba, C.; la Placa, S.; Saporito, L.; Corsello, G.; Ciccia, F.; Medaglia, A.; Romanin, B.; Serra, N.; di Carlo, P.; Cascio, A. Intestinal Involvement in Kawasaki Disease. *J. Pediatr.* **2018**, *202*, 186–193. [CrossRef] [PubMed]
9. Jafari, S.A.; Kiani, M.A.; Ahanchian, H.; Khakshour, A.; Partovi, S.; Kianifar, H.R.; Saeidi, M. Kawasaki Disease Presenting as Acute Clinical Hepatitis. *Int. J. Pediatr.* **2013**, *1*, 51–53. [CrossRef]
10. Singh, S.; Kawasaki, T. Kawasaki Disease in India–Lessons Learnt over the Last 20 Years. *Indian Pediatr.* **2016**, *53*, 119–124. [CrossRef]
11. Takahashi, K.; Oharaseki, T.; Yokouchi, Y.; Hiruta, N.; Naoe, S. Kawasaki Disease as a Systemic Vasculitis in Childhood. *Ann. Vasc. Dis.* **2010**, *3*, 173–181. [CrossRef] [PubMed]
12. Eladawy, M.; Dominguez, S.R.; Anderson, M.S.; Glodé, M.P. Abnormal Liver Panel in Acute Kawasaki Disease. *Pediatr. Infect. Dis. J.* **2011**, *30*, 141–144. [CrossRef] [PubMed]
13. Majumdar, I.; Wagner, S. Kawasaki Disease Masquerading as Hepatitis. *Clin. Pediatr.* **2016**, *55*, 73–75. [CrossRef] [PubMed]
14. Ohshio, G.; Furukawa, F.; Fujiwara, H.; Hamashima, Y. Hepatomegaly and Splenomegaly in Kawasaki Disease. *Pediatr. Pathol.* **1985**, *4*, 257–264. [CrossRef]
15. Yi, D.Y.; Kim, J.Y.; Choi, E.Y.; Choi, J.Y.; Yang, H.R. Hepatobiliary Risk Factors for Clinical Outcome of Kawasaki Disease in Children. *BMC Pediatr.* **2014**, *14*, 51. [CrossRef]
16. Taddio, A.; Pellegrin, M.C.; Centenari, C.; Filippeschi, I.P.; Ventura, A.; Maggiore, G. Acute Febrile Cholestatic Jaundice in Children. *J. Pediatr. Gastroenterol. Nutr.* **2012**, *55*, 380–383. [CrossRef]
17. Huang, S.-W.; Lin, S.-C.; Chen, S.-Y.; Hsieh, K.-S. Kawasaki Disease with Combined Cholestatic Hepatitis and Mycoplasma Pneumoniae Infection: A Case Report and Literature Review. *Front. Pediatr.* **2022**, *9*, 738215. [CrossRef]
18. Keeling, I.M.; Beran, E.; Dapunt, O.E. Kawasaki Disease and Hepatobiliary Involvement: Report of Two Cases. *Ital. J. Pediatr.* **2016**, *42*, 27. [CrossRef]

19. McMahon, M.A.; Wynne, B.; Murphy, G.M.; Kearns, G. Recurrence of Kawasaki Disease in an Adult Patient with Cholecystitis. *Ir. Med. J.* **2007**, *100*, 400–401.
20. Valentini, P.; Ausili, E.; Schiavino, A.; Angelone, D.F.; Focarelli, B.; de Rosa, G.; Ranno, O. Acute Cholestasis: Atypical Onset of Kawasaki Disease. *Dig. Liver Dis.* **2008**, *40*, 582–584. [CrossRef]
21. Vázquez Gomis, R.; Izquierdo Fos, I.; López Yañez, A.; Mendoza Durán, M.; Serrano Robles, M.I.; Vázquez Gomis, C.; Pastor Rosado, J. Hepatitis Colestásica En La Enfermedad de Kawasaki Resistente a Inmunoglobulinas. *Gastroenterol. Hepatol.* **2016**, *39*, 301–302. [CrossRef] [PubMed]
22. Sun, Q.; Zhang, J.; Yang, Y. Gallbladder Hydrops Associated with Kawasaki Disease: A Case Report and Literature Review. *Clin. Pediatr.* **2018**, *57*, 341–343. [CrossRef] [PubMed]
23. Jang, M.; Oh, M.S.; Oh, S.-C.; Kang, K.-S. Distribution of Diseases Causing Liver Function Test Abnormality in Children and Natural Recovery Time of the Abnormal Liver Function. *J. Korean Med. Sci.* **2016**, *31*, 1784. [CrossRef] [PubMed]
24. Paglia, P.; Nazzaro, L.; de Anseris, A.G.E.; Lettieri, M.; Colantuono, R.; Rocco, M.C.; Siano, M.A.; Biffaro, N.; VAJRO, P. Atypically Protracted Course of Liver Involvement in Kawasaki Disease. Case Report and Literature Review. *Pediatr. Rep.* **2021**, *13*, 357–362. [CrossRef]
25. Liu, L.; Yin, W.; Wang, R.; Sun, D.; He, X.; Ding, Y. The Prognostic Role of Abnormal Liver Function in IVIG Unresponsiveness in Kawasaki Disease: A Meta-Analysis. *Inflamm. Res.* **2016**, *65*, 161–168. [CrossRef]
26. Mat Bah, M.N.; Alias, E.Y.; Sapian, M.H.; Abdullah, N. Delayed Diagnosis of Kawasaki Disease in Malaysia: Who Is at Risk and What Is the Outcome. *Pediatr. Int.* **2022**, *64*, e15162. [CrossRef]
27. Lee, W.; Cheah, C.S.; Suhaini, S.A.; Azidin, A.H.; Khoo, M.S.; Ismail, N.A.S.; Ali, A. Clinical Manifestations and Laboratory Findings of Kawasaki Disease: Beyond the Classic Diagnostic Features. *Medicina* **2022**, *58*, 734. [CrossRef]
28. Muta, H.; Ishii, M.; Yashiro, M.; Uehara, R.; Nakamura, Y. Late Intravenous Immunoglobulin Treatment in Patients with Kawasaki Disease. *Pediatrics* **2012**, *129*, e291–e297. [CrossRef]
29. Bubp, J.; Jen, M.; Matuszewski, K. Caring for Glucose-6-Phosphate Dehydrogenase (G6PD)-Deficient Patients: Implications for Pharmacy. *Pharm. Ther.* **2015**, *40*, 572–574.
30. Chen, C.-H.; Lin, L.-Y.; Yang, K.D.; Hsieh, K.-S.; Kuo, H.-C. Kawasaki Disease with G6PD Deficiency—Report of One Case and Literature Review. *J. Microbiol. Immunol. Infect.* **2014**, *47*, 261–263. [CrossRef]

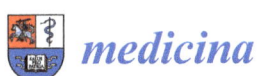

Article

Clinical Characteristics of Symptomatic Cholecystitis in Post-Gastrectomy Patients: 11 Years of Experience in a Single Center

Yun Suk Choi [1,†], Boram Cha [2,†], Sung Hoon Kim [1], Jin Wook Yi [1], Kyeong Deok Kim [1], Moon Suk Choi [1] and Yoon Seok Heo [1,*]

1. Department of Surgery, College of Medicine, Inha University Hospital, 27, Inhang-ro, Jung-gu, Inchon 22332, Korea
2. Department of Internal Medicine, College of Medicine, Inha University Hospital, 27, Inhang-ro, Jung-gu, Inchon 22332, Korea
* Correspondence: gshur@inha.ac.kr; Tel.: +82-32-890-3437; Fax: +82-32-890-3549
† These authors contributed equally to this work.

Abstract: *Background and Objectives*: Gallbladder (GB) stones, a major cause of symptomatic cholecystitis, are more likely to develop in post gastrectomy people. Our purpose is to evaluate characteristics of symptomatic cholecystitis after gastrectomy. *Materials and Method*: In January 2011–December 2021, total 1587 patients underwent operations for symptomatic cholecystitis at our hospital. We reviewed the patients' general characteristics, operation results, pathologic results, and postoperative complications. We classified the patients into non-gastrectomy and gastrectomy groups, further divided into subtotal gastrectomy and total gastrectomy groups. *Result*: The patients' ages, male proportion, and the open surgery rate were significantly higher (127/1543 (8.2%) vs. 17/44 (38.6%); $p < 0.001$), and the operation time was longer (102.51 ± 52.43 vs. 167.39 ± 82.95; $p < 0.001$) in the gastrectomy group. Extended surgery rates were significantly higher in the gastrectomy group (56/1543 (3.6%) vs. 12/44 (27.3%); $p < 0.001$). The period from gastrectomy to symptomatic cholecystitis was significantly shorter in the total gastrectomy group (12.72 ± 10.50 vs. 7.25 ± 4.80; $p = 0.040$). *Conclusion*: GB stones were more likely to develop in post-gastrectomy patients and extended surgery rates were higher. The period to cholecystitis was shorter in total gastrectomy. Efforts to prevent GB stones are considered in post-gastrectomy patients.

Keywords: cholecystectomy; cholecystitis; gastrectomy

1. Introduction

Gallbladder (GB) stones are the most common cause of symptomatic cholecystitis—one of the most common causes of abdominal emergency surgery—and of common bile duct stones that require endoscopic retrograde cholangiopancreatography (ERCP). The incidence of GB stones in the general population is known to be 2.2–5.0% [1,2], of which ~5% progress to symptomatic cholecystitis annually [3–5]. In Korea, >150,000 people are treated for cholelithiasis, and ~70,000 cholecystectomies are performed annually [6].

The reported incidence of GB stones after gastrectomy is 6.5–25%, which is higher than that in the general population [3,4,7,8]. The reasons for the high incidence of GB stones include hepatoduodenal lymph node dissection around the stomach, duodenum bypassing after gastrectomy, vagus nerve injury during gastrectomy, and rapid weight loss after surgery [4,9–11]. Due to these diverse causes, GB contraction decreases and bile salt concentration increases, leading to an increase in GB stone formation [12,13]. Several studies have recommended taking ursodeoxycholic acid (UDCA) to prevent post-gastrectomy GB stones and symptomatic cholecystitis [14–16].

Laparoscopic cholecystectomy was first performed in 1986 and is the gold standard for the treatment of symptomatic cholecystitis [17,18]. Postoperative adhesions can occur within the abdominal cavity in those who have undergone a gastrectomy, which can be particularly severe around the GB and in the Calot triangle due to hepatoduodenal ligament LN dissection. Therefore, cholecystectomy after gastrectomy is more difficult than cholecystectomy in the general population—the operation time is longer, the frequency of open cholecystectomy is higher, and the number of postoperative complications is higher [19,20]. The technique of laparoscopic surgery has been developed recently, and laparoscopic cholecystectomy is often performed even if there is a history of abdominal surgery [21,22].

Some investigators have attempted to perform prophylactic cholecystectomy together with gastrectomy, but this is not recommended [7,23–25]. The cholecystectomy is only performed at the same time as a gastrectomy if there is an abnormality within the GB before the preoperative evaluation. Although it is known that GB stones occur more frequently after gastrectomy, there are few reports on the association between GB stones and symptomatic cholecystitis. In addition, little is known about the differences in the clinical characteristics of symptomatic cholecystitis in patients with distal gastrectomy and total gastrectomy. In this study, we analyzed patients who visited the emergency room (ER) for symptomatic cholecystitis and underwent surgery at a single institution in South Korea over the past 11 years.

2. Materials and Methods

2.1. Data Collection and Patient Grouping

We retrospectively reviewed electric medical data for patients who visited the ER due to symptomatic cholecystitis at Inha University Hospital from January 2011 to December 2021. A total of 1587 patients were enrolled for the analysis. All patients were hospitalized for cholecystitis, and surgery was performed during hospitalization. We collected their clinical data, including patients' general characteristics (age, sex, and body mass index [BMI, kg/m^2]); personal history; operation-related variables such as the American Society of Anesthesiology [ASA] score; laboratory values—white blood cell (WBC), absolute neutrophil count (ANC), C-reactive protein (CRP), creatinine (Cr), hemoglobin (Hb), protein, albumin, bilirubin, aspartate aminotransferase (AST), alanine aminotransferase (ALT) and glucose—from the day of the operation to postoperative days 1 and 2; pathologic results; preoperative and postoperative clinical course, and medical and surgical complications related to cholecystectomy. Complications were evaluated as grades 0–V according to the Clavien–Dindo classification (CDC). We categorized the patients into two groups according to the CDC classification score: the mild complication group included CDC grades 0–III, and the severe complication group included CDC grades IV and V.

Patients who had undergone operations due to ulcer perforation, bariatric surgery, and other causes were excluded from the gastrectomy group. Only patients who underwent therapeutic gastrectomy for gastric cancer were included in the gastrectomy group. Since some patients underwent a gastrectomy at another hospital, all radiologic or endoscopic examinations before and after cholecystectomy were reviewed to evaluate the type of the previous gastrectomy.

2.2. Statistics and Ethics

Statistical analysis was performed using SPSS ver. 27.0 (SPSS Inc., Chicago, IL, USA). Either the chi-square test or Fisher's exact test was used for cross-table analysis depending on the sample size. Unpaired t-tests were used to compare the means between two clinical groups. This study were approved by the Institutional Review Board of Inha University Hospital (IRB number: INH 2022-05-007).

3. Results

Among the 1587 patients enrolled in the study, 1543 had no history of gastrectomy and 44 had undergone gastrectomy (Table 1). In the gastrectomy group, the patients' ages (57.58 ± 17.28 years vs. 66.98 ± 11.76 years; $p < 0.001$) and the proportion of men were significantly higher (802/1543 (52.0%) vs. 33/44 (75.0%); $p = 0.003$), while the patients' BMIs were significantly lower than in the non-gastrectomy group (25.31 ± 3.99 vs. 21.66 ± 3.20; $p < 0.001$). Among 44 patients in the gastrectomy group, 35 had underwent subtotal gastrectomy and 9 underwent total gastrectomy. The average duration of symptomatic cholecystitis after gastrectomy was 11.54 years. The proportion of patients who had underwent percutaneous transhepatic gallbladder drainage (PTGBD) insertion was significantly higher in the gastrectomy group than in the non-gastrectomy group (147/1543 (9.5%) vs. 9/44 (20.5%); $p = 0.016$), but there was no significant difference in the PTGBD insertion period. There was no difference in the duration from cholecystitis diagnosis in the ER to operation between the two groups, but the postoperative hospital stay was significantly longer in the gastrectomy group (5.19 ± 6.89 days vs. 8.20 ± 4.87 days; $p = 0.004$).

Table 1. Clinical characteristics of symptomatic cholecystitis patients.

Variable	Non-Gastrectomy (n = 1543)	Gastrectomy (n = 44)	p-Value
Age (years, mean ± sd)	57.58 ± 17.28	66.98 ± 11.78	<0.001
Gender			0.003
Male	802 (52.0%)	33 (75.0%)	
Female	741 (48.0%)	11 (25.0%)	
ASA score	2.54 ± 0.56	2.59 ± 0.58	0.650
I	18 (2.3%)	1 (3.4%)	
II	329 (42.2%)	10 (34.5%)	
III	428 (54.9%)	18 (62.1%)	
IV	5 (0.6%)	0 (0.0%)	
BMI (kg/m^2)	25.31 ± 3.99	21.66 ± 3.20	<0.001
ICU admission days	0.17 ± 1.37	0.07 ± 0.26	0.638
Operation time (min, mean ± sd)	102.51 ± 52.43	167.39 ± 82.95	<0.001
Stomach OP Hx			
Subtotal gastrectomy		35 (79.6%)	
Total gastrectomy		9 (20.4%)	
Stomach OP duration (years, mean ± sd)	-	11.54 ± 9.40	
PTGBD insertion			0.016
No	1396 (90.5%)	35 (79.5%)	
Yes	147 (9.5%)	9 (20.5%)	
PTGBD insertion (days, mean ± sd)	8.17 ± 6.79	7.33 ± 2.60	0.715
Post-op rescue (ERCP) procedure			0.892
No	1535 (99.5%)	44 (100.0%)	
Yes	8 (0.5%)	0 (0.0%)	
Remnant CBD stone removal	3 (0.2%)		
Bile leak	4 (0.25%)		
Bile duct stenosis	1 (0.05%)		
From ER to operation (days, mean ± sd)	4.05 ± 4.55	4.61 ± 4.63	0.415
Postoperative hospital stay (days, mean ± sd)	5.19 ± 6.89	8.20 ± 4.87	0.004
Hospital stay (days, mean ± sd)	9.24 ± 8.92	12.82 ± 6.66	0.008

ASA: American Society of Anesthesiology, ASA I: A normal healthy patient, ASA II: A patient with mild systemic disease, ASA III: A patient with severe systemic disease, ASA IV: A patient with severe, life-threatening systemic disease, BMI: body mass index, kg/m^2, ER: emergency room, NA: not applicable, PTGBD: percutaneous transhepatic gallbladder drainage, ERCP: endoscopic retrograde cholangiography, CBD: common bile duct.

Table 2 shows the pathologic and surgical results after surgery for the two groups. Among the patients diagnosed with cholecystitis on histological examination, the proportion of patients with severe cholecystitis showing gangrenous change, ulceration, and empyema as pathologic results was not different between the two groups (329/1519 (21.2%) vs. 11/43 (26.3%); $p = 0.683$). The rate of laparoscopic surgery was significantly lower in the gastrectomy group (1416/1538 (91.8%) vs. 27/44 (61.4%); $p < 0.001$). The proportion of patients who had undergone extended surgery for cholecystectomy combined with another surgery such as choledocolithotomy was significantly higher in the gastrectomy group (56/1543 (3.6%) vs. 12/44 (27.3%); $p < 0.001$), and the operation time was also significantly longer in the gastrectomy group (102.51 ± 52.43 min vs. 167.39 ± 82.95 min; $p < 0.001$). There was no difference in the postoperative surgical complication rates or the bile duct-related complications, which is one of the most significant complications, between the two groups. There was also no difference in the rates of postoperative medical complications, intensive care unit (ICU) hospitalizations, and mortality between the two groups. When the postoperative complications were classified by the Clavien–Dindo classification, there was no difference in the rates of postoperative severe complications between both groups.

Table 2. Pathologic and surgical characteristics of cholecystectomy patients.

Variable	Non-Gastrectomy (n = 1543)	Gastrectomy (n = 44)	p-Value
Cholecystitis severity according to pathologic results			
Gangrenous cholecystitis (gangrenous, ulceration, empyema)	329 (21.2%)	11 (26.3%)	0.683
Acute or chronic cholecystitis	1190 (78.4%)	32 (73.7%)	
Pathologic details			
Acute cholecystitis	462 (29.9%)	15 (34.1%)	NA
Chronic cholecystitis	728 (47.2%)	17 (38.6%)	
Gangrenous GB (gangrenous, ulceration, empyema)	329 (21.3%)	11 (25.0%)	
GB cancer	23 (1.5%)	1 (2.3%)	
Other	1 (0.1%)	0 (0.0%)	
Operation time (min, mean ± sd)	102.60 ± 52.82	164.87 ± 80.03	<0.001
Surgical approach			
Open surgery	127 (8.2%)	17 (38.6%)	<0.001
Laparoscopic surgery	1416 (91.8%)	27 (61.4%)	
Surgical extent			
Only cholecystectomy	1487 (96.4%)	32 (72.7%)	<0.001
Extended surgery	56 (3.6%)	12 (27.3%)	
Surgical method details			
Open cholecystectomy	93 (6.0%)	8 (18.2%)	NA
Laparoscopic cholecystectomy	1394 (90.3%)	24 (54.5%)	
OC + Choledocolithotomy	26 (1.7%)	9 (20.5%)	
LC + Choledocolithotomy	22 (1.4%)	3 (6.8%)	
Cholecystectomy with another operation (Small bowel resection, colon resection)	4 (0.3%)	0 (0.0%)	
Radical cholecystectomy	4 (0.3%)	0 (0.0%)	
Post-op bile duct problem (leak, stricture)			
No	1533 (99.4%)	44 (100.0%)	0.592
Yes	10 (0.6%)	0 (0.0%)	
Surgical complication			
No	1525 (98.8%)	44 (100.0%)	0.471
Yes	18 (1.2%)	0 (0.0%)	
Type of surgical complication			
Leak, fistula, perforation	12 (0.7%)	0 (0.0%)	N/A
Stricture, obstruction	1 (0.1%)	0 (0.0%)	
Ileus	1 (0.1%)	0 (0.0%)	
Bleeding	3 (0.2%)	0 (0.0%)	
Other	1 (0.1%)	0 (0.0%)	
ICU admission due to a medical problem			
No	1531 (99.2%)	44 (100.0%)	0.557
Yes	12 (0.8%)	0 (0.0%)	
ICU admission days (postoperative)	0.17 ± 1.37	0.07 ± 0.26	0.686
Area of medical problem			M/A
Lung	8 (0.5%)		
Renal	3 (0.2%)		
Infection	4 (0.3%)		
Cardio/Vascular	4 (0.3%)		
Death			
No	1531 (99.2%)	44 (100.0%)	0.557
Yes	12 (0.8%)	0 (0.0%)	
Clavien–Dindo Classification			
Mild complication (I–III)	1523 (98.6%)	44 (100.0%)	0.526
Severe complication (IV–V)	21 (1.4%)	0 (0.0%)	
IVa	7 (0.45%)	0 (0.0%)	
IVb	2 (0.12%)	0 (0.0%)	
V	12 (0.83%)	0 (0.0%)	

NA: not applicable, OC: open cholecystectomy, LC: laparoscopic cholecystectomy, ICU: intensive care unit.

A comparative analysis was performed between the two groups for laboratory tests performed on patients before and after surgery (Table 3 and Figure 1). Protein, albumin, and hemoglobin levels were significantly lower in the gastrectomy group before surgery. There was no difference in inflammatory markers such as WBC and CRP. However, bilirubin levels were higher in the gastrectomy group (1.67 ± 1.93 mg/dL vs. 2.44 ± 2.40 mg/dL; p = 0.055). On the postoperative day 1, WBC counts decreased in both groups, but the decrease was lower in the gastrectomy group, resulting in a significant difference between the two groups. Protein, albumin, and Hb levels were significantly lower in the gastrectomy group. Bilirubin was decreased in both groups, it was higher than normal in the gastrectomy group (1.09 ± 0.99 mg/dL vs. 1.51 ± 1.28 mg/dL; p = 0.052). On the postoperative day 2, WBC counts decreased in both groups. However, CRP levels continued to rise in the gastrectomy group, resulting in a significant difference between the two groups (11.80 ± 7.54 mg/L vs. 23.89 ± 1.35 mg/L; p = 0.026). Protein, albumin, and Hb levels were consistently and significantly lower in the gastrectomy group. Bilirubin levels were decreased in both groups, and there was no difference between the groups.

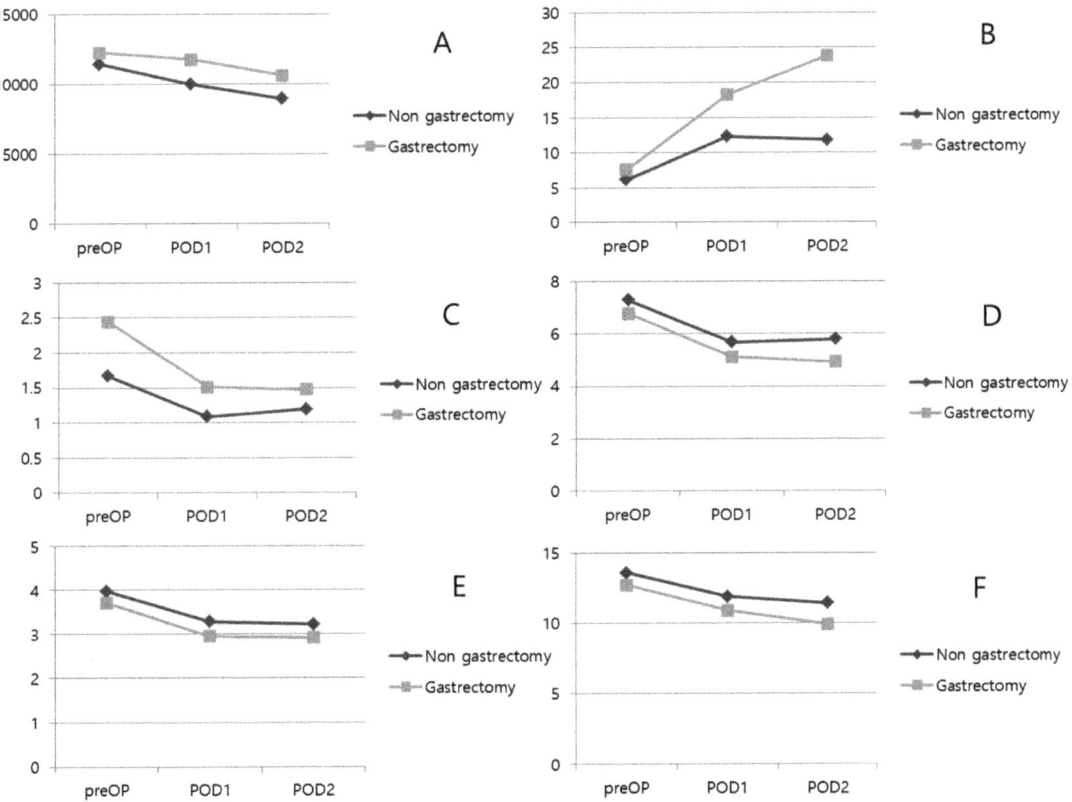

Figure 1. Perioperative laboratory results. (**A**): WBC. (**B**): CRP. (**C**): Total bilirubin. (**D**): Protein. (**E**): Albumin. (**F**): Hemoglobin. POD: postoperative day.

Table 3. Perioperative laboratory results.

Variable	Non-Gastrectomy (n = 1543)	Gastrectomy (n = 44)	p-Value
Pre-operative period			
WBC	11.45 ± 5.22	12.27 ± 7.21	0.497
CRP	6.18 ± 8.80	7.57 ± 9.57	0.332
ANC	9216.85 ± 5194.38	10,541.47 ± 7030.879	0.262
Hb	13.58 ± 1.78	12.69 ± 1.84	0.003
Protein	7.28 ± 0.63	6.78 ± 0.76	<0.001
Albumin	3.98 ± 0.53	3.71 ± 0.44	0.003
Creatinine	1.02 ± 0.85	0.94 ± 0.39	0.566
Bilirubin	1.67 ± 1.93	2.44 ± 2.40	0.059
AST	120.20 ± 200.23	211.38 ± 278.12	0.055
ALT	116.84 ± 186.69	145.76 ± 158.89	0.283
Post-operative day 1			
WBC	9.98 ± 3.88	11.76 ± 5.17	0.043
CRP	12.32 ± 8.64	18.20 ± 9.63	0.248
ANC	8003.79 ± 3919.72	10,115.22 ± 5161.68	0.017
Hb	11.89 ± 1.72	10.88 ± 1.75	<0.001
Protein	5.67 ± 0.66	5.11 ± 0.74	<0.001
Albumin	3.28 ± 0.52	2.95 ± 0.41	<0.001
Creatinine	0.98 ± 1.00	0.78 ± 0.28	0.421
Bilirubin	1.09 ± 0.99	1.51 ± 1.28	0.052
AST	66.39 ± 78.61	91.00 ± 103.28	0.154
ALT	71.80 ± 86.91	88.84 ± 93.23	0.280
Post-operative day 2			
WBC	8.94 ± 3.99	10.62 ± 5.25	0.190
CRP	11.80 ± 7.54	23.89 ± 1.35	0.026
ANC	6726.37 ± 3922.23	8878.00 ± 5091.63	0.088
Hb	11.42 ± 1.95	9.91 ± 1.62	0.015
Protein	5.80 ± 0.76	4.91 ± 0.60	<0.001
Albumin	3.22 ± 0.51	2.92 ± 0.37	0.048
Creatinine	0.95 ± 0.84	0.67 ± 0.28	0.328
Bilirubin	1.19 ± 1.20	1.47 ± 1.07	0.428
AST	53.20 ± 79.83	63.00 ± 44.18	0.685
ALT	72.70 ± 83.51	77.73 ± 73.84	0.843

WBC: White Blood Cell count X 1000 (/μL), Hb: Hemoglobin (g/dL), ANC: Absolute Neutrophil Count (/μL), CRP: C-reactive protein (mg/L).

To avoid statistical error, we analyzed only male patients separately (Table 4). A total of 802 patients in the non-gastrectomy group and 33 patients in the gastrectomy group were included. The rate of laparoscopic surgery was significantly lower in the gastrectomy group (725/802 (90.4%) vs. 21/33 (63.6%); $p < 0.001$). The proportion of patients who had undergone extended surgery for cholecystectomy combined with another surgery such as choledocolithotomy was significantly higher in the gastrectomy group (35/802 (4.4%) vs. 7/33 (21.2%); $p < 0.001$), and the operation time was also significantly longer in the gastrectomy group (109.02 ± 54.54 min vs. 157.41 ± 75.21 min; $p < 0.001$). The results of analyzing only male patients were similar to those of analyzing all patients.

Table 4. Clinical and pathologic characteristics of male cholecystitis patients.

Variable	Non-Gastrectomy (n = 802)	Gastrectomy (n = 33)	p-Value
Age (years, mean ± sd)	58.66 ± 16.19	65.07 ± 13.11	0.042
ASA score	2.55 ± 0.55	2.47 ± 0.62	0.544
BMI (kg/m^2)	25.50 ± 8.62	21.77 ± 2.57	0.025
Stomach OP Hx			
Subtotal gastrectomy		26 (78.8%)	
Total gastrectomy		7 (21.2%)	
Stomach OP duration (years, mean ± sd)	-	12.00 ± 10.48	
ICU admission days (days, mean ± sd)	0.25 ± 1.85	0.07 ± 0.27	0.612
Operation time (min, mean ± sd)	109.02 ± 54.54	157.41 ± 75.21	<0.001
Hospital stay (days, mean ± sd)	9.57 ± 9.15	11.22 ± 5.54	0.351
From ER to operation (days, mean ± sd)	4.18 ± 5.08	3.74 ± 3.21	0.653
Postoperative hospital stay (days, mean ± sd)	5.39 ± 6.31	7.48 ± 5.15	0.089
Clavien–Dindo Classification			
Mild complication (I–III)	789 (98.4%)	33 (100.0%)	
Severe complication (IV–V)	13 (1.6%)	0 (0.0%)	
Cholecystitis severity according to pathologic results			
Gangrenous cholecystitis (gangrenous, ulceration, empyema)	209 (26.1%)	8 (24.2%)	0.798
Acute or chronic cholecystitis	584 (72.8%)	25 (75.8%)	
Pathologic details			
Acute cholecystitis	242 (30.2%)	13 (39.4%)	NA
Chronic cholecystitis	342 (42.6%)	12 (36.4%)	
Gangrenous GB (gangrenous, ulceration, empyema)	209 (26.1%)	8 (24.2%)	
GB cancer	9 (1.1%)	0 (0.0%)	
Surgical approach			
Open surgery	77 (9.6%)	12 (36.4%)	<0.001
Laparoscopic surgery	725 (90.4%)	21 (63.6%)	
Surgical extent			
Only cholecystectomy	767 (95.6%)	26 (78.8%)	<0.001
Extended surgery	35 (4.4%)	7 (21.2%)	
Surgical method details			
Open cholecystectomy	54 (6.7%)	6 (18.2%)	NA
Laparoscopic cholecystectomy	713 (88.9%)	20 (60.6%)	
OC + Choledocolithotomy	20 (2.5%)	6 (18.2%)	
LC + Choledocolithotomy	12 (1.5%)	1 (3.0%)	
Cholecystectomy with another operation (Small bowel resection, colon resection)	1 (0.1%)	0 (0.0%)	
Radical cholecystectomy	2 (0.2%)	0 (0.0%)	

ASA: American Society of Anesthesiology, BMI: body mass index, kg/m^2, ICU: intensive care unit, ER: emergency room, NA: not applicable, OC: open cholecystectomy, LC: laparoscopic cholecystectomy.

A total of 44 patients who underwent gastrectomy were divided into subtotal gastrectomy and total gastrectomy groups for comparative analysis (Table 5). There were no differences in age, sex, and BMI between the two groups. In addition, there were no differences in surgical approach, surgical extent, and the severity of cholecystitis between the groups. The period from gastrectomy to symptomatic cholecystitis was significantly shorter in the total gastrectomy group than in the subtotal gastrectomy group (12.72 ± 10.50 years vs. 7.25 ± 4.80 years; p = 0.040).

Table 5. Clinical characteristics according to subtotal gastrectomy and total gastrectomy.

Variable	Subtotal Gastrectomy (n = 35)	Total Gastrectomy (n = 9)	p-Value
Age (years, mean ± sd)	65.51 ± 12.15	64.89 ± 10.59	0.557
Gender			
Male	25 (71.4%)	8 (88.9%)	0.281
Female	10 (28.6%)	1 (11.1%)	
BMI (kg/m^2)	21.76 ± 3.48	21.27 ± 1.81	0.572
Previous gastrectomy type			
Subtotal gastrectomy, Billroth I	11 (31.4%)		
Subtotal gastrectomy, Billroth II	19 (54.3%)		
Subtotal gastrectomy, Roux-en-Y	4 (11.4%)		
Proximal gastrectomy	1 (2.9%)		
Total gastrectomy, Roux-en-Y		9 (100%)	
Surgical approach			
Open	13 (37.1%)	4 (44.4%)	0.688
Laparoscopic	22 (62.9%)	5 (55.6%)	
Surgical extent			
Only cholecystectomy	26 (74.3%)	6 (66.7%)	0.647
Extended surgery	9 (25.7%)	3 (33.3%)	
ASA score	2.67 ± 0.48	2.20 ± 0.83	0.095
Pathologic diagnosis			
Gangrenous cholecystitis (gangrenous, ulceration, empyema)	9 (25.7%)	3 (33.3%)	0.647
Acute or chronic cholecystitis	26 (74.3%)	6 (66.7%)	
Operation time (min, mean ± sd)	169.57 ± 80.03	158.89 ± 98.29	0.735
Gastrectomy duration (years, mean ± sd)	12.72 ± 10.5	7.25 ± 4.80	0.040
From ER to operation (days, mean ± sd)	4.97 ± 4.99	3.22 ± 2.63	0.159
Postoperative hospital stay (days, mean ± sd)	8.43 ± 5.26	7.33 ± 3.00	0.554
Hospital stay (days, mean ± sd)	13.40 ± 7.34	10.56 ± 1.59	0.258

ASA: American Society of Anesthesiology, BMI: body mass index, kg/m^2, ER: emergency room, NA: not applicable.

4. Discussion

If there is any abnormality in the GB during gastrectomy, cholecystectomy is usually performed alongside it. This is because the incidence rate of GB stones after gastrectomy is significantly higher than that in the general population, and cholecystectomy is more difficult after gastrectomy. However, it is a general treatment principle not to perform cholecystectomy in patients without any GB abnormality [7,23–25]. As the symptomatic cholecystitis patients in the gastrectomy group were older than the general population, the GB stones could have formed after the gastrectomy and led to the development of symptoms such as cholecystitis after a certain period. The relatively high proportion of male patients in the gastrectomy group seems to correlate with the relatively high incidence of gastric cancer in males. According to South Korea's nationwide gastric cancer survey published in 2019, the prevalence of gastric cancer has approximately doubled in males over the past decade [26].

The proportion of patients who underwent gastrectomy among patients hospitalized in the ER for symptomatic cholecystitis was approximately 2.8%, which is similar to that reported in other studies [27,28]. It was determined that the gastrectomy did not affect the severity of inflammation or the pathology of the GB. Along to Tokyo guideline 2018, the severity of cholecystitis depends on the patient's condition and laboratory data rather than the pathologic results, it was difficult to evaluate the relationship between the gastrectomy and the severity of cholecystitis in this study [29]. However, inflammatory markers such as WBC and CRP levels were higher, recovery in the laboratory findings was slower, and hospital stay was longer in the gastrectomy group. As previously reported, when cholecystectomy was performed in the gastrectomy group, the operation time was longer and the open surgery rate was higher [19,20]. This is attributed to the effect of severe adhesions forming after gastrectomy around the GB and the hepatoduodenal ligament. Cholecystectomy combined with choledocolithotomy was performed more frequently in the gastrectomy group (56/1543 (3.6%) vs. 12/44 (27.3%); $p < 0.001$). In this study, choledocolithotomy was also performed for CBD stone removal in 10 patients and for bile duct injury in 2 patients in the gastrectomy group. Roux-en-Y and Billroth II reconstructions in gastrectomy patients, excluding Billroth I, had much lower ERCP success rates than in the general population [30]. Because of the difficulty of ERCP, there is a possibility that the rate of choledocolithotomy was increased to complete the surgery in one stage.

In this study, it was found that the gastrectomy increased the difficulty of the cholecystitis surgery, as evidenced by the long operation times and high rates of open surgery, but did not affect the surgical complications. In addition, there was no difference in bile duct leak or stricture, one of the most important complications, between the two groups. In this study, eight patients in the non-gastrectomy group who had remnant CBD stones, bile duct leakage, and stenosis underwent ERCP after surgery. Five patients underwent endoscopic retrograde biliary drainage (ERBD), and three patients underwent endoscopic nasobiliary drainage (ENBD) to eliminate the bile duct-related complications. Considering that ERCP is difficult after gastrectomy, more attention should be paid to prevent biliary problems, particularly during surgery. There was no difference medical complications after surgery between the two groups, but the gastrectomy group had a longer hospital stay after surgery and delayed recovery of laboratory inflammation markers such as WBC and CRP levels. Thus, these findings suggest that more careful treatment is required for postoperative management in gastrectomy group.

In this study, the postoperative period for patients who underwent gastrectomy was approximately 11 years. The lower BMI and lower protein, albumin, and Hb levels of the patients appeared to be long-term nutritional effects after gastrectomy. Nutritional parameters such as protein, albumin, and Hb were lower than those of the general population, but they are all within the normal range. The gastrectomy group patients had an average BMI of 22 kg/m^2, which was lower than that of the general cholecystitis patients. The BMI of gastrectomy group was within the normal range compared to general patients with grade I obesity. Although the average age of the patients in the gastrectomy group was higher, those patients had fewer severe complications, as evidenced by their CDC grades and ICU admission rates after surgery. There was no significant difference in the medical complication rates between general patients and the gastrectomy group. Thus, some nutritional deficits can occur after long-term gastrectomy, but they do not have much effect on the general condition of the patient.

In this study, it took an average of 11.13 years for patients to develop symptomatic cholecystitis after gastrectomy. In addition, the period from gastrectomy to symptomatic cholecystitis was approximately half in the total gastrectomy group (an average of 7.54 years) compared to the distal gastrectomy group (an average of 13.58 years). The posterior vagus nerve must be sacrificed after total gastrectomy. Due to the vagus nerve damage and food material bypassing the duodenum, GB contraction is reduced and bile concentration in the GB is increased. Therefore, GB stones are more likely to occur in total gastrectomy patients than in distal gastrectomy patients [4,11,13]. In addition, the proportion of patients who underwent total gastrectomy due to symptomatic cholecystitis was higher than the proportion of patients who underwent total gastrectomy for all types of gastric cancer [26]. Several studies have reported that GB stones are more likely to develop in patients who have undergone total gastrectomy than in those who have undergone distal gastrectomy [10,28,31]. Therefore, more attention should be paid to preventing GB stones after total gastrectomy.

5. Limitations

This study had several limitations. This was a retrospective review analysis, and the gastrectomy group contained a relatively small number of patients. Therefore, comparisons between the variables may also have limited statistical significance. There were inconsistencies because the surgeries were performed by various general surgeons who would also differ in their postoperative management practices; hence, these inconsistencies should be eliminated in future studies. Due to the small sample size, it was impossible to eliminate these differences in this study. A long-term follow-up prospective and large volume study on patients who underwent gastrectomy is needed to achieve better results.

6. Conclusions

The average duration from gastrectomy to surgery due to symptomatic cholecystitis was 11.13 years. In the case of total gastrectomy, this duration was shorter than that for distal gastrectomy. Endoscopic treatment such as ERCP is more difficult, and the rate of open surgery is high after gastrectomy. Therefore, efforts to prevent GB stones, such as UDCA, should be considered for post-gastrectomy patients, especially total gastrectomy patients.

Author Contributions: Conceptualization: Y.S.C., Data curation: Y.S.C., B.C. and K.D.K., Formal analysis: Y.S.C., B.C. and S.H.K., Funding acquisition: Y.S.H., Investigation: Y.S.C. and B.C., Methodology: Y.S.C. and J.W.Y. Project administration: Y.S.C., S.H.K., M.S.C. and K.D.K., Resources: Y.S.C. and Y.S.H., Supervision: Y.S.H., Writing-original draft: Y.S.C. and B.C.; Writing-review & editing: Y.S.H. All authors have read and agreed to the published version of the manuscript.

Funding: This work was supported by the Inha University Hospital Research Grant.

Institutional Review Board Statement: This study was approved by the Institutional Review Board of Inha University Hospital. (IRB number: INH 2022-05-007).

Informed Consent Statement: Patient consent was waived due to retrospective study with medical record.

Data Availability Statement: Data sharing not applicable.

Conflicts of Interest: The authors declare no conflict of interest.

References

1. Sakorafas, G.H.; Milingos, D.; Peros, G. Asymptomatic cholelithiasis: Is cholecystectomy really needed? A critical reappraisal 15 years after the introduction of laparoscopic cholecystectomy. *Dig. Dis. Sci.* **2007**, *52*, 1313–1325. [CrossRef] [PubMed]
2. Sanders, G.; Kingsnorth, A.N. Gallstones. *BMJ* **2007**, *335*, 295–299. [CrossRef]
3. Fukagawa, T.; Katai, H.; Saka, M.; Morita, S.; Sano, T.; Sasako, M. Gallstone formation after gastric cancer surgery. *J. Gastrointest. Surg.* **2009**, *13*, 886–889. [CrossRef] [PubMed]
4. Kobayashi, T.; Hisanaga, M.; Kanehiro, H.; Yamada, Y.; Ko, S.; Nakajima, Y. Analysis of risk factors for the development of gallstones after gastrectomy. *Br. J. Surg.* **2005**, *92*, 1399–1403. [CrossRef] [PubMed]
5. Li, V.K.; Pulido, N.; Martinez-Suartez, P.; Fajnwaks, P.; Jin, H.Y.; Szomstein, S.; Rosenthal, R.J. Symptomatic gallstones after sleeve gastrectomy. *Surg. Endosc.* **2009**, *23*, 2488–2492. [CrossRef]
6. Health Insurance Review and Assessment Service. *Korea Healthcare Bigdata Hub*; Health Insurance Review and Assessment Service: Wonju, Korea, 2021. Available online: http://opendata.hira.or.kr/ (accessed on 6 January 2020).
7. Kimura, J.; Kunisaki, C.; Takagawa, R.; Makino, H.; Ueda, M.; Ota, M.; Oba, M.; Kosaka, T.; Akiyama, H.; Endo, I. Is routine prophylactic cholecystectomy necessary during gastrectomy for gastric cancer? *World J. Surg.* **2017**, *41*, 1047–1053. [CrossRef]
8. Park, D.J.; Kim, K.H.; Park, Y.S.; Ahn, S.-H.; Park, D.J.; Kim, H.-H. Risk factors for gallstone formation after surgery for gastric cancer. *J. Gastric Cancer* **2016**, *16*, 98–104. [CrossRef]
9. Iglézias Brandão de Oliveira, C.; Adami Chaim, E.; da Silva, B.B. Impact of rapid weight reduction on risk of cholelithiasis after bariatric surgery. *Obes. Surg.* **2003**, *13*, 625–628. [CrossRef]
10. Jun, K.H.; Kim, J.H.; Kim, J.J.; Chin, H.M.; Park, S.M. Retrospective analysis on the gallstone disease after gastrectomy for gastric cancer. *Gastroenterol. Res. Pract.* **2015**, *2015*, 827864. [CrossRef]
11. Yi, S.Q.; Ohta, T.; Tsuchida, A.; Terayama, H.; Naito, M.; Li, J.; Wang, H.X.; Yi, N.; Tanaka, S.; Itoh, M. Surgical anatomy of innervation of the gallbladder in humans and Suncus murinus with special reference to morphological understanding of gallstone formation after gastrectomy. *World J. Gastroenterol.* **2007**, *13*, 2066–2071. [CrossRef]
12. Inoue, K.; Fuchigami, A.; Hosotani, R.; Kogire, M.; Huang, Y.S.; Miyashita, T.; Suzuki, T.; Tsuda, K.; Seino, Y.; Rayford, P.L.; et al. Release of cholecystokinin and gallbladder contraction before and after gastrectomy. *Ann. Surg.* **1987**, *205*, 27–32. [PubMed]
13. Pezzolla, F.; Lantone, G.; Guerra, V.; Misciagna, G.; Prete, F.; Giorgio, I.; Lorusso, D. Influence of the method of digestive tract reconstruction on gallstone development after total gastrectomy for gastric cancer. *Am. J. Surg.* **1993**, *166*, 6–10. [CrossRef]

14. Boerlage, T.C.C.; Haal, S.; Maurits de Brauw, L.; Acherman, Y.I.Z.; Bruin, S.; van de Laar, A.; Moes, D.E.; van Wagensveld, B.A.; de Vries, C.E.E.; van Veen, R.; et al. Ursodeoxycholic acid for the prevention of symptomatic gallstone disease after bariatric surgery: Study protocol for a randomized controlled trial (UPGRADE trial). *BMC Gastroenterol.* **2017**, *17*, 164. [CrossRef] [PubMed]
15. Haal, S.; Guman, M.S.S.; Boerlage, T.C.C.; Acherman, Y.I.Z.; de Brauw, L.M.; Bruin, S.; de Castro, S.M.M.; van Hooft, J.E.; van de Laar, A.; Moes, D.E.; et al. Ursodeoxycholic acid for the prevention of symptomatic gallstone disease after bariatric surgery (UPGRADE): A multicentre, double-blind, randomised, placebo-controlled superiority trial. *Lancet Gastroenterol. Hepatol.* **2021**, *6*, 993–1001. [CrossRef]
16. Lee, S.H.; Jang, D.K.; Yoo, M.W.; Hwang, S.H.; Ryu, S.Y.; Kwon, O.K.; Hur, H.; Man Yoon, H.; Eom, B.W.; Ahn, H.S.; et al. Efficacy and safety of ursodeoxycholic acid for the prevention of gallstone formation after gastrectomy in patients with gastric cancer: The PEGASUS-D randomized clinical trial. *JAMA Surg.* **2020**, *155*, 703–711. [CrossRef]
17. Reynolds, W., Jr. The first laparoscopic cholecystectomy. *JSLS* **2001**, *5*, 89–94.
18. Tazuma, S.; Unno, M.; Igarashi, Y.; Inui, K.; Uchiyama, K.; Kai, M.; Tsuyuguchi, T.; Maguchi, H.; Mori, T.; Yamaguchi, K.; et al. Evidence-based clinical practice guidelines for cholelithiasis 2016. *J. Gastroenterol.* **2017**, *52*, 276–300. [CrossRef]
19. Fraser, S.A.; Sigman, H. Conversion in laparoscopic cholecystectomy after gastric resection: A 15-year review. *Can. J. Surg.* **2009**, *52*, 463–466.
20. Sasaki, A.; Nakajima, J.; Nitta, H.; Obuchi, T.; Baba, S.; Wakabayashi, G. Laparoscopic cholecystectomy in patients with a history of gastrectomy. *Surg. Today* **2008**, *38*, 790–794. [CrossRef]
21. Ercan, M.; Bostanci, E.B.; Ulas, M.; Ozer, I.; Ozogul, Y.; Seven, C.; Atalay, F.; Akoglu, M. Effects of previous abdominal surgery incision type on complications and conversion rate in laparoscopic cholecystectomy. *Surg. Laparosc. Endosc. Percutan. Tech.* **2009**, *19*, 373–378. [CrossRef]
22. Zhang, M.-J.; Yan, Q.; Zhang, G.-L.; Zhou, S.-Y.; Yuan, W.-B.; Shen, H.-P. Laparoscopic cholecystectomy in patients with history of gastrectomy. *JSLS* **2016**, *20*, e2016.00075. [CrossRef] [PubMed]
23. Bencini, L.; Marchet, A.; Alfieri, S.; Rosa, F.; Verlato, G.; Marrelli, D.; Roviello, F.; Pacelli, F.; Cristadoro, L.; Taddei, A.; et al. The Cholegas trial: Long-term results of prophylactic cholecystectomy during gastrectomy for cancer-a randomized-controlled trial. *Gastric Cancer* **2019**, *22*, 632–639. [CrossRef] [PubMed]
24. Dakour-Aridi, H.N.; El-Rayess, H.M.; Abou-Abbass, H.; Abu-Gheida, I.; Habib, R.H.; Safadi, B.Y. Safety of concomitant cholecystectomy at the time of laparoscopic sleeve gastrectomy: Analysis of the American College of Surgeons National Surgical Quality Improvement Program database. *Surg. Obes. Relat. Dis.* **2017**, *13*, 934–941. [CrossRef]
25. Yardimci, S.; Coskun, M.; Demircioglu, S.; Erdim, A.; Cingi, A. Is concomitant cholecystectomy necessary for asymptomatic cholelithiasis during laparoscopic sleeve gastrectomy? *Obes. Surg.* **2018**, *28*, 469–473. [CrossRef] [PubMed]
26. Information Committee of the Korean Gastric Cancer Association. Korean Gastric Cancer Association-led nationwide survey on surgically treated gastric cancers in 2019. *J. Gastric Cancer* **2021**, *21*, 221–235. [CrossRef] [PubMed]
27. Harino, T.; Tomimaru, Y.; Yokota, Y.; Noguchi, K.; Shimizu, J.; Taguchi, T.; Yanagimoto, Y.; Suzuki, Y.; Hirota, M.; Tanida, T.; et al. Surgical outcome of laparoscopic cholecystectomy in patients with a history of gastrectomy. *Surg. Laparosc. Endosc. Percutaneous Tech.* **2020**, *31*, 170–174. [CrossRef]
28. Liang, T.J.; Liu, S.I.; Chen, Y.C.; Chang, P.M.; Huang, W.C.; Chang, H.T.; Chen, I.S. Analysis of gallstone disease after gastric cancer surgery. *Gastric Cancer* **2017**, *20*, 895–903. [CrossRef]
29. Yokoe, M.; Hata, J.; Takada, T.; Strasberg, S.M.; Asbun, H.J.; Wakabayashi, G.; Kozaka, K.; Endo, I.; Deziel, D.J.; Miura, F.; et al. Tokyo Guidelines 2018: Diagnostic criteria and severity grading of acute cholecystitis (with videos). *J. Hepatobiliary Pancreat. Sci.* **2018**, *25*, 41–54. [CrossRef]
30. Moreels, T.G. ERCP in the patient with surgically altered anatomy. *Curr. Gastroenterol. Rep.* **2013**, *15*, 343. [CrossRef]
31. Seo, G.H.; Lim, C.S.; Chai, Y.J. Incidence of gallstones after gastric resection for gastric cancer: A nationwide claims-based study. *Ann. Surg. Treat. Res.* **2018**, *95*, 87–93. [CrossRef]

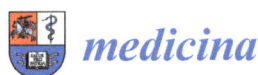

Article

Embryologic Origin of the Primary Tumor and RAS Status Predict Survival after Resection of Colorectal Liver Metastases

Sorin Tiberiu Alexandrescu [1,2], Ioana Mihaela Dinu [2,3,*], Andrei Sebastian Diaconescu [1,2], Alexandru Micu [1], Evelina Pasare [1], Cristiana Durdu [1,4], Bogdan Mihail Dorobantu [1,2] and Irinel Popescu [1]

1. Department of General Surgery, Fundeni Clinical Institute, 022328 Bucharest, Romania
2. Faculty of Medicine, Carol Davila University of Medicine and Pharmacy, 050474 Bucharest, Romania
3. Department of Oncology, Fundeni Clinical Institute, 022328 Bucharest, Romania
4. Filantropia Clinical Hospital, 011171 Bucharest, Romania
* Correspondence: dinu.zoe@drd.umfcd.ro; Tel.: +40-722461098

Citation: Alexandrescu, S.T.; Dinu, I.M.; Diaconescu, A.S.; Micu, A.; Pasare, E.; Durdu, C.; Dorobantu, B.M.; Popescu, I. Embryologic Origin of the Primary Tumor and RAS Status Predict Survival after Resection of Colorectal Liver Metastases. *Medicina* 2022, *58*, 1100. https://doi.org/10.3390/medicina58081100

Academic Editor: Maria Rosaria De Miglio

Received: 19 July 2022
Accepted: 12 August 2022
Published: 14 August 2022

Publisher's Note: MDPI stays neutral with regard to jurisdictional claims in published maps and institutional affiliations.

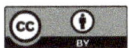

Copyright: © 2022 by the authors. Licensee MDPI, Basel, Switzerland. This article is an open access article distributed under the terms and conditions of the Creative Commons Attribution (CC BY) license (https://creativecommons.org/licenses/by/4.0/).

Abstract: *Background and objectives.* In colorectal cancers, the embryologic origin of the primary tumor determines important molecular dissimilarities between right-sided (RS) and left-sided (LS) carcinomas. Although important prognostic differences have been revealed between RS- and LS-patients with resected colorectal liver metastases (CLMs), it is still unclear if this observation depends on the RAS mutational status. To refine the impact of primary tumor location (PTL) on the long-term outcomes of patients with resected CLMs, the rates of overall survival (OS), relapse-free survival (RFS) and survival after recurrence (SAR) were compared between RS- vs. LS-patients, according to their RAS status. *Material and Methods.* All patients with known RAS status, operated until December 2019, were selected from a prospectively maintained database, including all patients who underwent hepatectomy for histologically-proven CLMs. A log-rank test was used to compare survival rates between the RS- vs. LS-group, in RAS-mut and RAS-wt patients, respectively. A multivariate analysis was performed to assess if PTL was independently associated with OS, RFS or SAR. *Results.* In 53 patients with RAS-mut CLMs, the OS, RFS and SAR rates were not significantly different ($p = 0.753$, 0.945 and 0.973, respectively) between the RS and LS group. In 89 patients with RAS-wt CLMs, the OS and SAR rates were significantly higher ($p = 0.007$ and 0.001, respectively) in the LS group vs. RS group, while RFS rates were similar ($p = 0.438$). The multivariate analysis performed in RAS-wt patients revealed that RS primary ($p = 0.009$), extrahepatic metastases ($p = 0.001$), N-positive ($p = 0.014$), age higher than 65 ($p = 0.002$) and preoperative chemotherapy ($p = 0.004$) were independently associated with worse OS, while RS location ($p < 0.001$) and N-positive ($p = 0.007$) were independent prognostic factors for poor SAR. *Conclusions.* After resection of CLMs, PTL had no impact on long-term outcomes in RAS-mut patients, while in RAS-wt patients, the RS primary was independently associated with worse OS and SAR.

Keywords: colorectal liver metastases; RAS mutational status; primary tumor sidedness; embryologic origin; liver resection; survival after recurrence

1. Introduction

Colorectal cancer is the most frequent digestive malignancy worldwide, accounting for almost 10% of cancer-related deaths [1]. The main cause of death in patients with colorectal cancer is metastatic disease. Although resection of primary tumor and metastases enables 5-year overall survival rates higher than 25% in most series reported so far, prognosis depends on clinical, pathologic, molecular and genetic factors. The embryologic origin of the primary colorectal cancer determines important molecular and pathologic dissimilarities between right-sided (RS) and left-sided (LS) carcinomas [2]. These biologic differences seem to have prognostic implications for tumors derived from midgut (RS tumors—located between caecum and splenic flexure) and those originating in the hindgut

(LS tumors—including descending and sigmoid colon, as well as rectum). During the last decade, most papers suggested that patients with unresectable metastatic RS colon carcinomas have lower overall survival (OS) rates compared to those with LS primaries [2–4]. In patients with resected colorectal liver metastases (CLMs), few reports failed to identify a significant impact of tumor sidedness on long-term outcomes [5–7]. Other studies, although they reported better OS rates after resection of CLMs in LS patients, revealed that LS tumors have similar [8,9] or even worse recurrence-free survival (RFS) rates compared to RS primaries [10]. In this fragmented landscape, some authors searched for a potential relationship between primary tumor location (PTL) and tumor mutational status. Although previous reports suggested that CLMs from RS colon cancer are associated with worse survival independent of KRAS mutational status [11–13], more recent studies suggested that a better prognostic stratification of patients with resected CLMs could be achieved by combining sidedness of the primary tumor and RAS mutational status [6,14,15]. RAS status is a well-known predictive factor for the response to anti-EGFR agents [16], but its prognostic value in patients with resected CLMs is still debatable. While some recent studies suggested that LS location is associated with better OS only in RAS-wt patients [14,17], the data about the impact of PTL on RFS rates according to the RAS status are lacking. Furthermore, the impact of primary tumor sidedness on survival after recurrence (SAR) in patients with resected CLMs has never been evaluated according to the RAS mutational status. To refine the impact of PTL on the long-term outcomes achieved by the resection of CLMs, we compared the rates of OS, RFS and SAR between LS and RS patients, according to their RAS status.

2. Materials and Methods

Since 2002, in our center, all patients who underwent curative-intent liver resection for suspected CLMs were prospectively enrolled in a database. The patients whose pathologic examination did not confirm the diagnosis of CLMs were excluded from the database. Preoperatively, the diagnosis of CLMs was established based on a contrast-enhanced CT scan, followed by a liver MRI when CT scan imaging was doubtful.

2.1. Selection of the Patients

All patients with a known RAS status, operated until December 2019, were selected from a prospectively maintained database, including all patients who underwent hepatectomy for histologically-proven CLMs in our center. Patients who died during the first 30 days post-surgery were excluded, because their death was most likely not secondary to cancer progression. Incomplete resection (R1/R2) and incomplete follow-up data were also exclusion criteria. Because the colon between the cecum and splenic flexure derives from midgut, patients with carcinomas with such a location were included in the right-sided group (RS group). Patients with primary colon tumors located distal to the splenic flexure and those with rectal carcinomas (which derive from hindgut) were included in the left-sided group (LS group). Patients with carcinomas located at the level of splenic flexure were excluded from the analysis. Similarly, patients with synchronous colorectal carcinomas located both on the right and left colon were excluded from analysis.

2.2. Molecular Diagnosis

Only mutations in exon 2 of the KRAS gene (at codons 12/13) were evaluated until 2013. After that, the tumors were subjected to full KRAS (exons 2, 3 and 4) and NRAS (exons 2, 3 and 4) analysis. Between 2006 and 2014, mutation detection was performed by High Resolution Melt Analysis (HRMA) and secondary confirmation by sequencing (ABI Prism 3130 sequencer). Since 2015, a targeted resequencing assay (Ion AmpliSeq© Panel, Thermo Fisher Scientific, Waltham, MA, USA) was used for mutation detection in exons 2, 3 and 4 of the KRAS and NRAS genes. Sequencing was carried out using the Next Generation Sequencing platform Ion proton (Thermo Fisher Scientific). Because treatment with monoclonal antibodies (either anti-EGFR or anti-VEGF agents) is recommended only in patients with unresectable metastatic colorectal cancer, in most patients RAS status was evaluated when they developed recurrence after resection of CLMs. Only in a small number of patients was RAS status evaluated immediately after liver resection (irrespective of recurrence development).

2.3. Treatment Allocation

Decisions regarding the timing of treatment were discussed in a multidisciplinary team. Patients with poor prognostic factors, such as extrahepatic disease, multiple, bilobar CLMs and initially unresectable or borderline resectable metastases, typically underwent neoadjuvant therapy. In contrast, patients with favorable prognostic factors were typically sent for up-front surgery. CLMs were considered resectable when complete clearance of the liver was anticipated before operation and the volume of the remnant liver parenchyma exceeded 30% of the total liver volume. In patients with concomitant extrahepatic metastases, surgery was recommended when complete resection of hepatic and extrahepatic metastases had been anticipated. When complete resection of metastatic disease (either hepatic or extrahepatic) could not be achieved by one or staged procedures, the operation was considered an incomplete resection and these patients were excluded from the current analysis.

Postoperative (adjuvant) chemotherapy was recommended to all the patients. Targeted therapies have never been used in the adjuvant setting for patients with completely resected CLMs, according to the international guidelines.

Only the patients with unresectable metastases from colorectal origin could benefit from the treatment with monoclonal antibodies. Thus, patients included in this study (who underwent complete resection of metastatic disease) received treatment with monoclonal antibodies associated to chemotherapy, according to the current guidelines, only after the disease's recurrence.

Although the patients enrolled in this study were treated during a long period of time (2006–2019), the oncologic therapy that was delivered to these patients was the same during this interval. Thus, chemotherapy consisted of a combination of 5-fluorouracil or capecitabine with oxaliplatin or irinotecan. During the entire period, targeted therapies consisted of anti-VEGF agent (bevacizumab) or anti-EGFR monoclonal antibodies (cetuximab or panitumumab). An assessment of the RAS status was specially performed to evaluate the possibility to give an anti-EGFR agent to the patient, because it was known since 2006 that tumors that have a RAS mutation do not respond to the anti-EGFR therapy. In such patients, the only targeted therapy available consisted of an anti-VEGF agent (bevacizumab).

2.4. Long-Term Outcomes

OS was calculated as the interval between liver resection and the date of patient's death or the last follow-up (performed by personal contact with the patient, the patient's family or the attending oncologist). RFS was calculated as the time period between hepatectomy and the date of malignancy recurrence or the last follow-up, if the patient was free of disease at that moment. SAR represents the interval between the recurrence of disease (after hepatectomy) and the death of the patient or the last follow-up (if the patient was alive at that moment). The patients who did not develop recurrent disease until the last follow-up were not included in the SAR analysis.

2.5. Prognostic Factors

To assess prognostic factors associated with long-term outcomes, the following parameters have been evaluated: age, sex, location of the primary tumor, presence of extrahepatic metastases, pathology data of colorectal tumor and liver metastases (pT, pN, maximum diameter, number and distribution of CLMs), tumor burden score (TBS), the association of ablative therapy concomitant with hepatectomy, the use of preoperative and postoperative chemotherapy as well as the presence and grade of postoperative complications. For patients with recurrent disease, the time interval between initial resection of metastases and the occurrence of recurrence was recorded. Furthermore, we recorded if the recurrent disease was resected or not. TBS was calculated according to the formula: $TBS^2 = $ (maximum tumor diameter)^2 + (number of tumors)^2, as previously published [18]. Postoperative complications were graded according to the Clavien–Dindo classification [19]. Minor complications were defined as Clavien–Dindo grades I or II, while major morbidity included complications graded III or higher according to the Clavien–Dindo classification.

2.6. Statistical Analysis

Categorical data are presented as absolute numbers and percentages. The association between categorical variables was analyzed with the Fischer exact test. Continuous data are presented as mean +/− standard deviation (SD) or as median and interquartile range [IQR25%-IQR75%], according to the tests used to evaluate the normality of distribution. Normality distribution was assessed by Shapiro–Wilk test and further comparison was performed with a t-test or Mann Whitney U test, accordingly. Survival rates were estimated with the Kaplan–Meier method and were compared between different groups by log-rank test. In a univariate analysis, the impacts of the previously mentioned parameters on OS, RFS and SAR were evaluated. The parameters that were associated with a p-value less than 0.10 at the univariate analysis were included in the multivariate analysis. A multivariate Cox proportional hazards regression analysis with a backward stepwise selection process was used to identify the independent prognostic factors associated with OS, RFS and SAR. A hazard ratio (HR) was reported with 95% confidence interval (CI). A p value lower than 0.05 was considered significant. The statistical analysis was performed using IBM SPSS software, version 23 (SPSS Inc, Chicago, IL, USA).

The study protocol, number 6571/1.02.2022, was approved by the local Institutional Review Board.

3. Results

There were 142 patients fulfilling the inclusion criteria and operated on between 2006 and 2019. Out of these, 53 had RAS-mut CLMs, while 89 had RAS-wt metastases.

3.1. RAS-Mut

There were 53 patients with resected RAS-wt CLMs fulfilling the inclusion criteria, with a mean age of 59.11 (+/−9.541) years old (p = 0.462, Shapiro–Wilk test). Out of these, 36 (67.9%) were male and 13 (24.5%) had RS primary tumors. In total, 7 patients (13.2%) had concomitant extrahepatic metastases (4—lymph nodes metastases, 2—limited peritoneal metastases and 1—ovarian metastases) that were completely resected concomitant with liver resection. Postoperative complications were recorded in 27 patients (50.9%), with 9 of them (17%) developing major morbidity. The comparative characteristics of patients with resected RAS-mut CLMs according to the primary sidedness are summarized in Table 1.

Table 1. Comparative characteristics of RAS-wt patients, according to the primary tumor location.

Clinico-Pathologic Characteristics	Right-Sided Group N (%)	Left-Sided Group N (%)	p Value (t test/Fischer's Exact Test)
Age (mean +/− SD)	58.47 (+/−10.81)	57.34 (+/−8.87)	0.6667
Sex			0.5731
Male	8 (53.3%)	32 (43.2%)	
Female	7 (46.7%)	42 (56.8%)	
Postoperative complications			1
No	8 (53.3%)	42 (56.8%)	
Yes	7 (46.7%)	32 (43.2%)	

Table 1. Cont.

Clinico-Pathologic Characteristics	Right-Sided Group N (%)	Left-Sided Group N (%)	p Value (t test/Fischer's Exact Test)
Major complications			1
No	13 (86.7%)	64 (86.5%)	
Yes	2 (13.3%)	10 (13.5%)	
Extrahepatic metastases			0.674
No	13 (86.7%)	66 (89.2%)	
Yes	2 (13.3%)	8 (10.8%)	
Extension of hepatectomy			1
Minor	12 (80%)	56 (78.4%)	
Major	3 (20%)	16 (21.6%)	
Associated ablation			0.3871
No	12 (80%)	66 (89.2%)	
Yes	3 (20%)	8 (10.8%)	
Maximum size of CLMs			0.219
≤5 cm	9 (60%)	56 (75.7%)	
>5 cm	6 (40%)	18 (24.3%)	
Maximum size of CLMs			0.2704
≤3 cm	5 (33.3%)	37 (50%)	
>3 cm	10 (66.7%)	37 (50%)	
Number of CLMS			0.7759
Single	7 (46.7%)	30 (40.5%)	
Multiple	8 (53.3%)	44 (59.5%)	
Number of CLMS			1
<4	11 (73.3%)	51 (68.9%)	
≥4	4 (26.7%)	23 (31.3%)	
TBS			1
≤4.47	7 (46.7%)	36 (48.6%)	
>4.47	8 (53.3%)	38 (51.4%)	
CLMs' distribution			0.5832
Unilobar	9 (60%)	38 (51.4%)	
Bilobar	6 (40%)	36 (48.6%)	
T-status			0.6786
T1–T3	12 (80%)	55 (74.3%)	
T4	1 (6.7%)	11 (14.9%)	
NA	2 (13.3%)	8 (10.8%)	
N-status			0.744
N−	3 (20%)	21 (28.4%)	
N+	10 (66.7%)	45 (60.8%)	
NA	2 (13.3%)	8 (10.8%)	

Table 1. Cont.

Clinico-Pathologic Characteristics	Right-Sided Group N (%)	Left-Sided Group N (%)	p Value (t test/Fischer's Exact Test)
Synchronous vs. Metachronous			0.5585
Synchronous	11 (73.3%)	46 (62.2%)	
Metachronous	4 (26.7%)	28 (37.8%)	
Initially resectable CLMs			0.4933
Yes	11 (73.3%)	60 (81.1%)	
No	4 (26.7%)	14 (18.9%)	
Preoperative chemotherapy			0.3958
No	10 (66.7%)	38 (51.4%)	
Yes	5 (33.3%)	36 (48.6%)	
Adjuvant chemotherapy			1
Yes	14 (93.3%)	68 (91.9%)	
No	1 (6.7%)	4 (5.4%)	
NA		2 (2.7%)	
Resection of recurrence *			0.1998
No	11 (84.6%)	40 (61.5%)	
Yes	2 (15.4%)	25 (38.5%)	
Time to recurrence *			0.526
≤12 months	10 (76.9%)	42 (64.6%)	
>12 months	3 (23.1%)	23 (35.4%)	

* Malignancy recurred in 78 patients (11 patients did not develop recurrence during follow-up).

Long-Term Outcomes

For the entire group, the median OS was 31 months, with 1-, 3- and 5-year OS rates of 92.4%, 48.1% and 17.8%, respectively. The 1-, 3- and 5-year OS rates were not significantly different ($p = 0.753$) between patients with LS primary tumors (94.9%, 48.8% and 15.8%, respectively) and those with RS colorectal tumors (84.6%, 46.2% and 23.1%, respectively) (Figure 1a).

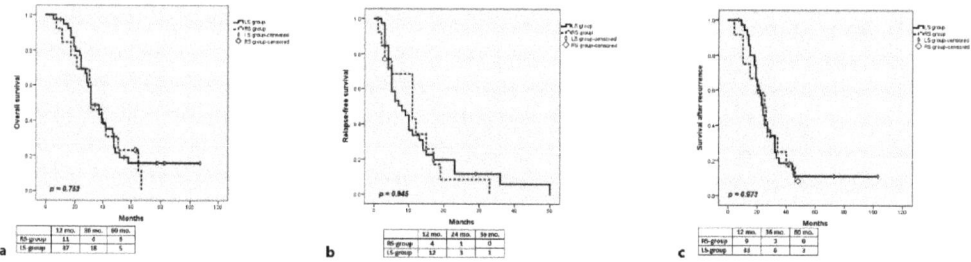

Figure 1. Comparative long-term outcomes between LS group and RS group in patients with RAS-mut CLMs; (a) overall survival; (b) relapse-free survival; (c) survival after recurrence.

After a median follow-up of 31 months, 48 patients developed recurrence: hepatic only—23 patients; hepatic and extrahepatic—10 patients; lung—7 patients; peritoneal—2 patients; lymph nodes—2 patients; local recurrence—2 patients; ovarian—1 patient; and bone—1 patient. For the entire group, the median RFS was 10 months, with 1- and 3-years RFS rates of 33.6%, and 3.6%, respectively. The RFS rates were not statistically significant different between the LS group and RS group (33.6% and 5.9% vs. 34.2% and 0% at 1- and 3-years, respectively, $p = 0.945$) (Figure 1b).

For all the patients who developed recurrence after the initial resection of CLMs, the 1-, 3- and 5-year SAR rates were 89.4%, 20.4% and 10.3%, respectively (median 24 months). The rate of SAR was similar in the LS group and RS group (94.3%, 18.6% and 11.1% vs. 75%, 25% and 0% at 1-, 3- and 5-years, respectively, $p = 0.973$) (Figure 1c).

3.2. RAS-Wt

There were 89 patients with resected RAS-wt CLMs fulfilling the inclusion criteria, with a median age of 57.53 (+/−9.169) years old ($p = 0.075$, Shapiro–Wilk test). Out of these, 50 were male (56.2%) and 15 (16.9%) had RS primary tumors. In total, 10 patients (11.2%) had concomitant extrahepatic metastases (5—limited peritoneal metastases, 3—hepatic pedicle lymph nodes metastases and 2—lung metastases) that were completely resected concomitant with CLMs (9 patients) or before hepatectomy (1 patient with lung metastases that were resected 3 months previous to liver resection). Postoperative complications were recorded in 39 patients (43.8%), with 12 of them developing major morbidity. The baseline characteristics of the patients are presented in Table 1. There were not significant differences between the LS group and RS group regarding baseline characteristics, the interval between resection of CLMs and disease recurrence or the resectability of recurrence (Table 1).

3.2.1. Long-Term Outcomes

For the entire group, the median OS was 45 months, with 1-, 3- and 5-year OS rates of 95.5%, 58.2% and 26.6%, respectively. In patients with LS primary tumors, the 1-, 3- and 5-year OS rates (97.3%, 62.5% and 28.4%, respectively) were significantly higher ($p = 0.007$) than those achieved by liver resection in the RS group (86.7%, 36.1% and 10.8%, respectively) (Figure 2a).

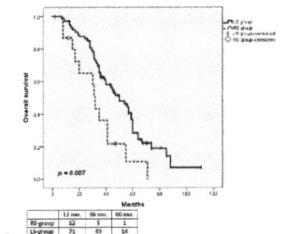
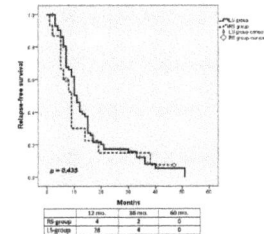
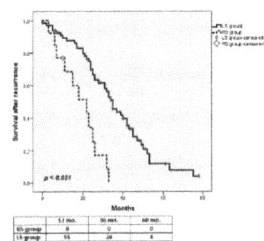

Figure 2. Comparative long-term outcomes between LS group and RS group in patients with RAS-wt CLMs; (**a**) overall survival; (**b**) relapse-free survival; (**c**) survival after recurrence.

After a median follow-up of 39 months, 78 patients developed recurrences: hepatic only—42 patients; hepatic and extrahepatic—15 patients; pulmonary—8 patients; peritoneal—4 patients; lymph nodes—4 patients; pelvic recurrence—3 patients; ovarian—1 patient; and bone—1 patient. The recurrence rate was not significantly different between the RS group (13/15) and LS group (65/74) ($p = 0.899$). For the entire group, the median RFS was 11 months, with 1- and 3-years RFS rates of 38.6% and 12.7%, respectively. The RFS rates were not statistically significant different between the LS group and RS group (40.2% and 8.1% vs. 30% and 15% at 1- and 3-years, respectively, $p = 0.438$) (Figure 2b).

Recurrent disease developed during the first year after initial resection of CLMs in 52 patients (66.7%) and after more than one year in 26 patients (33.3%). The recurrence was resected in 27 patients (34.6%): hepatic re-resection—17 patients; lung resection—6 patients; hepatic and extrahepatic resection—2 patients; oophorectomy—1 patient; and hepatic pedicle lymph nodes dissection—1 patient. Although the resectability rate of recurrence was higher in the LS group (25/65—38.4%) than in the RS group (2/13—15.3%), the difference was not statistically significant ($p = 0.199$).

For all the patients who developed recurrence after initial resection of CLMs, the 1-, 3- and 5-year SAR rates were 87.1%, 38.1% and 10%, respectively (median 33 months). The rates of SAR were significantly higher in the LS group vs. RS group (87.5%, 45.5% and 12% vs. 68.4%, 8.5% and 0% at 1-, 3- and 5-years, respectively, $p < 0.001$) (Figure 2c).

3.2.2. Univariate Analysis

Factors associated with a significantly worse OS in the univariate analysis were the RS location of the primary tumor ($p = 0.007$), extrahepatic metastases ($p = 0.014$) and metastatic lymph nodes around the primary tumor (N+) ($p = 0.004$). Age higher than 65 ($p = 0.095$) and the use of preoperative chemotherapy ($p = 0.084$) were marginally associated with poor OS in the univariate analysis (Table 2).

Table 2. Univariate and multivariate analysis for OS in RAS-wt patients.

Clinico-Pathologic Characteristics	p Value (Univariate, Log-Rank)	HR (Multivariate, Cox Regression)	95% CI (Multivariate, Cox Regression)	p Value (Multivariate, Cox Regression)
Age	0.095			*0.002*
≤65 y-o		1		
>65 y-o		0.292	0.133–0.640	
Sex	0.743			
Female				
Male				
Right vs. Left	*0.007*			*0.009*
Right-sided		0.398	0.199–0.794	
Left-sided		1		
Postoperative complications	0.672			
No				
Yes				
Major complications	0.305			
No				
Yes				
Extrahepatic metastases	*0.014*			*0.001*
No		1		
Yes		0.27	0.125–0.684	
Extension of hepatectomy	0.109			
Minor				
Major				
Associated ablation	0.463			
No				
Yes				
Maximum size of CLMs	0.394			
≤5 cm				
>5 cm				

Table 2. Cont.

Clinico-Pathologic Characteristics	p Value (Univariate, Log-Rank)	HR (Multivariate, Cox Regression)	95% CI (Multivariate, Cox Regression)	p Value (Multivariate, Cox Regression)
Maximum size of CLMs	0.88			
≤3 cm				
>3 cm				
Number of CLMS	0.324			
Single				
Multiple				
Number of CLMS	0.628			
<4				
≥4				
TBS	0.105			
≤4.47				
>4.47				
CLMs' distribution	0.765			
Unilobar				
Bilobar				
T-status	0.274			
T1-T3				
T4				
N-status	*0.004*			*0.014*
N−		1		
N+		0.426	0.216–0.841	
Synchronous vs. Metachronous	0.366			
Synchronous				
Metachronous				
Initially resectable CLMs	0.396			
Yes				
No				
Preoperative chemotherapy	0.084			*0.004*
No		1		
Yes		0.44	0.251–0.774	
Adjuvant chemotherapy	0.939			
Yes				
No				

Italic-bold: for all values lower than 0.05 (in this column).

The presence of postoperative complications ($p = 0.024$), extrahepatic disease ($p = 0.003$) and multiple CLMs ($p = 0.026$) were associated with significantly lower RFS rates in the univariate analysis (Table 3).

Table 3. Univariate and multivariate analysis for RFS in RAS-wt patients.

Clinico-Pathologic Characteristics	p Value (Univariate, Log-Rank)	HR (Multivariate, Cox Regression)	95% CI (Multivariate, Cox Regression)	p Value (Multivariate, Cox Regression)
Age	0.937			
≤65 y-o				
>65 y-o				
Sex	0.902			
Female				
Male				
Right vs. Left	0.438			
Right-sided				
Left-sided				
Postoperative complications	*0.024*			*0.024*
No		1		
Yes		0.587	0.370–0.932	
Major complications	0.441			
No				
Yes				
Extrahepatic metastases	*0.003*			*0.015*
No		1		
Yes		0.407	0.197–0.839	
Extension of hepatectomy	0.481			
Minor				
Major				
Associated ablation	0.918			
No				
Yes				
Maximum size of CLMs	0.636			
≤5 cm				
>5 cm				
Maximum size of CLMs	0.87			
≤3 cm				
>3 cm				
Number of CLMS	*0.026*			0.057
Single		1		
Multiple		0.627	0.387–1.015	
Number of CLMS	0.971			
<4				
≥4				
TBS	0.472			
≤4.47				
>4.47				

Table 3. Cont.

Clinico-Pathologic Characteristics	p Value (Univariate, Log-Rank)	HR (Multivariate, Cox Regression)	95% CI (Multivariate, Cox Regression)	p Value (Multivariate, Cox Regression)
CLMs' distribution	0.126			
Unilobar				
Bilobar				
T-status	0.903			
T1–T3				
T4				
N-status	0.188			
N−				
N+				
Synchronous vs. Metachronous	0.315			
Synchronous				
Metachronous				
Initially resectable CLMs	0.716			
Yes				
No				
Preoperative chemotherapy	0.123			
No				
Yes				
Adjuvant chemotherapy	0.383			
Yes				
No				

Italic-bold: for all values lower than 0.05 (in this column).

In the univariate analysis, the factors significantly associated with lower SAR rates were RS tumors ($p < 0.001$), N-positive primary tumor ($p = 0.011$), appearance of the recurrence during the first 12 months after resection of CLMs ($p = 0.048$) and resection of recurrence ($p = 0.007$) (Table 4).

Table 4. Univariate and multivariate analysis for SAR in RAS-wt patients.

Clinico-Pathologic Characteristics	p Value (Univariate, Log-Rank)	HR (Multivariate, Cox Regression)	95% CI (Multivariate, Cox Regression)	p Value (Multivariate, Cox Regression)
Age	0.248			
≤65 y-o				
>65 y-o				
Sex	0.796			
Female				
Male				
Right vs. Left	*<0.001*			*<0.001*
Right-sided		0.222	0.102–0.483	
Left-sided		1		

Table 4. Cont.

Clinico-Pathologic Characteristics	p Value (Univariate, Log-Rank)	HR (Multivariate, Cox Regression)	95% CI (Multivariate, Cox Regression)	p Value (Multivariate, Cox Regression)
Postoperative complications	0.415			
No				
Yes				
Major complications	0.343			
No				
Yes				
Extrahepatic metastases	0.237			
No				
Yes				
Extension of hepatectomy	0.187			
Minor				
Major				
Associated ablation	0.161			
No				
Yes				
Maximum size of CLMs	0.738			
≤5 cm				
>5 cm				
Maximum size of CLMs	0.419			
≤3 cm				
>3 cm				
Number of CLMS	0.784			
Single				
Multiple				
Number of CLMS	0.464			
<4				
≥4				
TBS	0.389			
≤4.47				
>4.47				
CLMs' distribution	0.496			
Unilobar				
Bilobar				
T-status	0.321			
T1-T3				
T4				
N-status	*0.011*			**0.007**
N−				
N+		0.407	0.211–0.786	

Table 4. Cont.

Clinico-Pathologic Characteristics	p Value (Univariate, Log-Rank)	HR (Multivariate, Cox Regression)	95% CI (Multivariate, Cox Regression)	p Value (Multivariate, Cox Regression)
Synchronous vs. Metachronous	0.447			
Synchronous				
Metachronous				
Initially resectable CLMs	0.192			
Yes				
No				
Preoperative chemotherapy	0.746			
No				
Yes				
Adjuvant chemotherapy	0.285			
Yes				
No				
Resection of recurrence	*0.007*			0.123
No		0.621	0.339–1.138	
Yes		1		
Time to recurrence	*0.048*			0.25
≤12 months		0.677	0.349–1.315	
>12 months		1		

Italic-bold: for all values lower than 0.05 (in this column).

3.2.3. Multivariate Analysis

To identify independent prognostic factors for poor long-term outcomes, characteristics that were associated with a p value < 0.01 in the univariate analysis were included in the multivariate analysis. Factors that were independently associated with poor OS were RS location of the primary tumor ($p = 0.009$), extrahepatic metastases ($p = 0.001$), N-positive primary tumor ($p = 0.014$), age higher than 65 years old ($p = 0.002$) and the use of preoperative chemotherapy ($p = 0.004$) (Table 2). For RFS, the factors independently associated with poor prognosis were postoperative complications ($p = 0.024$) and extrahepatic metastases ($p = 0.015$) (Table 3). RS tumors ($p < 0.001$) and N-positive status of the primary tumor ($p = 0.007$) were the only independent prognostic factors for poor SAR (Table 4).

4. Discussion

The data presented here argue that the prognostic stratification of patients with resected CLMs can be refined by using a combination of PTL and RAS status. Although some studies reported that liver resection achieved better OS rates in patients with LS primary tumors compared to those with RS colorectal carcinomas [8–13,20], other studies failed to identify a significant association between PTL and OS [5–7]. A meta-analysis revealed that although the RS location of the primary tumor was overall associated with poor OS, almost half of the included studies did not show significant associations between RS tumors and worse OS [21]. An explanation for these conflicting results has been suggested by a single center study published in 2020 [15], supported by a multi-center study published in 2021 [14] and strengthened by a meta-analysis published in 2022 [17], which revealed that the prognostic impact of PTL depends on the RAS status. Thus, the LS location of the primary tumor was associated with significantly better OS rates after hepatectomy for CLMs only in KRAS-wt tumors, while in patients with KRAS-mut CLMs there was not any significant difference in OS according to the PTL [14,15,17]. A similar result is reported in the present series, with PTL being independently associated with OS only in patients with resected RAS-wt CLMs. In contrast, in RAS-mut CLMs, we did not find a significant difference in OS rates in LS vs. RS patients. That observation can explain how different proportions of RAS-mut/RAS-wt patients included in previous studies which evaluated the impact of PTL regardless of the RAS status might induce a bias in the analysis of the impact of PTL on OS in these cohorts, resulting in the heterogeneous results that have been reported [22]. Thus, the higher proportion of RAS-wt CLMs observed in LS patients [6,7] might tip the scale toward higher OS rates in the LS group in those studies that evaluated the impact of PTL, irrespective of the RAS status.

Regarding the impact of PTL on RFS, previous studies generated even more conflicting results [8–10,23]. For example, 19 out of 25 studies included in a meta-analysis published in 2019 did not find a significant association between PTL and RFS [21]. Although the results of this meta-analysis revealed a marginally significant prognostic role of PTL regarding RFS, the authors concluded that the prognostic value of PTL on RFS should be regarded with caution, as long as its effect in predicting RFS was limited [21]. However, in the above-mentioned meta-analysis, the impact of PTL was not evaluated in correlation with RAS status. In light of the more recent evidence that the PTL impacts OS after resection of CLMs only in RAS-wt tumors, one may hypothesize that the results of this meta-analysis were altered by the inclusion of patients, irrespective of their RAS status. The present study refined the prognostic impact of PTL on RFS according to the RAS status, revealing that PTL has not a significant influence on RFS neither in RAS-mut CLMs, nor in RAS-wt ones. In the current study, the only factors which were independently associated with poor RFS in RAS-wt patients were the presence of extrahepatic metastases ($p = 0.015$) and development of complications after hepatectomy ($p = 0.024$). These two variables were also reported as independent prognostic factors for poor RFS in many other studies [5,24,25].

Although two previous studies revealed that patients with RS tumors had worse SAR, the authors did not investigate whether this observation is independent or not of RAS mutational status [8,10]. To address this question, the current study also investigated the impact of the embryologic origin of colorectal cancer on SAR in patients with resected CLMs, according to the RAS status. Although in RAS-mut patients the siddeness of the primary tumor had no impact on SAR, in patients with RAS-wt CLMs, the PTL had been independently associated with SAR ($p < 0.001$). One could hypothesize that better SAR rates in the LS group may be due to a higher resectability rate of the recurrence in these patients. This hypothesis cannot be supported by our results, as long as the resectability rates were not significantly different between the two groups. Moreover, although in the univariate analysis the resection of recurrent disease has been significantly associated ($p = 0.007$) with better SAR, it was not independently associated with SAR in the multivariate analysis. These observations rather suggest the reduced efficacy of current oncologic therapies in patients with RS primary colon cancer who develop recurrence after resection of RAS-wt CLMs, compared to those with LS tumors. A similar finding has been reported by a recent study, which revealed that in RAS-wt patients, primary tumor sidedness was strongly associated with OS, irrespective of the type of biological agent that was used (EGFR-inhibitor or bevacizumab) [26]. The above-mentioned study revealed that despite receipt of an EGFR-inhibitor or bevacizumab, sidedness plays the most important role in OS of patients with unresected CLMs [26]. These results are in line with those of a recent meta-analysis of 12 randomized trials, which found that in medically treated patients with unresectable metastatic colorectal cancer, the prognostic value of PTL was restricted to the KRAS wild-type population [27]. To the best of our knowledge, the current study is the first one that investigated the impact of tumor sidedness on SAR in patients with resected CLMs according to the RAS mutational status. Our results disclose for the first time that the better OS observed in the LS group after resection of RAS-wt CLMs is mainly attributable to a significantly higher SAR rate in this group of patients.

Since the RFS rates after hepatectomy are similar irrespective of PTL and RAS status, liver resection should not be discouraged in patients with RS primary tumors. The lower OS and SAR rates achieved by onco-surgical approaches in patients with RS primary tumors and RAS-wt CLMs rather emphasize the need for more efficient oncologic therapies in these patients.

Several observations could explain the worse long-term outcomes of patients with RS colon cancer and RAS-wt CLMs. Because RAS- and BRAF-mutations are typically mutually exclusive in patients with CLMs, it could be estimated that up to 10% of patients with RAS-wt CLMs from this series harbor a BRAF mutation [28,29]. In patients with metastatic colorectal cancer, BRAF-mut portends a significantly worse prognosis [11,28–30], and is associated with both a lack of response to anti-EGFR therapy [31] and a decreased resectability rate of recurrence after the initial resection of CLMs [32]. As RS primary tumors are more frequently associated with BRAF-mutations than the LS colorectal cancers [11,28], that can tip the balance of OS and SAR in favor of the LS group. Furthermore, RS carcinomas are more likely associated with microsatellite instability (MSI) than LS colorectal cancers [11,33]. Regarding the impact of MSI on the long-term outcomes of patients who underwent surgery for CLMs, a recent study including patients treated with resection and/or ablation for CLMs revealed that OS was significantly lower in the MSI group ($p < 0.001$), while local or distant progression-free survival rates were not significantly different between the MSI and MSS groups [34]. The lack of evaluation for other molecular alterations (e.g., BRAF status, MSI status, TP53, etc.) in the current series represent a limitation of this study. Thus, this study cannot draw a definitive conclusion on the mechanisms that determine a different prognosis in patients with resected CLMs according to the PTL, but could offer a basis for including patients with resected CLMs in distinct prognostic groups in future studies aiming to assess the molecular basis that determines dissimilar survival outcomes in LS vs. RS patients.

Another limitation of this study is its retrospective nature. For example, patients operated until 2013 were not tested for NRAS and KRAS exon 3,4 mutations, and consequently, some of them could be misclassified as RAS-wt. Because only 19 RAS-wt patients included in this study were operated on between 2006 and 2012 and the rate of additional RAS mutations is less than 15% in KRAS exon 2-wt patients [35], we estimate that up to 5 patients from this cohort might be misclassified as RAS-wt. It is unlikely that such a small proportion of misclassified patients (3.5%) could lead to an important bias in survival rates. Another limitation that could be perceived for this study is that the RAS mutational status was assessed, in most patients, at the time of recurrence development after initial hepatectomy. This is due to the fact that the use of monoclonal antibodies is not recommended in the adjuvant setting after the complete resection of CLMs, being indicated only in the palliative therapy of patients with CLMs. Thus, a lot of the patients operated in our center who did not develop recurrence after hepatectomy were not included in this study, as their RAS mutational status was not evaluated. That may explain the lower OS and RFS rates reported in this cohort, but had no influence on SAR rates. One could consider that another shortcoming of this study is the inclusion of the left colon cancers and rectal adenocarcinomas in the same group. The reason was their common embryologic origin and their similar outcomes compared to right-sided colon carcinomas. Although a recent study suggested that OS rates achieved by metastasectomy for CLMs were similar in patients with rectal cancers and right-sided primaries [15], most studies dealing with this subject reported similar long-term outcomes achieved by liver resection for CLMs in patients with left-sided colon cancers and rectal carcinomas [3,34,36]. Furthermore, a meta-analysis published in 2022 revealed that the variable effect of KRAS status on PTL persisted, regardless of whether the patients with rectal tumors were included or not in the LS group [17].

5. Conclusions

The effect of the embryologic origin of colorectal cancers on long-term outcomes after the resection of CLMs depends on the RAS mutational status. In RAS-mut CLMs, the primary tumor location has no impact on long-term outcomes. In RAS-wt patients, the

RS location of the primary is independently associated with poorer OS and SAR, but not with RFS. In patients with resected CLMs, PTL enables prognostic stratification only for RAS-wt tumors.

Author Contributions: Conceptualization: S.T.A., I.M.D. and I.P.; Data curation: C.D., I.M.D., A.S.D. and E.P.; Methodology: A.M. and A.S.D.; Formal analysis and investigation: B.M.D. and S.T.A.; Writing—original draft preparation: S.T.A. and E.P.; Writing—review and editing: I.M.D. and A.M.; Supervision: I.P. All authors have read and agreed to the published version of the manuscript.

Funding: This research received no external funding.

Institutional Review Board Statement: The study protocol was approved by the local Institutional Review Board (Ethics Council of Fundeni Clinical Institute) with the number 6571/1.02.2022.

Informed Consent Statement: Written informed consent was obtained from all the patients before the procedure, as part of our protocol for surgery.

Data Availability Statement: The datasets are not publicly available but are available from the corresponding author on reasonable request.

Conflicts of Interest: Author Alexandrescu Sorin Tiberiu has received speaker honoraria from the Merck company. Author Dinu Ioana Mihaela has received speaker honoraria from the Amgen, Merck and Roche companies. Authors Popescu Irinel, Diaconescu Andrei Sebastian, Micu Alexandru, Pasare Evelina, Durdu Cristiana and Dorobantu Bogdan Mihail declare they have no financial interests.

References

1. Sung, H.; Ferlay, J.; Siegel, R.L.; Laversanne, M.; Soerjomataram, I.; Jemal, A.; Bray, F. Global Cancer Statistics 2020: GLOBOCAN Estimates of Incidence and Mortality Worldwide for 36 Cancers in 185 Countries. *CA Cancer J. Clin.* **2021**, *71*, 209–249. [CrossRef]
2. Tejpar, S.; Stintzing, S.; Ciardiello, F.; Tabernero, J.; Van Cutsem, E.; Beier, F.; Esser, R.; Lenz, H.-J.; Heinemann, V. Prognostic and Predictive Relevance of Primary Tumor Location in Patients With RAS Wild-Type Metastatic Colorectal Cancer Retrospective Analyses of the CRYSTAL and FIRE-3 Trials. *JAMA Oncol.* **2017**, *3*, 194–201. [CrossRef]
3. Price, T.J.; Beeke, C.; Ullah, S.; Padbury, R.; Maddern, G.; Roder, D.; Townsend, A.R.; Moore, J.; Roy, A.; Tomita, Y.; et al. Does the primary site of colorectal cancer impact outcomes for patients with metastatic disease? *Cancer* **2014**, *121*, 830–835. [CrossRef]
4. Loupakis, F.; Yang, D.; Yau, L.; Feng, S.; Cremolini, C.; Zhang, W.; Maus, M.K.H.; Antoniotti, C.; Langer, C.; Scherer, S.J.; et al. Primary Tumor Location as a Prognostic Factor in Metastatic Colorectal Cancer. *JNCI J. Natl. Cancer Inst.* **2015**, *107*, dju427. [CrossRef] [PubMed]
5. Scherman, P.; Syk, I.; Holmberg, E.; Naredi, P.; Rizell, M. Influence of primary tumour and patient factors on survival in patients undergoing curative resection and treatment for liver metastases from colorectal cancer. *BJS Open* **2019**, *4*, 118–132. [CrossRef]
6. Wang, K.; Xu, D.; Yan, X.-L.; Poston, G.; Xing, B.-C. The impact of primary tumour location in patients undergoing hepatic resection for colorectal liver metastasis. *Eur. J. Surg. Oncol.* **2018**, *44*, 771–777. [CrossRef] [PubMed]
7. Marques, M.C.; Ribeiro, H.S.C.; Costa, W.L.; De Jesus, V.H.F.; De Macedo, M.P.; Diniz, A.L.; Godoy, A.; Farias, I.C.; Aguiar, S.; Riechelmann, R.S.P.; et al. Is primary sidedness a prognostic factor in patients with resected colon cancer liver metastases (CLM)? *J. Surg. Oncol.* **2018**, *117*, 858–863. [CrossRef] [PubMed]
8. Creasy, J.M.; Sadot, E.; Koerkamp, B.G.; Chou, J.F.; Gonen, M.; Kemeny, N.E.; Saltz, L.B.; Balachandran, V.P.; Kingham, T.P.; DeMatteo, R.P.; et al. The Impact of Primary Tumor Location on Long-Term Survival in Patients Undergoing Hepatic Resection for Metastatic Colon Cancer. *Ann. Surg. Oncol.* **2017**, *25*, 431–438. [CrossRef] [PubMed]
9. Gasser, E.; Braunwarth, E.; Riedmann, M.; Cardini, B.; Fadinger, N.; Presl, J.; Klieser, E.; Ellmerer, P.; Dupré, A.; Imai, K.; et al. Primary tumour location affects survival after resection of colorectal liver metastases: A two-institutional cohort study with international validation, systematic meta-analysis and a clinical risk score. *PLoS ONE* **2019**, *14*, e0217411. [CrossRef] [PubMed]
10. Sasaki, K.; Andreatos, N.; Margonis, G.A.; He, J.; Weiss, M.; Johnston, F.; Wolfgang, C.; Antoniou, E.; Pikoulis, E.; Pawlik, T.M. The prognostic implications of primary colorectal tumor location on recurrence and overall survival in patients undergoing resection for colorectal liver metastasis. *J. Surg. Oncol.* **2016**, *114*, 803–809. [CrossRef]
11. Missiaglia, E.; Jacobs, B.; D'Ario, G.; Di Narzo, A.; Soneson, C.; Budinska, E.; Popovici, V.; Vecchione, L.; Gerster, S.; Yan, P.; et al. Distal and proximal colon cancers differ in terms of molecular, pathological, and clinical features. *Ann. Oncol.* **2014**, *25*, 1995–2001. [CrossRef]
12. Yamashita, S.; Brudvik, K.W.; Kopetz, S.; Maru, D.; Clarke, C.N.; Passot, G.; Conrad, C.; Chun, Y.S.; Aloia, T.A.; Vauthey, J.-N. Embryonic Origin of Primary Colon Cancer Predicts Pathologic Response and Survival in Patients Undergoing Resection for Colon Cancer Liver Metastases. *Ann. Surg.* **2018**, *267*, 514–520. [CrossRef]
13. Goffredo, P.; Utria, A.F.; Beck, A.C.; Chun, Y.S.; Howe, J.R.; Weigel, R.J.; Vauthey, J.-N.; Hassan, I. The Prognostic Impact of KRAS Mutation in Patients Having Curative Resection of Synchronous Colorectal Liver Metastases. *J. Gastrointest. Surg.* **2018**, *23*, 1957–1963. [CrossRef]

14. Margonis, G.A.; Amini, N.; Buettner, S.; Kim, Y.; Wang, J.; Andreatos, N.; Wagner, D.; Sasaki, K.; Beer, A.; Kamphues, C.; et al. The Prognostic Impact of Primary Tumor Site Differs According to the KRAS Mutational Status: A Study By the International Genetic Consortium for Colorectal Liver Metastasis. *Ann. Surg.* **2019**, *273*, 1165–1172. [CrossRef]
15. Chen, T.-H.; Chen, W.-S.; Jiang, J.-K.; Yang, S.-H.; Wang, H.-S.; Chang, S.-C.; Lan, Y.-T.; Lin, C.-C.; Lin, H.-H.; Huang, S.-C.; et al. Effect of Primary Tumor Location on Postmetastasectomy Survival in Patients with Colorectal Cancer Liver Metastasis. *J. Gastrointest. Surg.* **2020**, *25*, 650–661. [CrossRef]
16. Lièvre, A.; Bachet, J.-B.; Le Corre, D.; Boige, V.; Landi, B.; Emile, J.-F.; Coôté, J.-F.; Tomasic, G.; Penna, C.; Ducreux, M.; et al. KRAS Mutation Status Is Predictive of Response to Cetuximab Therapy in Colorectal Cancer. *Cancer Res.* **2006**, *66*, 3992–3995. [CrossRef]
17. Belias, M.; Sasaki, K.; Wang, J.; Andreatos, N.; Kamphues, C.; Kyriakos, G.; Seeliger, H.; Beyer, K.; Kreis, M.E.; Margonis, G.A. Is Laterality Prognostic in Resected KRAS-Mutated Colorectal Liver Metastases? A Systematic Review and Meta-Analysis. *Cancers* **2022**, *14*, 799. [CrossRef]
18. Sasaki, K.; Morioka, D.; Conci, S.; Margonis, G.A.; Sawada, Y.; Ruzzenente, A.; Kumamoto, T.; Iacono, C.; Andreatos, N.; Guglielmi, A.; et al. The Tumor Burden Score: A New "Metro-ticket" Prognostic Tool For Colorectal Liver Metastases Based on Tumor Size and Number of Tumors. *Ann. Surg.* **2018**, *267*, 132–141. [CrossRef]
19. Dindo, D.; Demartines, N.; Clavien, P.-A. Classification of Surgical Complications: A new proposal with evaluation in a cohort of 6336 patients and results of a survey. *Ann. Surg.* **2004**, *240*, 205–213. [CrossRef]
20. Sawada, Y.; Sahara, K.; Endo, I.; Sakamoto, K.; Honda, G.; Beppu, T.; Kotake, K.; Yamamoto, M.; Takahashi, K.; Hasegawa, K.; et al. Long-term outcome of liver resection for colorectal metastases in the presence of extrahepatic disease: A multi-institutional Japanese study. *J. Hepato-Biliary-Pancreat. Sci.* **2020**, *27*, 810–818. [CrossRef]
21. Wang, X.-Y.; Zhang, R.; Wang, Z.; Geng, Y.; Lin, J.; Ma, K.; Zuo, J.-L.; Lu, L.; Zhang, J.-B.; Zhu, W.-W.; et al. Meta-analysis of the association between primary tumour location and prognosis after surgical resection of colorectal liver metastases. *Br. J. Surg.* **2019**, *106*, 1747–1760. [CrossRef]
22. Brudvik, K.W.; Kopetz, S.E.; Li, L.; Conrad, C.; Aloia, T.A.; Vauthey, J. Meta-analysis of KRAS mutations and survival after resection of colorectal liver metastases. *Br. J. Surg.* **2015**, *102*, 1175–1183. [CrossRef]
23. Dupré, A.; Malik, H.Z.; Jones, R.P.; Diaz-Nieto, R.; Fenwick, S.W.; Poston, G.J. Influence of the primary tumour location in patients undergoing surgery for colorectal liver metastases. *Eur. J. Surg. Oncol.* **2018**, *44*, 80–86. [CrossRef] [PubMed]
24. Dorcaratto, D.; Mazzinari, G.; Fernández-Moreno, M.-C.; Muñoz, E.; Garcés-Albir, M.; Ortega, J.; Sabater, L. Impact of Postoperative Complications on Survival and Recurrence After Resection of Colorectal Liver Metastases: Systematic Review and Meta-analysis. *Ann. Surg.* **2019**, *270*, 1018–1027. [CrossRef]
25. Viganò, L.; Gentile, D.; Galvanin, J.; Corleone, P.; Costa, G.; Cimino, M.; Procopio, F.; Torzilli, G. Very Early Recurrence After Liver Resection for Colorectal Metastases: Incidence, Risk Factors, and Prognostic Impact. *J. Gastrointest. Surg.* **2021**, *26*, 570–582. [CrossRef]
26. Kamran, S.C.; Clark, J.W.; Zheng, H.; Borger, D.R.; Blaszkowsky, L.S.; Allen, J.N.; Kwak, E.L.; Wo, J.Y.; Parikh, A.R.; Nipp, R.D.; et al. Primary tumor sidedness is an independent prognostic marker for survival in metastatic colorectal cancer: Results from a large retrospective cohort with mutational analysis. *Cancer Med.* **2018**, *7*, 2934–2942. [CrossRef]
27. Yin, J.; Cohen, R.; Jin, Z.; Liu, H.; Pederson, L.; Adams, R.; Grothey, A.; Maughan, T.S.; Venook, A.; Van Cutsem, E.; et al. Prognostic and Predictive Impact of Primary Tumor Sidedness for Previously Untreated Advanced Colorectal Cancer. *JNCI J. Natl. Cancer Inst.* **2021**, *113*, 1705–1713. [CrossRef] [PubMed]
28. Margonis, G.A.; Buettner, S.; Andreatos, N.; Kim, Y.; Wagner, D.; Sasaki, K.; Beer, A.; Schwarz, C.; Loes, I.M.; Smolle, M.; et al. Association of BRAF Mutations With Survival and Recurrence in Surgically Treated Patients With Metastatic Colorectal Liver Cancer. *JAMA Surg.* **2018**, *153*, e180996. [CrossRef]
29. Schirripa, M.; Bergamo, F.; Cremolini, C.; Casagrande, M.; Lonardi, S.; Aprile, G.; Yang, D.; Marmorino, F.; Pasquini, G.; Sensi, E.; et al. BRAF and RAS mutations as prognostic factors in metastatic colorectal cancer patients undergoing liver resection. *Br. J. Cancer* **2015**, *112*, 1921–1928. [CrossRef]
30. Gagnière, J.; Dupré, A.; Gholami, S.S.; Pezet, D.; Boerner, T.; Gönen, M.; Kingham, T.P.; Allen, P.J.; Balachandran, V.P.; De Matteo, R.P.; et al. Is Hepatectomy Justified for BRAF Mutant Colorectal Liver Metastases?: A Multi-institutional Analysis of 1497 Patients. *Ann. Surg.* **2020**, *271*, 147–154. [CrossRef]
31. Hsu, H.-C.; Thiam, T.K.; Lu, Y.-J.; Yeh, C.Y.; Tsai, W.-S.; You, J.F.; Hung, H.Y.; Tsai, C.-N.; Hsu, A.; Chen, H.-C.; et al. Mutations of KRAS/NRAS/BRAF predict cetuximab resistance in metastatic colorectal cancer patients. *Oncotarget* **2016**, *7*, 22257–22270. [CrossRef]
32. Kobayashi, S.; Takahashi, S.; Takahashi, N.; Masuishi, T.; Shoji, H.; Shinozaki, E.; Yamaguchi, T.; Kojima, M.; Gotohda, N.; Nomura, S.; et al. Survival Outcomes of Resected BRAF V600E Mutant Colorectal Liver Metastases: A Multicenter Retrospective Cohort Study in Japan. *Ann. Surg. Oncol.* **2020**, *27*, 3307–3315. [CrossRef] [PubMed]
33. Fujiyoshi, K.; Yamamoto, G.; Takenoya, T.; Takahashi, A.; Arai, Y.; Yamada, M.; Kakuta, M.; Yamaguchi, K.; Akagi, Y.; Nishimura, Y.; et al. Metastatic Pattern of Stage IV Colorectal Cancer with High-Frequency Microsatellite Instability as a Prognostic Factor. *Anticancer Res.* **2017**, *37*, 239–248. [CrossRef] [PubMed]

34. Dijkstra, M.; Nieuwenhuizen, S.; Puijk, R.; Timmer, F.; Geboers, B.; Schouten, E.; Opperman, J.; Scheffer, H.; de Vries, J.; Versteeg, K.; et al. Primary Tumor Sidedness, RAS and BRAF Mutations and MSI Status as Prognostic Factors in Patients with Colorectal Liver Metastases Treated with Surgery and Thermal Ablation: Results from the Amsterdam Colorectal Liver Met Registry (AmCORE). *Biomedicines* **2021**, *9*, 962. [CrossRef] [PubMed]
35. Schirripa, M.; Cremolini, C.; Loupakis, F.; Morvillo, M.; Bergamo, F.; Zoratto, F.; Salvatore, L.; Antoniotti, C.; Marmorino, F.; Sensi, E.; et al. Role of NRAS mutations as prognostic and predictive markers in metastatic colorectal cancer: NRAS mutations as prognostic and predictive markers in mCRC. *Int. J. Cancer* **2014**, *136*, 83–90. [CrossRef] [PubMed]
36. Bingmer, K.; Ofshteyn, A.; Bliggenstorfer, J.T.; Kethman, W.; Ammori, J.B.; Charles, R.; Stein, S.L.; Steinhagen, E. Primary tumor location impacts survival in colorectal cancer patients after resection of liver metastases. *J. Surg. Oncol.* **2020**, *122*, 745–752. [CrossRef] [PubMed]

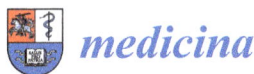

Review

Mental Illnesses in Inflammatory Bowel Diseases: *mens sana in corpore sano*

Bianca Bartocci [1,2], Arianna Dal Buono [1], Roberto Gabbiadini [1], Anita Busacca [1], Alessandro Quadarella [1], Alessandro Repici [2], Emanuela Mencaglia [3], Linda Gasparini [4] and Alessandro Armuzzi [1,2,*]

1 IBD Center, Humanitas Research Hospital-IRCCS, Via Manzoni 56, Rozzano, 20089 Milan, Italy
2 Department of Biomedical Sciences, Humanitas University, Pieve Emanuele, 20072 Milan, Italy
3 Medical Oncology and Haematology Unit, Humanitas Cancer Center, Humanitas Research Hospital IRCCS, Via Manzoni 56, Rozzano, 20089 Milan, Italy
4 Child Neuropsychiatry Unit, Niguarda Hospital, 20162 Milan, Italy
* Correspondence: alessandro.armuzzi@hunimed.eu

Abstract: *Background and aims*: Inflammatory bowel diseases (IBD) are chronic disorders associated with a reduced quality of life, and patients often also suffer from psychiatric comorbidities. Overall, both mood and cognitive disorders are prevalent in chronic organic diseases, especially in the case of a strong immune component, such as rheumatoid arthritis, multiple sclerosis, and cancer. Divergent data regarding the true incidence and prevalence of mental disorders in patients with IBD are available. We aimed to review the current evidence on the topic and the burden of mental illness in IBD patients, the role of the brain–gut axis in their co-existence, and its implication in an integrated clinical management. *Methods*: PubMed was searched to identify relevant studies investigating the gut–brain interactions and the incidence and prevalence of psychiatric disorders, especially of depression, anxiety, and cognitive dysfunction in the IBD population. *Results*: Among IBD patients, there is a high prevalence of psychiatric comorbidities, especially of anxiety and depression. Approximately 20–30% of IBD patients are affected by mood disorders and/or present with anxiety symptoms. Furthermore, it has been observed that the prevalence of mental illnesses increases in patients with active intestinal disease. Psychiatric comorbidities continue to be under-diagnosed in IBD patients and remain an unresolved issue in the management of these patients. *Conclusions*: Psychiatric illnesses co-occurring in IBD patients deserve acknowledgment from IBD specialists. These comorbidities highly impact the management of IBD patients and should be studied as an adjunctive therapeutic target.

Keywords: mental illnesses; inflammatory bowel disease; disability; anxiety; quality of life

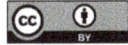

1. Introduction

Inflammatory bowel diseases (IBDs), including ulcerative colitis (UC) and Crohn's disease (CD), are chronic conditions affecting the intestinal wall with a relapsing–remitting behavior [1,2]. The pathogenesis of IBDs remain unknown, but a variety of risks and triggering factors have been recognized, including host genetics, immune dysregulation, and gut microbiota alterations [3]. The natural history of IBD is characterized by periods of quiescence interspersed with episodic flares of disease activity [1–3]. IBD markedly impacts the quality of life (QoL) and lifestyle of the affected patients [4], and it is known that patients with IBD might frequently present mental disorders, such as anxiety and depression [5]. However, the biological basis and explanation of the burden of mental illnesses in IBD patients is not fully established, and it is still unclear to what extent these diseases co-occur and in what sequence they mutually develop [6]. The relationship between IBD and psychological factors is a rather old issue: as early as 1930, it was noted that emotional factors and personal experiences were correlated with the severity of the disease, to the point of considering IBDs psychosomatic disorders [7]. The effects of living with the diagnosis of CD or UC on the patients' psychosocial sphere and QoL has been assessed throughout the last decades [8].

Indeed, in IBD patients, the worsening of the QoL is mainly attributable to the juvenile onset, the chronic nature of the disease, and the unpredictable severity of symptoms and their significant impact on social life [7,8]. These factors have a detrimental effect on the ability of the affected person to carry out routine daily activities, resulting in lower working capacity, a higher likelihood of being unemployed, and diminished economic capacity [9]. Therefore, on the one hand, the diagnosis of IBD itself significantly impacts the mental health of the subject; on the other hand, once intestinal disease develops, the unpredictability, uncertainty, and chronic course of the disease can lead to additional consequences for the patient, such as social isolation, stigmatization, shame of one's condition, dissatisfaction with one's body image, and a feeling of poor body hygiene and sexual inadequacy [9,10].

In the management of IBD, psychological distress deserves particular consideration since it does not only affect patient's QoL, but is also associated with increased disease activity, higher frequency of relapse, and greater use of health services [11].

It has been recognized that the individual response to stress depends on the personal perception of the stressful event, which is more heightened in subjects with IBD [7,12]. In fact, several studies have demonstrated that psychological distress and its personal perception by IBD patients can influence worse health outcomes [12]. In a prospective study of patients with UC in clinical remission, long-term perceived stress tripled the risk of exacerbation of disease [13], and, interestingly, this association remained after adjusting for possible confounding factors (i.e., shorter sleep, shorter remission) [13].

Among psychiatric illnesses, anxiety and depression are the disorders most frequently associated with IBD [3]. In the attempt to causatively link IBD and psychiatric disorders, a great body of research focused on the central role of the gut–brain axis [6].

In the last years, the relationship between mental illness and IBD has received considerable interest; observational studies have shown that pre-existing psychiatric morbidity is associated with adverse outcomes during IBD longitudinal follow-up, and the inflammatory activity is associated with the de novo development of psychological disorders [14]. Psychological stress has been addressed as a possible cause of the altered permeability of the intestinal mucosa, with subsequent cytokine secretion [15]; this mechanism possibly influences the risk of relapse and disease severity of IBD. Among the potential predictors of mental illness, a history of previous surgery, female gender, extra-intestinal manifestations, and the use of tobacco have been identified [16].

Moreover, patients with IBD are probably more vulnerable to the effects of stress; the identification of potential markers of individual vulnerability to stress for the use of psychological interventions to reduce stress appears to be an accessible therapeutic strategy [17].

Whether gastrointestinal inflammation favors the development of mental illnesses, or rather the opposite, remains an open question that will be addressed in our review. In this review, we aim to summarize the current evidence on neural interactions driven by intestinal inflammation and to examine the burden of mental illnesses in IBD.

2. Materials and Methods

We searched PubMed until January 2023 using the following terms: "Inflammatory Bowel Diseases", "Crohn Disease", "Ulcerative Colitis", "Depression", "Anxiety", "Mood Disorders", "Stress", and "Cognitive disorders" to recognize relevant publications exploring the implications of the brain–gut axis in patients with IBD, the association between mental illnesses and IBD, and any related therapeutic applications. Both animal and human studies were included.

3. Neural Mechanisms Implied

The mutual association between IBD and psychological illnesses can be explained by a bidirectional communication via the gut–brain axis. The term "gut–brain axis" refers to the complex interactions between neuroendocrine pathways, the central nervous system (CNS), the peripheral nervous system, and the gastrointestinal tract through the enteral nervous system, as well as paracrine regulations [18,19]. Mental disorders, especially depression, partially share some pathophysiological mechanisms of IBD, including oxidative stress, increased proinflammatory cytokines and C-reactive protein (CRP), dysbiosis, and gut permeability [20]. Moreover, many inflammatory signaling pathways (i.e., IL-1–6, IL-23, and CRP) depend on a parasympathetic and hypothalamus–pituitary–adrenal (HPA) axis dysregulation, which has been proven to participate in triggering mental disorders, including depression, schizophrenia, and bipolar disorders [20,21].

In detail, increased levels of stress induce the activation of the HPA axis, favoring the release of the corticotropin-releasing factor (CRF), which in turn stimulates the anterior pituitary gland to release adrenocorticotropic hormone (ACTH) with direct effects on the intestine, such as an increase in intestinal permeability [22].

At the same time, stress promotes the activation of the sympathetic nervous system, resulting in the release of catecholamines from the adrenal medulla and a reduction in parasympathetic activity [23–26]. These factors lead to a massive secretion of proinflammatory cytokines, determining inflammation in the intestinal tract [22–25].

In addition, the immune system itself can affect afferents of the vagus nerve, and circulating cytokines can induce the cerebral production of prostaglandins and nitric oxide, activating leukocytes to enter the brain through circumventricular organs [26,27].

The vagus nerve performs a modulating action of inflammation through different pathways, making the vagal nerve stimulation a catching point in the management of IBD [28]. The role of the HPA axis, the importance of catecholamines in inflammatory pathways, and the vagus nerve action underline the importance in the connection between inflammatory illness and neural mechanism [28].

In detail, Ghia et al. demonstrated that, in mice, depression induces an exaggerated response to inflammatory stimuli in the gut and increases susceptibility to intestinal inflammation thorough the impairment of the parasympathetic system (i.e., tonic vagal inhibition) [29]. Vagotomized mice displayed severe colitis, and, after the administration of tricyclic antidepressants, a restoration of the vagal function was observed, as well as a reduced intestinal inflammation [29].

Summarizing these data, we can conclude that both acute and chronic stress, to which IBD patients are exposed, during their disease course increases intestinal permeability, weakens tight junctions, and increases bacterial translocation through the intestinal wall [30]. Several studies investigating the causative mechanisms shared by intestinal inflammation and psychiatric illnesses have been conducted in mouse models.

It was demonstrated that in adult male mice models of colitis induced by intrarectal injection of DNBS (dinitrobenzene sulfonic acid), depressive and anxious behaviors were associated with increased expression of inflammatory genes and abnormal mitochondrial function in the hippocampus [31]. These results suggest that the peripheral inflammation can, to some extent, increase the transcriptional levels of the genes in the toll-like receptor pathway, and these negative effects may be involved in the co-occurrence of anxiety and depression in the early stages of colitis, especially CD [31].

Furthermore, a study by Carloni et al. identified the presence of a vascular barrier of the choroid plexus in the CNS, which closes during acute phases of intestinal inflammation as a defense strategy through the wingless-type, catenin-beta 1 (Wnt/β-catenin) signaling pathway, explaining the behavioral change consistent with depression and anxiety in mice after induced colitis [31]. This mechanism leads to the production of pro-inflammatory cytokines, especially in the hippocampus [32].

Additional evidence on the impact of inflammation on the CNS derives from recent studies on dextran sodium sulfate mouse IBD models: it was demonstrated that chronic intestinal inflammation, through increased plasma levels of IL-6 and TNF-α, modifies and reduces the neurogenesis, specifically in the hippocampus [33]. In similar experiments, it was shown that numerous inflammatory-related genes (TGF-β, Smad-3, IL-6, IL-1β, and S-100) are upregulated in the CNS, causing microgliosis and astrocyte activation [34].

These studies endorse an impaired neurogenesis and an altered CNS homeostasis as a possible biological basis of psychiatric illnesses in patients with IBD.

Several observations have also been made in human studies, mainly derived from neurofunctional studies. In a study including 74 patients affected by UC investigating global and local networks with functional brain imaging, a significantly lower neural modularity was observed compared to healthy controls ($p = 0.015$), as well as significantly enhanced connectivities in somatomotor, dorsal attention and the visual subnetwork in UC patients compared to healthy controls [35]. Major differences in structural brain measures have been described in patients with CD, even those in clinical remission, as compared to age- and gender-matched controls, such as an increased average left hemisphere cortical thickness (mean, 2.68 mm ± 0.17 SD, $p < 0.01$), including in the left superior frontal region, a functional area implicated both in cognitive and affective processes [36]. In Figure 1, the interactions between chronic intestinal inflammation and the CNS are presented.

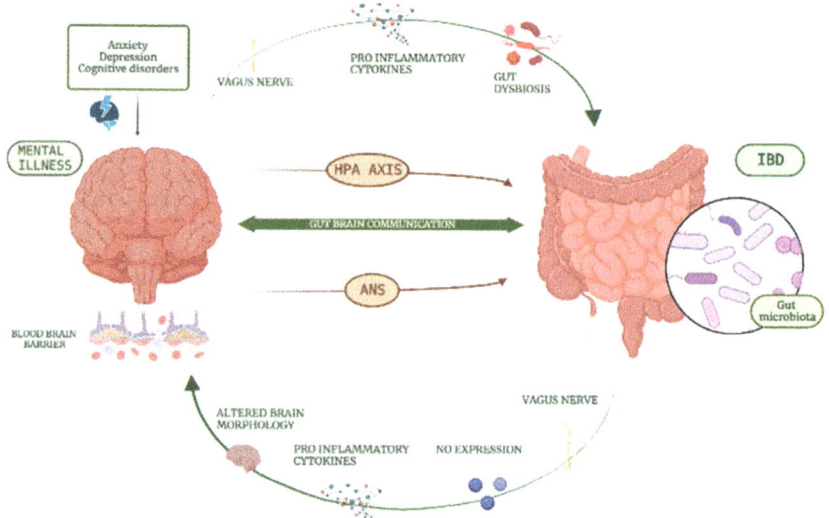

Figure 1. Interactions between chronic intestinal inflammation and the central nervous system. HPA: hypothalamus–pituitary–adrenal, IBD: inflammatory bowel diseases, ANS: autonomous nervous system.

Figure 1 shows the bidirectional communication between the gastrointestinal tract and the central nervous system via the gut–brain axis, vagus nerve, and hypothalamus–pituitary–adrenal axis.

4. Incidence and Prevalence

Overall, both mood and cognitive disorders present higher rates of prevalence among patients affected by IBD compared to a healthy population [37]. Additionally, higher rates of mental illnesses are reported, particularly in concomitance with flares of disease activity [37]. Below, we report summarized epidemiological data of psychiatric comorbidities in IBD divided into subgroups. Table 1 shows the main data on incidence and prevalence of mental illnesses in IBD.

4.1. Depression

Estimated prevalence rates, derived from systematic reviews and cohort studies, of depressive disorders among patients with IBD range from 15% to 40% [38,39]. Notably, a significant association between disease activity and both depression and anxiety are reported (p = 0.01) [40]. The prevalence of psychiatric illnesses in IBD has been examined in different studies with different methodologies: many studies adopted the International Classification of Diseases 9 (ICD-9) or ICD-10 codes to evaluate depression and/or anxiety, while most studies employed several questionnaires, among which the most common is the Hospital Anxiety and Depression Scale (HADS).

Regarding the prevalence, currently robust data on the prevalence of depression in the IBD population have been endorsed by three meta-analyses, where a pooled prevalence of depressive symptoms ranged from 21.0% to 25.2% [5,37,38], with recurring observation of a higher prevalence in patients with active intestinal disease [5,39,40].

In a recent nationwide, population-based study, Choi et al. estimated an incidence rate of depression of 14.99 per 1000 persons/year in the CD patients' group, while for UC, an incidence rate of 19.63 per 1000 persons/year was assessed, both significantly higher compared to the non-IBD controls (p = 0.01) [41]. The authors reported, over a mean follow-up of 6 years, a cumulative incidence of depression of 8% vs. of 4% in unaffected controls [41]. Further data have shown depression incidence rates of 0.89 (0.84–0.95), and 1.61 (1.48–1.75) over a period of 5 years after the diagnosis of IBD and over a mean follow-up of 9.6 years, respectively [42,43]. Additional data worth mentioning concern the high prevalence of suicidal ideation, suicide attempts, and suicide: the risk appears higher in specific groups (i.e., Crohn's disease subtypes, female IBD, pediatric-onset IBD, young adult IBD, and elderly-onset IBD). In addition, suicide itself appears to be more strongly associated with CD [44–46].

4.2. Anxiety

According to current evidence, anxiety is the most frequently associated psychiatric condition in patients with IBD [5,39,40]. An incidence rate of anxiety of 20.88 per 1000 persons/year in CD patients and an incidence rate of 31.19 per 1000 persons/year in UC patients were assessed vs. 14.31 in non-CD controls and 21.55 in non-UC controls, respectively (p = 0.01) [41]. As reported in meta-analyses, the pooled prevalence of anxious symptoms varies from 19.1% to 32.1% [5,37,38]. Concerning lifetime prevalence, in the Manitoba IBD cohort study, markedly higher rates of anxiety disorders among IBD patients were found. More precisely, lifetime prevalence of major depression was assessed at 27.2% (vs. 12.3% in healthy controls, OR 2.20, 95% CI 1.64–2.95), and the lifetime prevalence of any anxiety or mood disorder was assessed as 35.8% (vs. 22.1 in healthy controls, OR 1.24, 95% CI 0.96–1.59) [47]. Additionally, the same study reported that, for patients with IBD and anxiety, in around 80% of the cases, the first episode of anxiety anticipated the diagnosis of IBD by 2 years or more [47].

4.3. Bipolar Disorder

Bipolar disorder is defined by irregular cycles of mania, hypomania, depression, and/or mixed mood states, proven to be rather prevalent in IBD patients [48]. Data from an Asian population-based cross-sectional study show that bipolar disorder was more frequent in IBD patients than in matched comparison patients without IBD, and that the adjusted odds ratio of IBD patients developing a bipolar disorder was 2.10 (95% CI 1.30–3.38) [49]. Moreover, with specific respect to UC patients, the adjusted odds ratio appeared higher (OR 2.23, 95% CI 1.31–3.82) compared to the comparison population [49]. Similarly, the estimated incidence of bipolar disorder in a Canadian population-based study was significantly higher in the IBD group compared to the matched cohort (IRR, 3.80, 95% CI 2.29–6.30; vs. 1.56, 95% CI 1.09–2.23), with concordant higher incidence rate ratios (IRR, 1.82; 95% CI, 1.44–2.30) [50].

4.4. Cognitive Disorders

The term 'cognitive' refers to thought and numerous related processes; the corresponding disorders are characterized by an acquired impairment to one or more among learning and memory, complex attention, language, pre-conceptual motor functions, executive functions, and social cognition [51]. Cognitive impairment has been suggested as a potential extraintestinal manifestation of IBD. Indeed, data derived from meta-analyses have shown that IBD patients exhibit objective deficits in attention and executive functions, especially in working memory, compared with healthy controls [52,53]. Nevertheless, the cognitive impairment in IBD appears to be less frequent than mood disorders, and mild compared to other chronic conditions (i.e., multiple sclerosis) [52,53].

As shown in a recent cross-sectional multicenter study including CD patients, the disease activity was linearly correlated with age- and education-adjusted cognitive function scores [54]. As revealed by Ascertain Dementia 8 (AD8) and MFI questionnaires, approximately 50% of the included patients reported that their subjective cognitive capabilities were declining or reported extreme cognitive fatigue [55]; objective cognitive scores below one standard deviation of age and education expected average were then confirmed in nearly 37% of the patients [54]. Crohn's disease activity index and nutritional risk index significantly correlated with cognitive scores ($r = -0.34, 0.39, 0.33, p < 0.05$), and both significances remained independent of associated depression ($p < 0.05$) [4].

Concerning dementia, preclinical models of Alzheimer's disease (AD) also showed that IBD itself aggravated the AD course [55]. In a population-based cohort analyzing more the 1700 IBD patients and 17,000 controls, an overall higher incidence of dementia, mostly AD, as well as an earlier age of presentation among patients with IBD was observed compared with controls: 5.5% vs. 1.4% and 76 vs. 83 years, respectively [56].

Nevertheless, meta-analyses have underlined that, despite the available data on the association of IBD with subsequent dementia development, the exact risk of dementia in IBD cannot be precisely established due to high heterogeneity in the study design of the available studies [57]. Finally, from observational analyses, the causal role of IBD in triggering AD appears unlikely, as it may result from confounding factors, and the evidence remains weak [58].

4.5. Schizophrenia

Among patients with schizophrenia, the risk of developing IBD is higher than in the general population (1.14% vs. 0.25%) [59]. The connection between schizophrenia and IBD also has genetic fundamentals, as shown by a Mendelian randomization analysis which provided causal effects of schizophrenia on IBD but not vice versa [60]. Patients with schizophrenia have been demonstrated to show higher gut permeability, defined as a lactulose/mannitol ratio ≥ 0.1, than controls (22.7% vs. 5.8%, OR 4.8, 95%, CI 1.2–18.3, $p = 0.03$) [61]. In the etiopathogenesis of schizophrenia, the impaired intestinal permeability with subsequent inflammation may have a triggering role [62], and it was shown that the serum zonulin levels, which regulate intestinal and blood–brain barrier tight junctions [63], were significantly higher in patients with schizophrenia than in the unaffected population [64].

Table 1. Data on incidence and prevalence of mental illnesses in IBD. IBD: inflammatory bowel disease; UC: ulcerative colitis; CD: Crohn's disease.

Reference	Year	Study Design	Observation Time	Incidence/Prevalence of Depression	Incidence/Prevalence of Anxiety	Incidence/Prevalence of Bipolar Disorder	Incidence/Prevalence of Dementia
Barberio et al. [5]	2021	Meta-analysis		Pooled prevalence of depressive symptoms: 25.2%	Pooled prevalence of anxiety symptoms: 32.1%		
Mikocka-Walus et al. [37]	2016	Systematic review		Pooled prevalence of depression in IBD vs. healthy control: 21.2% vs. 13.4%, in active vs. inactive disease: 34.7% vs. 19.9%	Pooled prevalence of anxiety in IBD vs. healthy control: 19.1% vs. 9.6%, in active vs. inactive disease: 66.4% vs. 28.2%		
Neuendorf et al. [38]	2014	Systematic review		Pooled prevalence of depression disorders: 15.2%, depressive symptoms: 21.6%, pooled prevalence of depressive symptoms in active vs. inactive disease: 40.7% vs. 16.5%	Pooled prevalence of anxiety disorders: 20.5%, anxiety symptoms: 35.1%, pooled prevalence of anxiety symptoms in active vs. inactive disease: 75.6% vs. 31.4%		
Choi et al. [41]	2019	Cohort study	6 years	Incidence rate (per 1000 persons/year) in CD vs. non-CD controls: 14.99 vs. 7.75 In UC vs. non-UC controls: 19.63 vs. 11.28 Prevalence in IBD vs. non-IBD controls: 8.0% vs. 3.7%	Incidence rate (per 1000 persons/year) in CD vs. non-CD controls: 20.88 vs. 14.31, in UC vs. non-UC controls: 31.19 vs. 21.55 Prevalence in IBD vs. non-IBD controls: 12.2% vs. 8.7%		
Marrie et al. [42]	2017	Cohort study	9.6 years	Incidence rate ratio of depression in IBD of 1.61	Incidence rate ratio of anxiety in IBD of 1.37		
Walker et al. [43]	2008	Cohort study		Lifetime prevalence of major depressive disorder in IBD vs. control: 27.2% vs. 12.3%	Lifetime prevalence of any anxiety or mood disorder in IBD vs. control: 35.8% vs. 22.1%		
Kao et al. [48]	2019	Population-based cohort study				Adjusted odds ratio of developing a bipolar disorder of 2.10 (95% CI 1.30–3.38)	
Bernstein et al. [50]	2019	Population-based cohort study				Incidence in the IBD group as compared to the matched cohort (3.80, 95% CI 2.29–6.30; vs. 1.56, 95% CI 1.09–2.23), higher incidence rate ratios (IRR, 1.82; 95% CI, 1.44–2.30)	
Zhang et al. [56]	2021	Cohort study	16 years				Incidence (per 1700 persons) of dementia in IBD vs. healthy control: 5.5% vs. 1.4%

5. Compliance to Therapy and Role of Psychotherapeutic Intervention

Nonadherence to maintenance therapy, either oral or biologic, in patients with IBD is a significant healthcare problem and can lead to unnecessary therapy escalation.

Overall, medication nonadherence can occur in up to 45% of patients with IBD and is markedly influenced by psychological factors, particularly psychological distress, and patients' beliefs [65].

Compliance has been repeatedly demonstrated to inversely correlate with the presence of psychiatric disorders in IBD cohorts [66,67]; the co-occurrence of anxiety and mood disorders significantly increased the risk of discontinuation in the first year following anti-TNF initiation (hazard ratio, 1.50; 95% CI, 1.15–1.94) and the overall risk of discontinuation of anti-TNF therapy (adjusted hazard ratio, 1.28; 95%, CI, 1.03–1.59) [67]. Concerning anti-TNF, further data have shown that depressive symptoms at baseline significantly led to noncompliance over a 2-year period of follow-up (HR 2.28, CI 1.1–4.6, $p < 0.05$) [68].

However, the effect of psychiatric disorders on non-compliance is not limited to parenteral administration; indeed, in the early 2000s, it was also observed with aminosalicylates and thiopurines [69–71].

Psychological interventions can also address disease acceptance and pain misrepresentation and misreporting. Among the possible psychotherapeutic interventions, cognitive behavioral therapy, hypnotherapy, and mindfulness therapy are included. In a prospective multicenter study, the adoption of structured personalized counseling sessions led to significantly increased medication acceptance rates in nonadherent IBD patients over a follow-up of 24 months [72].

However, the available meta-analyses did not endorse this evidence: a first systematic review with meta-analysis, in 2011, found that psychotherapy had no effect on the QoL, emotional status, or disease activation in adult patients with IBD, while in adolescents, psychological interventions appeared to be beneficial, despite limited evidence [73]. With respect to adolescent IBD patients, in a randomized controlled trial (RCT) investigating the effect of cognitive behavioral therapy on disease course, the time to relapse did not differ between the intervention group and the controls ($p = 0.915$), or in the course of clinical disease activity over time between the two groups [62]. Regardless, the psychotherapy duration significantly affected fecal calprotectin (β, -0.11, 95% CI, -0.195 to -0.031; $p = 0.008$) [74]. Importantly, behavioral interventions have been demonstrated to improve medication adherence in adolescent IBD patients [75].

A later analysis confirmed no effect of individual psychological therapies either on psychological wellbeing scores or on disease activity indices [64], except for cognitive behavioral therapy, which was proven to have small short-term beneficial effects on depression scores and QoL in patients with IBD [76].

Notably, the heterogeneity of psychological interventions and the design of the included studies may have created bias in the results of these meta-analyses, and more RCTs are required to accurately address the role of psychological therapies in the management of IBD.

According to the results of a latter prospective study, among those IBD patients who accepted psychological intervention, the frequency and number of emergency visits significantly decreased over the year after the start of psychotherapy, compared with the year before psychotherapy ($p < 0.05$) [76]. Psychotherapy was associated with a net saving of resources in the cost–benefit analysis [76].

Finally, evidence from studies conducted in operated IBD patients, specifically those undergoing stoma surgery, supports perioperative psychological support in order to reduce patients' distress and anxiety related to surgery, as well as to ameliorate psychological and surgical outcomes in the postoperative follow-up [77,78].

As for mindfulness strategies, an RCT conducted by Jedel S et al. including patients with UC in remission examined the efficacy of mindfulness-based stress reduction (MBSR) to reduce disease flares and improve QoL [79]. Lower stress and an improved QoL while in active disease were observed compared to flared patients in the control group ($p = 0.04$

and $p < 0.01$, respectively); however, no effect on inflammatory markers and disease course was observed [79]. Further RCTs have reported an improvement in QoL and depression scores in IBD patients under mindfulness-based stress reduction therapy [80,81]; notably, disease course, disease activity, and inflammatory markers of the intestinal disease were not ameliorated [81,82].

6. Discussion

What emerges from our review is that the prevalence of mental illnesses in IBD patients is high, ranging from 15% to 40%, particularly anxiety [5,6,37–39]. The association between IBD and mood disorders is relevant, while the link with other psychiatric illnesses, such as dementia and schizophrenia, appears lower [50,58].

Considering their high prevalence, mental illnesses can be regarded as proper extra-intestinal comorbidities in these patients (Figure 2) [5,6,37–39].

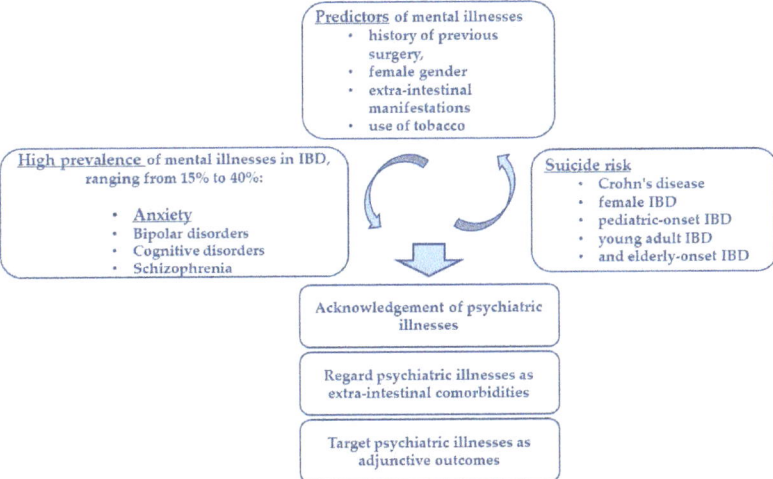

Figure 2. Integration of mental illnesses in the management of IBD.

Despite this evidence, psychiatric comorbidities remain under-recognized and inadequately treated. Our review highlights the limitation of systematically summarizing the true magnitude of mental illnesses in IBD due to the lack of prospective, large, and population-based studies.

Concerning the pathophysiology of mental illnesses in IBD, it appears clear that the central role of the vagal nerve is regulating signals from the depressed brain areas to the gastrointestinal tract, and vice versa [26,27,34] (Figure 1). The involvement of the vagal nerve together with the role of inflammatory mediators is also endorsed by pre-clinical data on the development of depression subsequent to induced colitis, and conversely, the occurrence of colitis after induced depressive symptoms in animal models [26,27,34].

Many open questions remain regarding the temporal relationship between IBD and depression and/or anxiety, any possible genetic correlation between IBD and psychiatric diseases, the true benefit of psychological interventions in regard to IBD disease severity, and the possible influence of IBD therapies on the occurrence of depression and/or anxiety. Since long-term medication is crucial for maintaining remission in IBD patients, a close collaboration between gastroenterologists, psychiatrists, and family members is advised.

Notably, most of the studies have demonstrated the usefulness of psychotherapeutic intervention on quality of life, perception of stress, and adherence to therapies [74–76], as well as on more concrete indicators such as emergency visits and saving of resources [77], though it seems reasonable to exclude the true impact of the available psychotherapeutic approaches on disease severity, course, natural history, and surgery rates, where the biology alone mostly impacts. However, there may be advantages in targeting specific subgroups of IBD patients, including youths and adolescents, and those with significant psychiatric comorbidity [74–76].

In our view, it would be helpful to immediately integrate a psychiatric consultation and potential psychotherapy into the clinical management of these specific patients, and particular long-term psychological support should be considered for patients with pediatric-onset IBD.

In conclusion, it is essential for dedicated physicians managing IBD patients not only to acknowledge the psychiatric illnesses co-occurring in these patients, but also to consider these comorbidities as part of the medical context and as adjunctive outcomes (Figure 2). The separation between physical and mental health appears misleading and outdated when caring for patients with IBD.

Author Contributions: B.B., A.D.B. and R.G. performed the research and wrote the manuscript. A.A., A.B., L.G., E.M., A.Q. and A.R. critically reviewed the content of the paper. A.A. conceived the subject of the paper, contributed to the critical interpretation, and supervised the project. Guarantor of the article: Alessandro Armuzzi. All authors have read and agreed to the published version of the manuscript.

Funding: This research received no external funding.

Institutional Review Board Statement: Not applicable.

Informed Consent Statement: Not applicable.

Data Availability Statement: No new data were created or analyzed in this study. Data sharing is not applicable to this article.

Conflicts of Interest: A Armuzzi has received consulting fees from: AbbVie, Allergan, Amgen, Arena, Biogen, Boehringer Ingelheim, Bristol-Myers Squibb, Celgene, Celltrion, Eli-Lilly, Ferring, Galapagos, Gilead, Janssen, MSD, Mylan, Pfizer, Protagonist Therapeutics, Roche, Samsung Bioepis, Sandoz, and Takeda; speaker's fees from: AbbVie, Amgen, Arena, Biogen, Bristol-Myers Squibb, Eli-Lilly, Ferring, Galapagos, Gilead, Janssen, MSD, Novartis, Pfizer, Roche, Samsung Bioepis, Sandoz, Takeda, and Tigenix; and research support from: MSD, Takeda, Pfizer, and Biogen. R Gabbiadini has received speaker's fees from Pfizer. A Dal Buono has received speaker's fees from Abbvie. A Repici received consultancy fees from Medtronic and Fujifilm. B Bartocci, A Busacca, E Mencaglia, A Quadarella, and L Gasparini declare no conflicts of interest.

References

1. Roda, G.; Chien, N.S.; Kotze, P.G.; Argollo, M.; Panaccione, R.; Spinelli, A.; Kaser, A.; Peyrin-Biroulet, L.; Danese, S. Crohn's disease. *Nat. Rev. Dis. Primers* **2020**, *6*, 22. [CrossRef] [PubMed]
2. Kobayashi, T.; Siegmund, B.; Le Berre, C.; Wei, S.C.; Ferrante, M.; Shen, B.; Bernstein, C.N.; Danese, S.; Peyrin-Biroulet, L.; Hibi, T. Ulcerative colitis. *Nat. Rev. Dis. Primers* **2020**, *6*, 74. [CrossRef]
3. Ananthakrishnan, A.N.; Bernstein, C.N.; Iliopoulos, D.; Macpherson, A.; Neurath, M.F.; Ali, R.A.R.; Vavricka, S.R.; Fiocchi, C. Environmental triggers in IBD: A review of progress and evidence. *Nat. Rev. Gastroenterol. Hepatol.* **2018**, *15*, 39–49. [CrossRef] [PubMed]
4. Armuzzi, A.; Liguori, G. Quality of life in patients with moderate to severe ulcerative colitis and the impact of treatment: A narrative review. *Dig. Liver Dis.* **2021**, *53*, 803–808. [CrossRef] [PubMed]
5. Barberio, B.; Zamani, M.; Black, C.J.; Savarino, E.V.; Ford, A.C. Prevalence of symptoms of anxiety and depression in patients with inflammatory bowel disease: A systematic review and meta-analysis. *Lancet Gastroenterol. Hepatol.* **2021**, *6*, 359–370. [CrossRef] [PubMed]
6. Bisgaard, T.H.; Allin, K.H.; Keefer, L.; Ananthakrishnan, A.N.; Jess, T. Depression and anxiety in inflammatory bowel disease: Epidemiology, mechanisms and treatment. *Nat. Rev. Gastroenterol. Hepatol.* **2022**, *19*, 717–726. [CrossRef]
7. Keefer, L.; Keshavarzian, A.; Mutlu, E. Reconsidering the methodology of "stress" research in inflammatory bowel disease. *J. Crohns Colitis* **2008**, *2*, 193–201. [CrossRef]
8. Ghosh, S.; Mitchell, R. Impact of inflammatory bowel disease on quality of life: Results of the European Federationof Crohn's and ulcerative colitis associations (EFCCA) patient survey. *J. Crohns Colitis* **2007**, *1*, 10–20. [CrossRef]
9. Eugenicos, M.P.; Ferreira, N.B. Psychological factors associated with inflammatory bowel disease. *Br. Med. Bull.* **2021**, *138*, 16–28. [CrossRef]

10. Park, K.T.; Allen, J.I.; Meadows, P.; Szigethy, E.M.; Henrichsen, K.; Kim, S.C.; Lawton, R.C.; Murphy, S.M.; Regueiro, M.; Rubin, D.T.; et al. The Cost of Inflammatory Bowel Disease: An Initiative From the Crohn's & Colitis Foundation. *Inflamm. Bowel Dis.* **2020**, *26*, 1–10.
11. Casati, J.; Toner, B.B. Psychosocial aspects of inflammatory bowel disease. *Biomed. Pharmacother.* **2000**, *54*, 388–393. [CrossRef] [PubMed]
12. Sewitch, M.J.; Abrahamowicz, M.; Bitton, A.; Daly, D.; Wild, G.E.; Cohen, A.; Katz, S.; Szego, P.L.; Dobkin, P.L. Psychological distress, social support, and disease activity in patients with inflammatory bowel disease. *Am. J. Gastroenterol.* **2001**, *96*, 1470–1479. [CrossRef] [PubMed]
13. Levenstein, S.; Prantera, C.; Varvo, V.; Scribano, M.L.; Andreoli, A.; Luzi, C.; Arcà, M.; Berto, E.; Milite, G.; Marcheggiano, A. Stress and exacerbation in ulcerative colitis: A prospective study of patients enrolled in remission. *Am. J. Gastroenterol.* **2000**, *95*, 1213–1220. [CrossRef] [PubMed]
14. Ananthakrishnan, A.N.; Gainer, V.S.; Perez, R.G.; Cai, T.; Cheng, S.C.; Savova, G.; Chen, P.; Szolovits, P.; Xia, Z.; De Jager, P.L.; et al. Psychiatric co-morbidity is associated with increased risk of surgery in Crohn's disease. *Aliment. Pharmacol. Ther.* **2013**, *37*, 445–454. [CrossRef] [PubMed]
15. Oligschlaeger, Y.; Yadati, T.; Houben, T.; Condello Oliván, C.M.; Shiri-Sverdlov, R. Inflammatory Bowel Disease: A Stressed "Gut/Feeling". *Cells* **2019**, *8*, 659. [CrossRef] [PubMed]
16. Navabi, S.; Gorrepati, V.S.; Yadav, S.; Chintanaboina, J.; Maher, S.; Demuth, P.; Stern, B.; Stuart, A.; Tinsley, A.; Clarke, K.; et al. Influences and Impact of Anxiety and Depression in the Setting of Inflammatory Bowel Disease. *Inflamm. Bowel Dis.* **2018**, *24*, 2303–2308. [CrossRef]
17. Maunder, R.G.; Levenstein, S. The role of stress in the development and clinical course of inflammatory bowel disease: Epidemiological evidence. *Curr. Mol. Med.* **2008**, *8*, 247–252. [CrossRef]
18. Gracie, D.J.; Hamlin, P.J.; Ford, A.C. The influence of the brain-gut axis in inflammatory bowel disease and possible implications for treatment. *Lancet Gastroenterol. Hepatol.* **2019**, *4*, 632–642. [CrossRef]
19. Stuart, M.J.; Baune, B.T. Chemokines and chemokine receptors in mood disorders, schizophrenia, and cognitive impairment: A systematic review of biomarker studies. *Neurosci. Biobehav. Rev.* **2014**, *42*, 93–115. [CrossRef]
20. Frolkis, A.D.; Vallerand, I.A.; Shaheen, A.A.; Lowerison, M.W.; Swain, M.G.; Barnabe, C.; Patten, S.B.; Kaplan, G.G. Depression increases the risk of inflammatory bowel disease, which may be mitigated by the use of antidepressants in the treatment of depression. *Gut* **2019**, *68*, 1606–1612. [CrossRef]
21. Santos, J.; Saunders, P.R.; Hanssen, N.P.; Yang, P.C.; Yates, D.; Groot, J.A.; Perdue, M.H. Corticotropin-releasing hormone mimics stress-induced colonic epithelial pathophysiology in the rat. *Am. J. Physiol.* **1999**, *277*, G391–G399. [CrossRef] [PubMed]
22. Johnson, J.D.; Campisi, J.; Sharkey, C.M.; Kennedy, S.L.; Nickerson, M.; Greenwood, B.N.; Fleshner, M. Catecholamines mediate stress-induced increases in peripheral and central inflammatory cytokines. *Neuroscience* **2005**, *135*, 1295–1307. [CrossRef] [PubMed]
23. Farhadi, A.; Keshavarzian, A.; Van de Kar, L.D.; Jakate, S.; Domm, A.; Zhang, L.; Shaikh, M.; Banan, A.; Fields, J.Z. Heightened responses to stressors in patients with inflammatory bowel disease. *Am. J. Gastroenterol.* **2005**, *100*, 1796–1804. [CrossRef] [PubMed]
24. Brzozowski, B.; Mazur-Bialy, A.; Pajdo, R.; Kwiecien, S.; Bilski, J.; Zwolinska-Wcislo, M.; Mach, T.; Brzozowski, T. Mechanisms by which Stress Affects the Experimental and Clinical Inflammatory Bowel Disease (IBD): Role of Brain-Gut Axis. *Curr. Neuropharmacol.* **2016**, *14*, 892–900. [CrossRef]
25. Dal Buono, A.; Caldirola, D.; Allocca, M. Genetic susceptibility to inflammatory bowel disease: Should we be looking to the hypothalamus? *Expert Rev. Clin. Immunol.* **2021**, *17*, 803–806. [CrossRef]
26. Murayama, S.; Kurganov, E.; Miyata, S. Activation of microglia and macrophages in the circumventricular organs of the mouse brain during TLR2-induced fever and sickness responses. *J. Neuroimmunol.* **2019**, *334*, 576973. [CrossRef]
27. McCusker, R.H.; Kelley, K.W. Immune-neural connections: How the immune system's response to infectious agents influences behavior. *J. Exp. Biol.* **2013**, *216 Pt 1*, 84–98. [CrossRef]
28. Fornaro, R.; Actis, G.C.; Caviglia, G.P.; Pitoni, D.; Ribaldone, D.G. Inflammatory Bowel Disease: Role of Vagus Nerve Stimulation. *J. Clin. Med.* **2022**, *11*, 5690. [CrossRef]
29. Ghia, J.E.; Blennerhassett, P.; Collins, S.M. Impaired parasympathetic function increases susceptibility to inflammatory bowel disease in a mouse model of depression. *J. Clin. Investig.* **2008**, *118*, 2209–2218. [CrossRef]
30. Camilleri, M. Leaky gut: Mechanisms, measurement and clinical implications in humans. *Gut* **2019**, *68*, 1516–1526. [CrossRef]
31. Haj-Mirzaian, A.; Amiri, S.; Amini-Khoei, H.; Hosseini, M.J.; Haj-Mirzaian, A.; Momeny, M.; Rahimi-Balaei, M.; Dehpour, A.R. Anxiety- and Depressive-Like Behaviors are Associated with Altered Hippocampal Energy and Inflammatory Status in a Mouse Model of Crohn's Disease. *Neuroscience* **2017**, *366*, 124–137. [CrossRef] [PubMed]
32. Carloni, S.; Bertocchi, A.; Mancinelli, S.; Bellini, M.; Erreni, M.; Borreca, A.; Braga, D.; Giugliano, S.; Mozzarelli, A.M.; Manganaro, D.; et al. Identification of a choroid plexus vascular barrier closing during intestinal inflammation. *Science* **2021**, *374*, 439–448. [CrossRef] [PubMed]
33. Zonis, S.; Pechnick, R.N.; Ljubimov, V.A.; Mahgerefteh, M.; Wawrowsky, K.; Michelsen, K.S.; Chesnokova, V. Chronic intestinal inflammation alters hippocampal neurogenesis. *J. Neuroinflamm.* **2015**, *12*, 65. [CrossRef] [PubMed]

34. Vitali, R.; Prioreschi, C.; Lorenzo Rebenaque, L.; Colantoni, E.; Giovannini, D.; Frusciante, S.; Diretto, G.; Marco-Jiménez, F.; Mancuso, M.; Casciati, A.; et al. Gut-Brain Axis: Insights from Hippocampal Neurogenesis and Brain Tumor Development in a Mouse Model of Experimental Colitis Induced by Dextran Sodium Sulfate. *Int. J. Mol. Sci.* **2022**, *23*, 11495. [CrossRef]
35. Wang, H.; Labus, J.S.; Griffin, F.; Gupta, A.; Bhatt, R.R.; Sauk, J.S.; Turkiewicz, J.; Bernstein, C.N.; Kornelsen, J.; Mayer, E.A. Functional brain rewiring and altered cortical stability in ulcerative colitis. *Mol. Psychiatry* **2022**, *27*, 1792–1804. [CrossRef]
36. Nair, V.A.; Beniwal-Patel, P.; Mbah, I.; Young, B.M.; Prabhakaran, V.; Saha, S. Structural Imaging Changes and Behavioral Correlates in Patients with Crohn's Disease in Remission. *Front. Hum. Neurosci.* **2016**, *10*, 460. [CrossRef]
37. Mikocka-Walus, A.; Knowles, S.R.; Keefer, L.; Graff, L. Controversies Revisited: A Systematic Review of the Comorbidity of Depression and Anxiety with Inflammatory Bowel Diseases. *Inflamm. Bowel Dis.* **2016**, *22*, 752–762. [CrossRef]
38. Neuendorf, R.; Harding, A.; Stello, N.; Hanes, D.; Wahbeh, H. Depression and anxiety in patients with Inflammatory Bowel Disease: A systematic review. *J. Psychosom. Res.* **2016**, *87*, 70–80. [CrossRef]
39. Panara, A.J.; Yarur, A.J.; Rieders, B.; Proksell, S.; Deshpande, A.R.; Abreu, M.T.; Sussman, D.A. The incidence and risk factors for developing depression after being diagnosed with inflammatory bowel disease: A cohort study. *Aliment. Pharmacol. Ther.* **2014**, *39*, 802–810. [CrossRef]
40. Byrne, G.; Rosenfeld, G.; Leung, Y.; Qian, H.; Raudzus, J.; Nunez, C.; Bressler, B. Prevalence of Anxiety and Depression in Patients with Inflammatory Bowel Disease. *Can. J. Gastroenterol. Hepatol.* **2017**, *2017*, 6496727. [CrossRef]
41. Choi, K.; Chun, J.; Han, K.; Park, S.; Soh, H.; Kim, J.; Lee, J.; Lee, H.J.; Im, J.P.; Kim, J.S. Risk of Anxiety and Depression in Patients with Inflammatory Bowel Disease: A Nationwide, Population-Based Study. *J. Clin. Med.* **2019**, *8*, 654. [CrossRef] [PubMed]
42. Marrie, R.A.; Walld, R.; Bolton, J.M.; Sareen, J.; Walker, J.R.; Patten, S.B.; Singer, A.; Lix, L.M.; Hitchon, C.A.; El-Gabalawy, R.; et al. Rising incidence of psychiatric disorders before diagnosis of immune-mediated inflammatory disease. *Epidemiol. Psychiatr. Sci.* **2019**, *28*, 333–342. [CrossRef] [PubMed]
43. Marrie, R.A.; Walld, R.; Bolton, J.M.; Sareen, J.; Walker, J.R.; Patten, S.B.; Singer, A.; Lix, L.M.; Hitchon, C.A.; El-Gabalawy, R.; et al. Increased incidence of psychiatric disorders in immune-mediated inflammatory disease. *J. Psychosom. Res.* **2017**, *101*, 17–23. [CrossRef] [PubMed]
44. Ludvigsson, J.F.; Olén, O.; Larsson, H.; Halfvarson, J.; Almqvist, C.; Lichtenstein, P.; Butwicka, A. Association Between Inflammatory Bowel Disease and Psychiatric Morbidity and Suicide: A Swedish Nationwide Population-Based Cohort Study With Sibling Comparisons. *J. Crohns Colitis* **2021**, *15*, 1824–1836. [CrossRef] [PubMed]
45. Xiong, Q.; Tang, F.; Li, Y.; Xie, F.; Yuan, L.; Yao, C.; Wu, R.; Wang, J.; Wang, Q.; Feng, P. Association of inflammatory bowel disease with suicidal ideation, suicide attempts, and suicide: A systematic review and meta-analysis. *J. Psychosom. Res.* **2022**, *160*, 110983. [CrossRef]
46. Butwicka, A.; Olén, O.; Larsson, H.; Halfvarson, J.; Almqvist, C.; Lichtenstein, P.; Serlachius, E.; Frisén, L.; Ludvigsson, J.F. Association of Childhood-Onset Inflammatory Bowel Disease With Risk of Psychiatric Disorders and Suicide Attempt. *JAMA Pediatr.* **2019**, *173*, 969–978. [CrossRef]
47. Walker, J.R.; Ediger, J.P.; Graff, L.A.; Greenfeld, J.M.; Clara, I.; Lix, L.; Rawsthorne, P.; Miller, N.; Rogala, L.; McPhail, C.M.; et al. The Manitoba IBD cohort study: A population-based study of the prevalence of lifetime and 12-month anxiety and mood disorders. *Am. J. Gastroenterol.* **2008**, *103*, 1989–1997. [CrossRef]
48. Nikolova, V.L.; Pelton, L.; Moulton, C.D.; Zorzato, D.; Cleare, A.J.; Young, A.H.; Stone, J.M. The Prevalence and Incidence of Irritable Bowel Syndrome and Inflammatory Bowel Disease in Depression and Bipolar Disorder: A Systematic Review and Meta-Analysis. *Psychosom. Med.* **2022**, *84*, 313–324. [CrossRef]
49. Kao, L.T.; Lin, H.C.; Lee, H.C. Inflammatory bowel disease and bipolar disorder: A population-based cross-sectional study. *J. Affect. Disord.* **2019**, *247*, 120–124. [CrossRef]
50. Bernstein, C.N.; Hitchon, C.A.; Walld, R.; Bolton, J.M.; Sareen, J.; Walker, J.R.; Graff, L.A.; Patten, S.B.; Singer, A.; Lix, L.M.; et al. Increased Burden of Psychiatric Disorders in Inflammatory Bowel Disease. *Inflamm. Bowel Dis.* **2019**, *25*, 360–368. [CrossRef]
51. Sachdev, P.S.; Blacker, D.; Blazer, D.G.; Ganguli, M.; Jeste, D.V.; Paulsen, J.S.; Petersen, R.C. Classifying neurocognitive disorders: The DSM-5 approach. *Nat. Rev. Neurol.* **2014**, *10*, 634–642. [CrossRef] [PubMed]
52. Hopkins, C.W.P.; Powell, N.; Norton, C.; Dumbrill, J.L.; Hayee, B.; Moulton, C.D. Cognitive Impairment in Adult Inflammatory Bowel Disease: A Systematic Review and Meta-Analysis. *J. Acad. Consult. Liaison Psychiatry* **2021**, *62*, 387–403. [CrossRef] [PubMed]
53. Whitehouse, C.E.; Fisk, J.D.; Bernstein, C.N.; Berrigan, L.I.; Bolton, J.M.; Graff, L.A.; Hitchon, C.A.; Marriott, J.J.; Peschken, C.A.; Sareen, J.; et al. Comorbid anxiety, depression, and cognition in MS and other immune-mediated disorders. *Neurology* **2019**, *92*, e406–e417. [CrossRef]
54. Golan, D.; Gross, B.; Miller, A.; Klil-Drori, S.; Lavi, I.; Shiller, M.; Honigman, S.; Almog, R.; Segol, O. Cognitive Function of Patients with Crohn's Disease is Associated with Intestinal Disease Activity. *Inflamm. Bowel Dis.* **2016**, *22*, 364–371. [CrossRef]
55. Wang, D.; Zhang, X.; Du, H. Inflammatory bowel disease: A potential pathogenic factor of Alzheimer's disease. *Prog. Neuropsychopharmacol. Biol. Psychiatry* **2022**, *119*, 110610. [CrossRef] [PubMed]
56. Zhang, B.; Wang, H.E.; Bai, Y.M.; Tsai, S.J.; Su, T.P.; Chen, T.J.; Wang, Y.P.; Chen, M.H. Inflammatory bowel disease is associated with higher dementia risk: A nationwide longitudinal study. *Gut* **2021**, *70*, 85–91. [CrossRef]
57. Liu, N.; Wang, Y.; He, L.; Sun, J.; Wang, X.; Li, H. Inflammatory bowel disease and risk of dementia: An updated meta-analysis. *Front. Aging Neurosci.* **2022**, *4*, 962681. [CrossRef]

58. Huang, J.; Su, B.; Karhunen, V.; Gill, D.; Zuber, V.; Ahola-Olli, A.; Palaniswamy, S.; Auvinen, J.; Herzig, K.H.; Keinänen-Kiukaanniemi, S.; et al. Inflammatory Diseases, Inflammatory Biomarkers, and Alzheimer Disease: An Observational Analysis and Mendelian Randomization. *Neurology* **2023**, *100*, e568–e581. [CrossRef]
59. Sung, K.Y.; Zhang, B.; Wang, H.E.; Bai, Y.M.; Tsai, S.J.; Su, T.P.; Chen, T.J.; Hou, M.C.; Lu, C.L.; Wang, Y.P.; et al. Schizophrenia and risk of new-onset inflammatory bowel disease: A nationwide longitudinal study. *Aliment. Pharmacol. Ther.* **2022**, *55*, 1192–1201. [CrossRef]
60. Qian, L.; He, X.; Gao, F.; Fan, Y.; Zhao, B.; Ma, Q.; Yan, B.; Wang, W.; Ma, X.; Yang, J. Estimation of the bidirectional relationship between schizophrenia and inflammatory bowel disease using the mendelian randomization approach. *Schizophrenia* **2022**, *8*, 31. [CrossRef]
61. Ishida, I.; Ogura, J.; Aizawa, E.; Ota, M.; Hidese, S.; Yomogida, Y.; Matsuo, J.; Yoshida, S.; Kunugi, H. Gut permeability and its clinical relevance in schizophrenia. *Neuropsychopharmacol. Rep.* **2022**, *42*, 70–76. [CrossRef] [PubMed]
62. Gokulakrishnan, K.; Nikhil, J.; Vs, S.; Holla, B.; Thirumoorthy, C.; Sandhya, N.; Nichenametla, S.; Pathak, H.; Shivakumar, V.; Debnath, M.; et al. Altered Intestinal Permeability Biomarkers in Schizophrenia: A Possible Link with Subclinical Inflammation. *Ann. Neurosci.* **2022**, *29*, 151–158. [CrossRef] [PubMed]
63. Maes, M.; Sirivichayakul, S.; Kanchanatawan, B.; Vodjani, A. Upregulation of the Intestinal Paracellular Pathway with Breakdown of Tight and Adherens Junctions in Deficit Schizophrenia. *Mol. Neurobiol.* **2019**, *56*, 7056–7073. [CrossRef] [PubMed]
64. Usta, A.; Kılıç, F.; Demirdaş, A.; Işık, Ü.; Doğuç, D.K.; Bozkurt, M. Serum zonulin and claudin-5 levels in patients with schizophrenia. *Eur. Arch. Psychiatry Clin. Neurosci.* **2021**, *271*, 767–773. [CrossRef]
65. Jackson, C.A.; Clatworthy, J.; Robinson, A.; Horne, R. Factors associated with non-adherence to oral medication for inflammatory bowel disease: A systematic review. *Am. J. Gastroenterol.* **2010**, *105*, 525–539. [CrossRef]
66. Nigro, G.; Angelini, G.; Grosso, S.B.; Caula, G.; Sategna-Guidetti, C. Psychiatric predictors of noncompliance in inflammatory bowel disease: Psychiatry and compliance. *J. Clin. Gastroenterol.* **2001**, *32*, 66–68. [CrossRef]
67. Dolovich, C.; Bernstein, C.N.; Singh, H.; Nugent, Z.; Tennakoon, A.; Shafer, L.A.; Marrie, R.A.; Sareen, J.; Targownik, L.E. Anxiety and Depression Leads to Anti-Tumor Necrosis Factor Discontinuation in Inflammatory Bowel Disease. *Clin. Gastroenterol. Hepatol.* **2021**, *19*, 1200–1208.e1. [CrossRef]
68. Calloway, A.; Dalal, R.; Beaulieu, D.B.; Duley, C.; Annis, K.; Gaines, L.; Slaughter, C.; Schwartz, D.A.; Horst, S. Depressive Symptoms Predict Anti-tumor Necrosis Factor Therapy Noncompliance in Patients with Inflammatory Bowel Disease. *Dig. Dis. Sci.* **2017**, *62*, 3563–3567. [CrossRef]
69. Kane, S.V.; Accortt, N.A.; Magowan, S.; Brixner, D. Predictors of persistence with 5-aminosalicylic acid therapy for ulcerative colitis. *Aliment. Pharmacol. Ther.* **2009**, *29*, 855–862. [CrossRef]
70. Shale, M.J.; Riley, S.A. Studies of compliance with delayed-release mesalazine therapy in patients with inflammatory bowel disease. *Aliment. Pharmacol. Ther.* **2003**, *18*, 191–198. [CrossRef]
71. Goodhand, J.R.; Kamperidis, N.; Sirwan, B.; Macken, L.; Tshuma, N.; Koodun, Y.; Chowdhury, F.A.; Croft, N.M.; Direkze, N.; Langmead, L.; et al. Factors associated with thiopurine non-adherence in patients with inflammatory bowel disease. *Aliment. Pharmacol. Ther.* **2013**, *38*, 1097–1108. [CrossRef] [PubMed]
72. Tiao, D.K.; Chan, W.; Jeganathan, J.; Chan, J.T.; Perry, J.; Selinger, C.P.; Leong, R.W. Inflammatory Bowel Disease Pharmacist Adherence Counseling Improves Medication Adherence in Crohn's Disease and Ulcerative Colitis. *Inflamm. Bowel Dis.* **2017**, *23*, 1257–1261. [CrossRef]
73. Timmer, A.; Preiss, J.C.; Motschall, E.; Rücker, G.; Jantschek, G.; Moser, G. Psychological interventions for treatment of inflammatory bowel disease. *Cochrane Database Syst. Rev.* **2011**. [CrossRef]
74. Van den Brink, G.; Stapersma, L.; Bom, A.S.; Rizopolous, D.; van der Woude, C.J.; Stuyt, R.J.L.; Hendriks, D.M.; van der Burg, J.A.T.; Beukers, R.; Korpershoek, T.A.; et al. Effect of Cognitive Behavioral Therapy on Clinical Disease Course in Adolescents and Young Adults With Inflammatory Bowel Disease and Subclinical Anxiety and/or Depression: Results of a Randomized Trial. *Inflamm. Bowel Dis.* **2019**, *25*, 1945–1956. [CrossRef] [PubMed]
75. Hommel, K.A.; Hente, E.A.; Odell, S.; Herzer, M.; Ingerski, L.M.; Guilfoyle, S.M.; Denson, L.A. Evaluation of a group-based behavioral intervention to promote adherence in adolescents with inflammatory bowel disease. *Eur. J. Gastroenterol. Hepatol.* **2012**, *24*, 64–69. [CrossRef] [PubMed]
76. Gracie, D.J.; Irvine, A.J.; Sood, R.; Mikocka-Walus, A.; Hamlin, P.J.; Ford, A.C. Effect of psychological therapy on disease activity, psychological comorbidity, and quality of life in inflammatory bowel disease: A systematic review and meta-analysis. *Lancet Gastroenterol. Hepatol.* **2017**, *2*, 189–199. [CrossRef]
77. Spinelli, A.; Carvello, M.; D'Hoore, A.; Pagnini, F. Psychological perspectives of inflammatory bowel disease patients undergoing surgery: Rightful concerns and preconceptions. *Curr. Drug Targets* **2014**, *15*, 1074–1078. [CrossRef]
78. Polidano, K.; Chew-Graham, C.A.; Farmer, A.D.; Saunders, B. Access to Psychological Support for Young People Following Stoma Surgery: Exploring Patients' and Clinicians' Perspectives. *Qual. Health Res.* **2021**, *31*, 535–549. [CrossRef]
79. Lores, T.; Goess, C.; Mikocka-Walus, A.; Collins, K.L.; Burke, A.L.J.; Chur-Hansen, A.; Delfabbro, P.; Andrews, J.M. Integrated Psychological Care Reduces Health Care Costs at a Hospital-Based Inflammatory Bowel Disease Service. *Clin. Gastroenterol. Hepatol.* **2021**, *19*, 96–103.e3. [CrossRef]

80. Jedel, S.; Hoffman, A.; Merriman, P.; Swanson, B.; Voigt, R.; Rajan, K.B.; Shaikh, M.; Li, H.; Keshavarzian, A. A randomized controlled trial of mindfulness-based stress reduction to prevent flare-up in patients with inactive ulcerative colitis. *Digestion* **2014**, *89*, 142–155. [CrossRef]
81. Neilson, K.; Ftanou, M.; Monshat, K.; Salzberg, M.; Bell, S.; Kamm, M.A.; Connell, W.; Knowles, S.R.; Sevar, K.; Mancuso, S.G.; et al. A Controlled Study of a Group Mindfulness Intervention for Individuals Living with Inflammatory Bowel Disease. *Inflamm. Bowel Dis.* **2016**, *22*, 694–701. [CrossRef]
82. Boye, B.; Lundin, K.E.; Jantschek, G.; Leganger, S.; Mokleby, K.; Tangen, T.; Jantschek, I.; Pripp, A.H.; Wojniusz, S.; Dahlstroem, A.; et al. INSPIRE study: Does stress management improve the course of inflammatory bowel disease and disease-specific quality of life in distressed patients with ulcerative colitis or Crohn's disease? A randomized controlled trial. *Inflamm. Bowel Dis.* **2011**, *17*, 1863–1873. [CrossRef]

Disclaimer/Publisher's Note: The statements, opinions and data contained in all publications are solely those of the individual author(s) and contributor(s) and not of MDPI and/or the editor(s). MDPI and/or the editor(s) disclaim responsibility for any injury to people or property resulting from any ideas, methods, instructions or products referred to in the content.

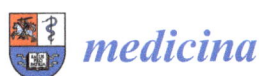

Review

Metabolic-Dysfunction-Associated Fatty Liver Disease and Gut Microbiota: From Fatty Liver to Dysmetabolic Syndrome

Ludovico Abenavoli [1,*], Giuseppe Guido Maria Scarlata [1], Emidio Scarpellini [2], Luigi Boccuto [3,4], Rocco Spagnuolo [1], Bruno Tilocca [1], Paola Roncada [1] and Francesco Luzza [1]

1 Department of Health Sciences, University "Magna Graecia", 88100 Catanzaro, Italy
2 Translationeel Onderzoek van Gastro-enterologische Aandoeningen (T.A.R.G.I.D.), Gasthuisberg University Hospital, KU Leuven, Herestraat 49, 3000 Leuven, Belgium
3 School of Nursing, Healthcare Genetics Program, Clemson University, Clemson, SC 29634, USA
4 School of Health Research, Clemson University, Clemson, SC 29634, USA
* Correspondence: l.abenavoli@unicz.it; Tel.: +39-0961-369-4387

Abstract: Metabolic-dysfunction-associated fatty liver disease (MAFLD) is the recent nomenclature designation that associates the condition of non-alcoholic fatty liver disease (NAFLD) with metabolic dysfunction. Its diagnosis has been debated in the recent period and is generally associated with a diagnosis of steatosis and at least one pathologic condition among overweight/obesity, type 2 diabetes mellitus, and metabolic dysregulation. Its pathogenesis is defined by a "multiple-hit" model and is associated with alteration or dysbiosis of the gut microbiota. The pathogenic role of dysbiosis of the gut microbiota has been investigated in many diseases, including obesity, type 2 diabetes mellitus, and NAFLD. However, only a few works correlate it with MAFLD, although common pathogenetic links to these diseases are suspected. This review underlines the most recurrent changes in the gut microbiota of patients with MAFLD, while also evidencing possible pathogenetic links.

Keywords: fatty liver; gut microbiota; dysbiosis; obesity; type 2 diabetes mellitus

1. Introduction

Metabolic dysfunction-associated fatty liver disease (MAFLD) is a recent nomenclature that associates non-alcoholic fatty liver disease (NAFLD) with a condition of systemic metabolic dysfunction [1]. The diagnosis of MAFLD follows specific criteria, such as the detection of hepatic steatosis (with a diagnosis conducted by imaging, biomarkers, or histology) and at least one characteristic among overweight/obesity, type 2 diabetes mellitus (T2DM), and metabolic dysregulation. The last criterion requires the presence of at least two characteristics, including increased waist circumference, hypertension, hypertriglyceridemia, low high-density lipoprotein cholesterol (HDL-C), pre-diabetes, insulin resistance, and subclinical inflammation [2]. Lin and colleagues [3] were the first to compare the diagnostic criteria of MAFLD and NAFLD in 13,083 cases identified from the NHANES III database. Their data showed that the MAFLD population had higher liver enzymes and more glucose and lipid-metabolism-related disorders. According to the authors, this new definition of MAFLD can specifically identify more patients at risk of developing cirrhosis and liver cancer, as they are affected by metabolic syndrome [3]. Further investigations corroborated the important role of this new MAFLD definition, as it better identified patients with significant hepatic fibrosis (93.9% MAFLD vs. 73.0% NAFLD) [4] or high liver stiffness (adjusted beta 0.116, $p < 0.001$ MAFLD vs. adjusted beta 0.006, $p = 0.90$ NAFLD), with respect to the NAFLD criteria [5]. Furthermore, in 2306 subjects with fatty liver, MAFLD (Hazard Ratio; HR 1.08, 95% CI 1.02–1.15, $p = 0.014$) and alcohol consumption (20–39 g/day; HR 1.73, 95% CI 1.26–2.36, $p = 0.001$) were independently associated with the worsening of the Suita score to predict the progression of atherosclerotic cardiovascular risk vs. the NAFLD group (HR 0.70, 95% CI 0.50–0.98, $p = 0.042$) [6]. This important evidence led to

Citation: Abenavoli, L.; Scarlata, G.G.M.; Scarpellini, E.; Boccuto, L.; Spagnuolo, R.; Tilocca, B.; Roncada, P.; Luzza, F. Metabolic-Dysfunction-Associated Fatty Liver Disease and Gut Microbiota: From Fatty Liver to Dysmetabolic Syndrome. *Medicina* **2023**, *59*, 594. https://doi.org/10.3390/medicina59030594

Academic Editor: Giovanni Tarantino

Received: 17 February 2023
Revised: 10 March 2023
Accepted: 15 March 2023
Published: 17 March 2023

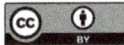

Copyright: © 2023 by the authors. Licensee MDPI, Basel, Switzerland. This article is an open access article distributed under the terms and conditions of the Creative Commons Attribution (CC BY) license (https://creativecommons.org/licenses/by/4.0/).

the acceptance of the definition of MAFLD nomenclature in 2022 by the "Global multi-stakeholder consensus on the redefinition of fatty liver disease", which includes more than 1000 signatories with different expertise backgrounds, from over 134 different countries [7]. From an epidemiological point of view, the prevalence of MAFLD varies between 26% and 39% [8–11] in the general population, up to 42% in inflammatory bowel diseases (IBD) [11], and 50.7% in overweight/obese adults [12]. This great heterogeneity relates to the use of different diagnostic techniques applied to various populations under investigation [11]. Finally, an imbalance of the gut microbiota composition, defined as dysbiosis, is involved in the development of MAFLD [13]. The present review underlines the most recurrent changes in the gut microbiota of patients with MAFLD, and hypothesizes their possible pathogenic links.

2. Materials and Methods

Literature Review

A review of the literature was performed through PubMed, NCBI and Scopus search engines. Mesh terms were the keywords: "MAFLD", "gut microbiota", "probiotic", "prebiotic", "postbiotic", "diet", and "dysbiosis". The search included English papers published in each period. All types of papers were included, i.e., reviews, retrospective analyses, and experimental studies. Figure 1 details a PRISMA flow diagram summarizing the short-listing procedure and reasons for exclusion of articles.

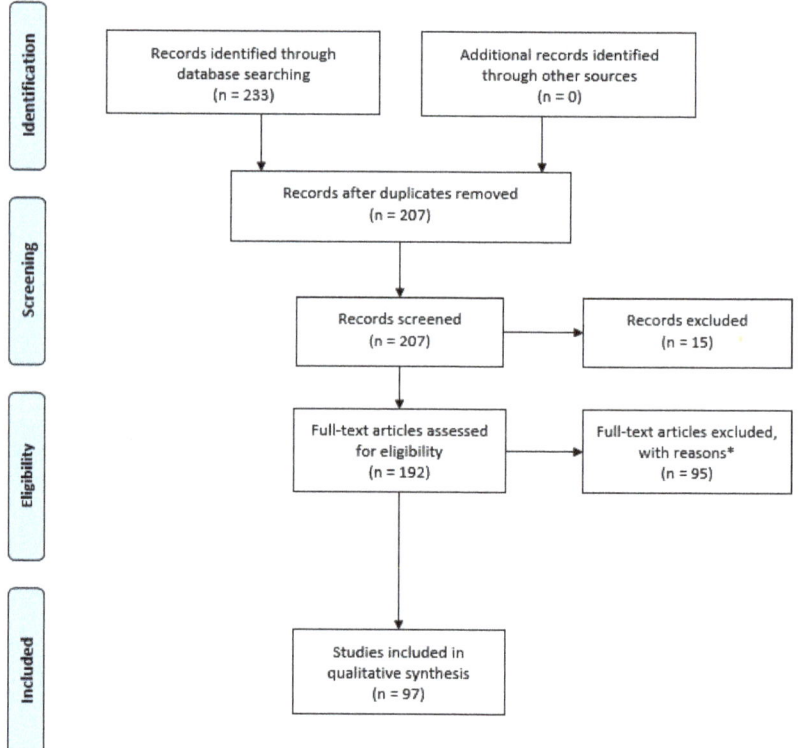

Figure 1. PRISMA flow diagram. * Full-text articles were excluded due to the following reasons: (1) the articles did not report data for individual comparison groups; (2) the articles did not distinguish NAFLD and MAFLD.

3. Gut Microbiota Changes in MAFLD Patients

Gut microbiota is an ecosystem composed of over 35,000 bacterial species, and performs several functions, such as nutrient and drug metabolism and antimicrobial protection, and it is involved in immunomodulation and the integrity of the gut barrier [14]. *Firmicutes* and *Bacteroidetes* constitute 90% of the microbial *Phyla* that characterize this ecosystem, while the remaining 10% are *Actinobacteria, Proteobacteria, Fusobacteria*, and *Verrucomicrobia* [15]. Specifically, the *phylum Firmicutes* is further characterized by more than 200 different genera, such as *Lactobacillus, Bacillus, Clostridium* (with a 95% abundance), *Enterococcus*, and *Ruminicoccus* [16]. On the other hand, the *Phylum Bacteroidetes* is characterized by fewer genera, such as *Bacteroides, Parabacteroides, Prevotella, Porphyromonas*, and *Alistipes* [17]. The two main phyla are in a delicate balance (measured as *Firmicutes/Bacteroidetes* ratio) with each other, thus maintaining the proper homeostasis of the gastrointestinal tract. This balance changes at various stages of life, from 0.4 in infants to 10.9 in adults and 0.6 in the elderly [18], and in dysmetabolic conditions, such as T2DM [19] and obesity [20]. For this reason, the *Firmicutes/Bacteroidetes* ratio is being studied as a biomarker of gut dysbiosis [21]. As previously reported, a condition of dysbiosis is involved in the development of MAFLD [13]. Few studies have analyzed the composition of the gut microbiota in MAFLD patients and healthy control subjects. In a retrospective cross-sectional study conducted by Zhang and colleagues, the authors analyzed the gut microbiota of 17 MAFLD patients with liver stiffness (LSM) $\geq$ 7.4 kPa (case group) and 68 control subjects with an LSM < 7.4 kPa (control group) [22]. Whole-genome sequencing from stool samples showed that *Bacteroidetes, Firmicutes*, and *Actinobacteria* were the most dominant *phyla* in the case group. At the genus and species level, *Prevotella copri, Phascolarctobacterium succinatutens, Eubacterium biforme*, and *Collinsella aerofaciens* were all more abundant in the case group than in the control group ($p < 0.05$). Furthermore, *Bacteroides coprocola* and *Bacteroides stercoris* were all reduced in the case group ($p < 0.05$). However, there was no statistically significant difference between the case and control groups ($p > 0.05$) using two different diversity indexes (α and β diversity, respectively). Regarding the correlation between dysbiosis and LSM, the levels of *Phascolarctobacterium succinatutens, Eubacterium biforme*, and *Collinsella aerofaciens* were also positively correlated with LSM ($p < 0.05$), while the levels of *Bacteroides stercoris* were inversely correlated with LSM ($p < 0.05$).

In another case-control study conducted by Yang and colleagues, the gut microbiota of 32 MAFLD patients and 30 healthy controls was analyzed using 16S ribosomal RNA (16S rRNA) sequencing from stool samples [23]. At the *phylum* level, the relative abundance of *Bacteroidetes, Proteobacteria*, and *Fusobacteria* increased, and *Firmicutes* decreased in MAFLD patients as compared to healthy control subjects. At the genus level, the relative abundances of *Prevotella, Bacteroides, Escherichia shigella, Megamonas, Fusobacterium*, and *Lachnoclostridium* increased, while *Clostridium, Agathobacter, Romboutsia, Faecalibacterium*, and *Blautia* decreased in MAFLD patients vs. healthy control subjects. Furthermore, the metabolomic analysis from stool and sera samples showed a reduction of hypoxanthine, propionyl carnitine, tyrosyl-alanine, hesperetin, methionine, and neohesperidin. As reported by the authors, flavonoids, such as hesperetin and neohesperidine, can reduce inflammatory cell infiltrations, hepatic steatosis and fibrosis, body weight, and insulin resistance in mice models. Finally, the authors set the inter-individual variability in the composition of the gut microbiota that is influenced by diet as a limitation of the study. The subjects enrolled did not follow the same diet before undergoing this study, so more standardized studies in patient selection are needed.

In a single-center prospective study conducted by Oh et al., the gut microbiota of 66 MAFLD patients and healthy controls was analyzed using 16S rRNA sequencing from stool samples [24]. The two groups showed different compositions of the gut microbiota. A statistically significant decrease of *Firmicutes* was observed in patients with MAFLD (50.08% in the MAFLD group and 60.15% in the healthy group; $p < 0.001$). *Proteobacteria* (10.69% vs. 3.09%; $p < 0.001$) and *Actinobacteria* (7.68% vs. 2.54%; $p < 0.001$) were significantly increased in patients with MAFLD compared to those in healthy control subjects. Finally, α-

diversity showed statistically significant differences between the two groups ($p < 0.001$). In addition, a reduction in bacterial diversity for butyrate-producing microorganisms, such as *Anaerostipes, Coprococcus, Eubacterium, Roseburia, Faecalibacterium, Odoribacter, Oscillibacter, Subdoligranulum, Butyricimonas, Alistipes, Pseudoflavonifractor, Clostridium, Butyricicoccus,* and *Flavonifractor* was also shown in MAFLD patients. A reduction in the abundance of butyrate-producing bacteria implies an increase in intestinal permeability, with possible translocation of microorganisms to the liver, promoting the onset of MAFLD. The main limitation of the study includes not assessing the physical activity and lifestyle of the few subjects enrolled, as these factors play a key role in the composition of the gut microbiota and certainly need to be evaluated in further studies.

Yang et al. compared the gut microbiota of 20 patients with MAFLD, 20 patients with MAFLD and T2DM, and 19 healthy control subjects, using 16S rRNA sequencing from stool samples [25]. *Bacteroidetes, Firmicutes,* and *Proteobacteria* were the most abundant *phyla* in case groups (MAFLD and MAFLD + T2DM, respectively) vs. healthy control subjects ($p < 0.05$). This study showed significant differences among the groups regarding *Prevotellaceae, Cyanobacteria, Ruminococcaceae, Oscillospirales,* and *Clostridia* genera ($p < 0.05$). Finally, α and β diversity index analyses showed moderate differences in species among the groups under investigation. As previously reported, the diversity in the composition of the gut microbiota in the case population compared with the control population induces increased intestinal permeability, resulting in liver damage. Overall, although the cohort under review is rather small, this is one of the few case-control studies correlating T2DM and MAFLD. Indeed, according to the authors, assessment of the composition of the gut microbiota and its metabolites could be a reliable biomarker in the future.

Dorofeyev A. et al. analyzed the gut microbiota of 111 patients and 30 healthy control subjects, using 16S rRNA sequencing from stool samples [26]. The main group included 56 MAFLD + T2DM patients, the first group included 28 patients with MAFLD without T2DM and the second group included 27 patients with T2DM without MAFLD. The main group of patients, compared to healthy control subjects, showed a significant increase in levels of *Actinobacteria* (28.6% vs. 14.1%; $p < 0.05$), a decrease in *Bacteroidetes* (13.7% vs. 41.7%; $p < 0.05$) and an increase in the ratio of *Firmicutes/Bacteroidetes* (3.16% vs. 0.88%; $p < 0.05$). Significantly higher levels of *Actinobacteria* were found in the main group, as compared to the first group (28.6% vs. 19.8%; $p < 0.05$). When these groups were compared against the second group, the data revealed higher levels of *Actinobacteria* (28.6% vs. 17.1%; $p < 0.05$), lower levels of *Bacteroidetes* (13.7% vs. 32.4%; $p < 0.05$) and an increased *Firmicutes/Bacteroidetes* ratio (3.16% vs. 1.06%; $p < 0.05$). The comparison between the first group and healthy controls showed significantly lower levels of *Bacteroidetes* (21.1% vs. 41.7%; $p < 0.05$) and an increase in the ratio of *Firmicutes/Bacteroidetes* (2.26% vs. 0.88%; $p < 0.05$). Regarding the second group, the authors found only a significant increase in "other" microorganisms compared to the control group (15.8% vs. 6.9%; $p < 0.05$). According to the authors, the composition of the gut microbiota is strongly influenced by the population under investigation. Indeed, these changes in the composition of the gut microbiota in cases from Ukraine, compared to controls, could be associated with genetic characteristics, dietary habits, and the use of hypoglycemic drugs. A schematic representation of gut microbiota dysbiosis in MAFLD patients and MAFLD patients with T2DM is shown in Figure 2.

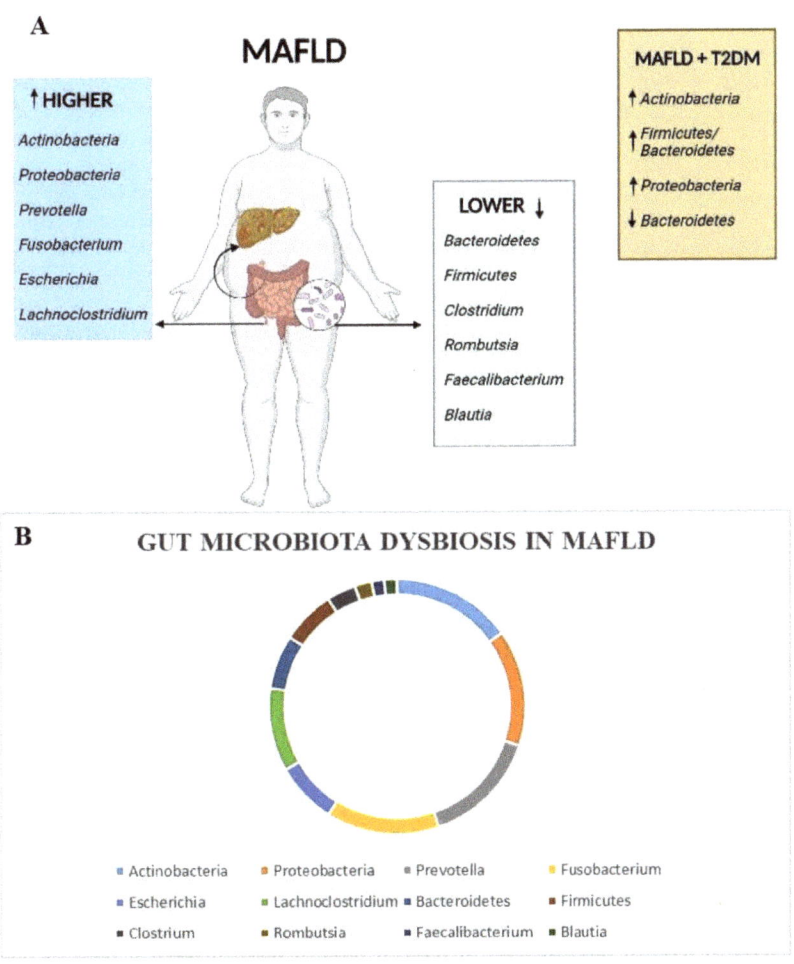

Figure 2. Schematic representation of gut microbiota dysbiosis in MAFLD patients (light blue and green boxes; panel (A,B)) and MAFLD + T2DM patients (orange box; panel (A)).

4. MAFLD and Gut Microbiota: Possible Pathogenetic Ways

Although the pathogenetic link between gut microbiota and NAFLD has been widely investigated [27,28], its relationship with MAFLD is poorly known. It is well known that MAFLD is a "multiple-hit" disease, which has obesity, diabetes, insulin resistance, genetic and environmental factors, and a dysbiosis of the gut microbiota as risk factors [29], as shown in Figure 3.

The human gut, after being colonized by microorganisms, manages to maintain a state of homeostasis due to continuous regulation by the immune system [30]. In addition, the diet can facilitate this delicate balance, promoting the integrity of the mucosal barrier and disfavoring the translocation of intestinal pathogens [31]. The structure of the intestinal barrier is maintained strong by tight junctions consisting of transmembrane single-span (such as junctional adhesion molecules) or tetraspan proteins (such as occludin, claudin, and tricellulin) [32]. Additional proteins that serve as scaffolds are *zonula occludens* proteins [33]. The junctional adhesion molecule A (JAM-A) was studied by Rahman et al. in mouse models, with interruption of the *F11r* gene encoding for JAM-A. Male C57BL/6 (control) or $F11r^{-/-}$ mice were fed differently for 8 weeks: first a normal diet, then a diet with a high content of saturated fat, fructose, and cholesterol. The diet rich in saturated fat, fructose, and cholesterol increased the abundance of *Proteobacteria* and *Firmicutes* and reduced the abundance of *Bacteroidetes* in the lumen of control and $F11r^{-/-}$ mice. Furthermore, after being fed a diet rich in saturated fat, fructose, and cholesterol, the $F11r^{-/-}$ mice showed histological evidence of severe steatosis and lobular inflammation, in contrast to the moderate steatosis developed by control mice that had been fed the same diet. In addition, decreased expression of JAM-A was correlated with increased mucosal inflammation. This event, according to the authors, is related to a compensatory mechanism in the maintenance of the intestinal barrier function in the absence of JAM-A, corroborated by the increased expression of occludin and claudin-4 in the colon of $F11r^{-/-}$ mice fed a normal diet, as compared to control mice [34]. Clinical trials showed that the reduced levels of bacteria of the genus *Akkermansia* found in MAFLD patients compared to healthy controls are the consequence of a reduction in fermentation products, including butyrate and acetate. These short-chain fatty acids are critical in maintaining the homeostasis of the microbiota and in the structure of the gut [35,36]. Overall, the role of *Akkermasia* in obesity and metabolic disorders warrants further investigation using clinical models. In fact, in pre-clinical models with an abundance of this bacterium, prebiotics, and polyphenols have been shown to have positive effects on metabolic disorders [37]. Similar events result in increased intestinal permeability, known as "leaky gut" [38], with a transition of lipopolysaccharide (LPS), a component of the Gram-negative outer wall, to the liver via the portal vein [39]. The interaction between LPS and Toll-like receptor 4 (TLR4) expressed by Kupffer cells, activates the nuclear factor kappa-light-chain enhancer of activated B cells (NF-κB) and subsequently an inflammatory cascade, which is a pathogenetic mechanism shared with NAFLD [40].

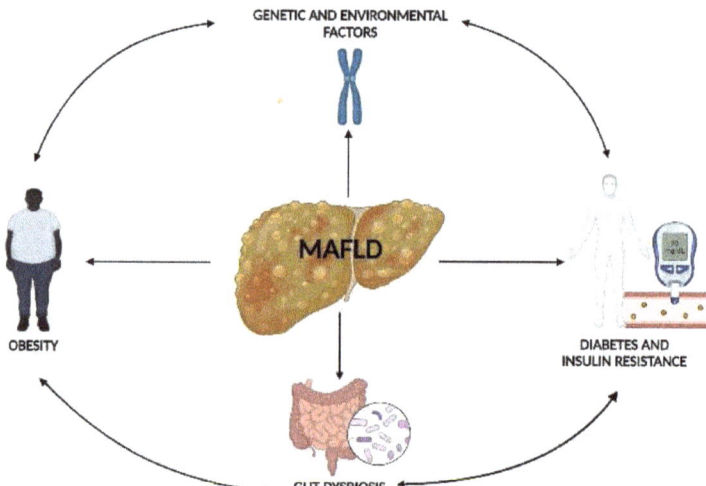

Figure 3. "Multiple-hit" hypothesis in MAFLD pathogenesis.

4.1. Gut Microbiota Dysbiosis and Obesity

Dysbiosis of the gut microbiota is related to other pathogenic factors that contribute to the development of MAFLD. It is known how the gut microbiota regulates certain mechanisms that lead to obesity [41]. The gut microbiota ferments carbohydrates into short-chain fatty acids (SCFAs), which, after intestinal absorption, promote energy homeostasis [42]. In the enterocyte, the three main SCFAs, acetate, butyrate, and propionate, are converted to acetyl-CoA by acetyl-CoA carboxylase to produce adenosine triphosphate (ATP) through the Krebs cycle. This pathway contributes to maintaining cellular homeostasis, consequently strengthening tight-junction function and intestinal barrier integrity [43]. Despite this "beneficial" role, a dysbiosis of the gut microbiota can lead to increased SCFA production, resulting in lipid accumulation in the liver [44]. This mechanism could support a possible pathogenetic link between gut dysbiosis, obesity, and MAFLD. In addition, microorganisms in the gastrointestinal tract are involved in the production of hormones that positively or negatively regulate satiety, such as leptin, insulin, and ghrelin [45]. Specifically, neurons that express pro-opiomelanocortin (POMC) and cocaine- and amphetamine-regulated transcript (CART) in the hypothalamic arcuate nucleus are the targets of leptin binding to them to inhibit hunger signals [46]. Ghrelin is a 28-amino-acid peptide present in our organism in two different iso-forms: n-octanoyl modified ghrelin, and des-acyl ghrelin [47]. The acylated form is mainly involved in the orexigenic role by stimulating the synthesis of neuropeptide Y (NPY) and agouti-related protein (AgRP) in neurons in the arcuate nucleus of the hypothalamus and cerebellum, which promote increased food intake [48]. Insulin-like peptide 5 (Insl5) is a two-chains peptide hormone member of the relaxin family of peptides, with a structure similar to insulin [49]. Its biochemical pathway involves the G-protein-coupled relaxin/insulin-like family peptide receptor 4 (Rxfp4) to carry out its orexigenic action [50]. In pre-clinical models, Insl5 increased food intake in wild-type mice with respect to mice models without the Rxfp4 receptor. Furthermore, plasmatic Insl5 levels were increased in fasting, but decreased with feeding [51]. Although further studies in clinical and pre-clinical models are needed, the regulation of these hormones could be used to improve body weight or metabolism [52]. Table 1 summarizes case-control studies regarding metabolite production and obesity.

Table 1. Summary table of case-control studies regarding metabolite production and obesity.

Sample Size	Metabolites Involved	Biological Samples Analyzed	Results	References
208 obese subjects vs. 191 normal-weight subjects	Acetate, propionate, valerate, butyrate	Serum and stool	Higher concentrations of acetate (SMD = 0.87, 95% CI = 0.24–1.50), propionate (SMD = 0.86, 95% CI = 0.35–1.36), valerate (SMD = 0.32, 95% CI = 0.00–0.64) and butyrate (SMD = 0.78, 95% CI = 0.29–1.27) in obese subjects vs. normal-weight subjects	Kim KN et al., 2019 [53]
13 obese subjects vs. 13 normal-weight subjects	Acetate, butyrate	Stool	Acetate and butyrate were significantly higher in the group of obese patients compared to normal-weight patients ($p = 0.033$ and $p = 0.004$, respectively)	Martínez-Cuesta et al., 2021 [54]
92 obese adults vs. 92 normal-weight subjects	Leptin	Serum	Higher levels of leptin (51.24 ± 18.12 vs. 9.10 ± 2.99: $p < 0.0001$) in obese adults as compared to healthy control subjects	Kumar et al., 2020 [55]
35 obese adults vs. 20 normal-weight subjects	Leptin	Serum	Significant difference ($p < 0.001$) in leptin between the obese group (34.78 ± 13.96 ng/mL) and the non-obese control subjects (10.6 ± 4.2 ng/mL)	Al Maskari MY et al., 2006 [56]

Table 1. Cont.

Sample Size	Metabolites Involved	Biological Samples Analyzed	Results	References
1125 obese adults vs. 738 normal-weight subjects	Ghrelin	Serum	Lower levels of acyl ghrelin at baseline (SMD: −0.85; 95% CI: −1.13 to −0.57; $p < 0.001$) and postprandial at different time points (SMD 30 min: −0.85, 95% CI: −1.18 to −0.53, $p < 0.001$; SMD 60 min: −1.00, 95% CI: −1.37 to −0.63, $p < 0.001$; SMD 120 min: −1.21, 95% CI: −1.59 to −0.83, $p < 0.001$) in obese patients in respect to healthy control subjects	Wang Y. et al., 2022 [57]

Overall, studies have focused on characterizing the diversity in the composition of the gut microbiota non-lean NAFLD, lean NAFLD, and healthy control subjects. A recent review showed the following differences in gut microbiota composition: (i) both NAFLD groups had a decrease in *Firmicutes* and *Ruminococcaceae*, but a decrease in *Leuconostocaceae* was only observed in obese NAFLD; (ii) an increase in the *Bacteroidetes/Firmicutes* ratio in lean and obese NAFLD patients compared to healthy control subjects; (iii) lean NAFLD patients showed an increase in *Ruminococcaceae* compared to obese NAFLD, and an increase in *Dorea* and a decrease in *Marvinbryantia* and *Christensellenaceae* compared to healthy control subjects [58]. However, there is a lack of case-control studies regarding MAFLD, obesity, and gut microbiota composition.

4.2. Gut Microbiota Dysbiosis, T2MD, and Insulin Resistance

Another support for the pathogenesis of MAFLD may be the close correlation between gut microbiota, T2DM, and insulin resistance. T2DM is associated with an over-production of pro-inflammatory cytokines, such as interleukin (IL)-1α, IL-6, IL-10, and IL-22 [59]. The role of the gut microbiota is to modulate the inflammatory response by secreting anti-inflammatory cytokines. For example, *Roseburia intestinalis* promotes the production of IL-22, a cytokine with anti-inflammatory action, while reducing insulin resistance and diabetes initiation [60]. *Bacteroides fragilis* polysaccharide A induces IL-10 secretion by B and T cells obtaining the reduced inflammatory process in the gut [61]. In knockout mouse models of the IL-6 gene, the absence of this cytokine led to significantly increased expression of defensins α3 and α4 in the gut, promoting microbiota remodeling and subsequent inflammatory response [62]. Similarly, in IL-1α-deficient mice, dysbiosis of the gut microbiota had been found, resulting in an inflammatory intestinal state vs. wild-type mouse models [63]. The gut microbiota is closely related to T2DM, as it can regulate insulin clearance [64]. Foley et al. found impaired insulin clearance after 6 weeks in mouse models lacking gut microbes and after a fat-rich obesogenic diet, compared with generally healthy mice treated with a control diet [65]. Additionally, insulin resistance is associated with increased intestinal permeability under conditions of dysbiosis, without necessarily being influenced by obesity [46]. Reduced adiponectin concentrations and increased leptin concentrations were associated ($p < 0.05$) with obesity, while Zonulin expression is positively associated ($p < 0.05$) with body mass index and insulin concentration. In addition, elevated insulin production was associated with increased intestinal barrier permeability [66]. Overall, dysbiosis of the gut microbiota that promotes T2DM and insulin resistance may lead to considering MAFLD a hepatic phenotype of systemic insulin resistance [67].

4.3. Gut Microbiota Dysbiosis and Genetic Factors

Lastly, genetic and environmental factors are continuously investigated regarding the predisposition and pathogenesis of MAFLD. Certainly, the mechanism by which specific single nucleotide polymorphisms (SNPs) are inherited plays a key role in susceptibility to the development of the disease. These include *Patatin-like Phospholipase Domain -containing 3 (PNPLA3)* and *Membrane-Bound O-acyltransferase Domain-containing 7 (MBOAT7)* [68]. Specifically, the rs641738 variant of the *MBOAT7* gene, which promotes the regulation of insulinemia, has been evaluated as a predisposing factor of hepatocellular carcinoma (HCC), even in the absence of cirrhosis in MAFLD patients [69]. A recent study conducted on 564 MAFLD patients and healthy control subjects showed that the CC genotype of the *PNPLA3* gene (encoding for a triacylglycerol lipase that mediates the hydrolysis of triacylglycerol in adipocytes) rs738409 and the TT genotype of the *MBOAT7* gene rs64173 are risk factors for the occurrence of MAFLD [70]. Another case-control study, conducted by Liao S. et al. on 286 MAFLD patients and 250 healthy control subjects, showed a correlation between the *PNPLA3* rs738409 variant and MAFLD (odds ratio [OR] = 1.791 and 1.377, respectively, p = 0.038 and 0.027, respectively) and with aspartate aminotransferase (AST) levels [71]. On the other hand, dysbiosis of the gut microbiota in association with genetic mutations is called "genetic dysbiosis" [72]. This is characterized by two possible events: (i) mutation of genes encoding pattern recognition receptors (PRRs) failing bacterial recognition [73]; (ii) mutations in genes involved in the regulation of the immune response, resulting in stimulation of pro-inflammatory cytokines and diffuse inflammation in the gut, affecting the composition of the microbiota [74]. Moreover, they are certainly related to the onset of IBD, which in turn is closely related to MAFLD [71]. Overall, genetic factors that promote dysbiosis of the gut microbiota may contribute to the pathogenesis of MAFLD.

4.4. Dysmetabolic Comorbidities and MAFLD Progression

The evidence cited so far underlines the pathogenic multifactorial nature of MAFLD, in which inter-individual factors and dysmetabolic comorbidities promote its onset and progression. Alteration in the composition of the gut microbiota is an important factor in its occurrence, through pathways that disfavor the production of metabolites by affecting the integrity of the gut barrier and increasing its permeability. The passage of microorganisms and Gram-negative LPS via the portal vein to the liver is carried out by an inflammatory process. In addition, the cascade mechanism of pro-inflammatory cytokines is already widely represented in patients with dysmetabolic diseases such as T2DM, insulin resistance, and obesity. Moreover, the overproduction of SCFA under dysbiosis conditions is responsible for the accumulation of liver fat in these patients. All these interconnected mechanisms could explain the etiopathogenesis of MAFLD, which still deserves further investigation.

5. Therapeutic Approaches

Possible therapeutic approaches are related to re-establishing the eubiosis condition of the gut microbiota, and thus the correct balance of the microbial community within [75]. Diet is an important factor that influences the composition of the gut microbiota, which is the reason why a balanced diet can promote its eubiosis [76]. The Mediterranean diet was purposed as a possible therapeutic approach [77]. However, studies aimed at investigating proper dietary intake are needed for better management of MAFLD patients [78]. We know more about the preventive role of the Mediterranean diet in NAFLD [79]. This dietary regimen is composed mainly of a higher intake of fish and vegetables than of meat and dairy products, which disadvantages the onset of many diseases, such as T2DM, obesity, and NAFLD [80]. The antioxidants (such as polyphenols) in this diet promote the reduction of the inflammatory state typical of these diseases [81,82], acting at different levels: (i) modulating the pathway of mitogen-activated protein kinases (MAPKs), resulting in reduced production of pro-inflammatory cytokines [83]; (ii) inhibiting NF-κB-induced pro-inflammatory gene expression at multiple levels [84]; and (iii) inhibiting cyclo-oxygenases (COX) with reduced prostaglandin synthesis [85]. This dietary approach—rich in vegetables and antioxidants—has "healthy" consequences on the remodeling of the gut microbiota by promoting the growth of good bacteria that promote SCFA synthesis and degrade toxic metabolites [86]. Overall, the prevention of these diseases may be related to the prevention of MAFLD progression [87].

As reported by The International Scientific Association for Probiotics and Prebiotics, probiotics are defined as "live microorganisms that, when administered in adequate amounts, confer a health benefit to the host" [88], while prebiotics are "a selectively fermented ingredient that results in specific changes in the composition and/or activity of the gastrointestinal microbiota, thus conferring benefit(s) upon host health" [89]. Subsequently, the same International Scientific Association defined postbiotics as "a preparation of inanimate microorganisms and/or their components that confers a health benefit on the host" [90]. While the preventive and therapeutic role of probiotics in NAFLD is quite clear in clinical [91,92] and pre-clinical models [93,94], further investigations are needed in patients with MAFLD. A recent meta-analysis showed that the use of probiotics holds promise for reducing liver enzyme levels in patients with MAFLD. Among a total of 772 patients, the use of probiotics for therapeutic purposes could reduce the levels of alanine aminotransferase (mean difference (MD): -11.76 (-16.06, -7.46), $p < 0.00001$), aspartate aminotransferase (MD: -9.08 (-13.60, -4.56), $p < 0.0001$), γ-glutamyltransferase (MD: -5.67 (-6.80, -4.54), $p < 0.00001$) and homeostasis model assessment of insulin resistance (MD: -0.62 (-1.08, -0.15), $p = 0.01$) in patients with MAFLD, compared to control patients. Indeed, this study did not show statistical significance for levels of total cholesterol, triglycerides, low-density lipoproteins (LDL), C-reactive protein (PCR), and tumor necrosis factor-α (TNF-α) [95]. Regarding prebiotics, their use, in combination with probiotics, is recommended, as suggested by a recent review that underlines the importance of this combined approach that showed a significant reduction in the levels of hepatic steatosis, alanine aminotransferase (ALT), AST, HDL, LDL, triglyceride and cholesterol levels in 782 MAFLD patients compared to healthy controls [96]. Finally, the use of postbiotics in mouse models promoted insulin sensitivity, whereas the use of ursodeoxycholic acid in human models showed a reduction in transaminases and insulin resistance [97]. Despite this, the literature about clinical trials that promote the use of postbiotics in MAFLD patients is still lacking. Overall, while the diagnostic approach regarding MAFLD has been clarified, international guidelines for the treatment of this disease are needed.

6. Conclusions and Future Directions

MAFLD is generally related to other disease states, such as T2DM, obesity, and insulin resistance, and constitutes a serious public health burden. A dysbiosis of the gut microbiota plays a key role in this context. Specifically, the increased permeability of the intestinal barrier, known as "leaky gut," allows the passage of toxic products, such as LPS from Gram-negative bacteria, through the portal vein to the liver. However, the complex pathways involved in such dysbiosis deserve further investigation via the planning of new case-control studies. On the other hand, the preventive and therapeutic use of a diet rich in polyphenols, such as the Mediterranean diet, and the combined use of probiotics and prebiotics are widely recommended in the management of MAFLD patients. However, the literature on clinical trials related to these patients is still poor. For this reason, although the treatment of NAFLD patients is the subject of specific international guidelines, the therapeutic approach to be used with MAFLD patients is still under investigation. Expanding our knowledge of the active role that the gut microbiota can play in the pathogenesis of MAFLD could also facilitate the development of international guidelines for the prevention and treatment of this disease.

Author Contributions: Conceptualization, L.A. and E.S.; methodology, G.G.M.S.; resources, E.S. and B.T.; writing—original draft preparation, L.A. and G.G.M.S.; writing—review and editing, E.S. and L.B.; visualization, L.B. and R.S.; supervision, P.R. and F.L. All authors have read and agreed to the published version of the manuscript.

Funding: This research received no external funding.

Institutional Review Board Statement: Not applicable.

Informed Consent Statement: Not applicable.

Data Availability Statement: Not applicable.

Conflicts of Interest: The authors declare no conflict of interest.

References

1. Eslam, M.; Newsome, P.N.; Sarin, S.K.; Anstee, Q.M.; Targher, G.; Romero-Gomez, M.; Zelber-Sagi, S.; Wai-Sun Wong, V.; Dufour, J.F.; Schattenberg, J.M.; et al. A new definition for metabolic dysfunction-associated fatty liver disease: An international expert consensus statement. *J. Hepatol.* **2020**, *73*, 202–209. [CrossRef]
2. Bianco, C.; Romeo, S.; Petta, S.; Long, M.T.; Valenti, L. MAFLD vs. NAFLD: Let the contest begin! *Liver Int.* **2020**, *40*, 2079–2081. [CrossRef]
3. Lin, S.; Huang, J.; Wang, M.; Kumar, R.; Liu, Y.; Liu, S.; Wu, Y.; Wang, X.; Zhu, Y. Comparison of MAFLD and NAFLD diagnostic criteria in real world. *Liver Int.* **2020**, *40*, 2082–2089. [CrossRef]
4. Yamamura, S.; Eslam, M.; Kawaguchi, T.; Tsutsumi, T.; Nakano, D.; Yoshinaga, S.; Takahashi, H.; Anzai, K.; George, J.; Torimura, T. MAFLD identifies patients with significant hepatic fibrosis better than NAFLD. *Liver Int.* **2020**, *40*, 3018–3030. [CrossRef]
5. van Kleef, L.A.; Ayada, I.; Alferink, L.J.M.; Pan, Q.; de Knegt, R.J. Metabolic dysfunction-associated fatty liver disease improves detection of high liver stiffness: The Rotterdam Study. *Hepatology* **2022**, *75*, 419–429. [CrossRef]
6. Tsutsumi, T.; Eslam, M.; Kawaguchi, T.; Yamamura, S.; Kawaguchi, A.; Nakano, D.; Koseki, M.; Yoshinaga, S.; Takahashi, H.; Anzai, K.; et al. MAFLD better predicts the progression of atherosclerotic cardiovascular risk than NAFLD: Generalized estimating equation approach. *Hepatol. Res.* **2021**, *5*, 1115–1128. [CrossRef]
7. Méndez-Sánchez, N.; Bugianesi, E.; Gish, R.G.; Lammert, F.; Tilg, H.; Nguyen, M.H.; Sarin, S.K.; Fabrellas, N.; Zelber-Sagi, S.; Fan, J.G.; et al. Global multi-stakeholder endorsement of the MAFLD definition. *Lancet Gastroenterol. Hepatol.* **2022**, *7*, 388–390. [CrossRef]
8. Ciardullo, S.; Perseghin, G. Prevalence of NAFLD, MAFLD and associated advanced fibrosis in the contemporary United States population. *Liver Int.* **2021**, *41*, 1290–1293. [CrossRef]
9. Chen, Y.L.; Li, H.; Li, S.; Xu, Z.; Tian, S.; Wu, J.; Liang, X.Y.; Li, X.; Liu, Z.L.; Xiao, J.; et al. Prevalence of and risk factors for metabolic associated fatty liver disease in an urban population in China: A cross-sectional comparative study. *BMC Gastroenterol.* **2021**, *21*, 212. [CrossRef]
10. Yuan, Q.; Wang, H.; Gao, P.; Chen, W.; Lv, M.; Bai, S.; Wu, J. Prevalence and Risk Factors of Metabolic-Associated Fatty Liver Disease among 73,566 Individuals in Beijing, China. *Int. J. Environ. Res. Public Health* **2022**, *19*, 2096. [CrossRef]
11. Rodriguez-Duque, J.C.; Calleja, J.L.; Iruzubieta, P.; Hernández-Conde, M.; Rivas-Rivas, C.; Vera, M.I.; Garcia, M.J.; Pascual, M.; Castro, B.; García-Blanco, A.; et al. Increased risk of MAFLD and Liver Fibrosis in Inflammatory Bowel Disease Independent of Classic Metabolic Risk Factors. *Clin. Gastroenterol. Hepatol.* **2022**, *21*, 406–414. [CrossRef]
12. Liu, J.; Ayada, I.; Zhang, X.; Wang, L.; Li, Y.; Wen, T.; Ma, Z.; Bruno, M.J.; de Knegt, R.J.; Cao, W.; et al. Estimating Global Prevalence of Metabolic Dysfunction-Associated Fatty Liver Disease in Overweight or Obese Adults. *Clin. Gastroenterol. Hepatol.* **2022**, *20*, e573–e582. [CrossRef]
13. Hrncir, T.; Hrncirova, L.; Kverka, M.; Hromadka, R.; Machova, V.; Trckova, E.; Kostovcikova, K.; Kralickova, P.; Krejsek, J.; Tlaskalova-Hogenova, H. Gut Microbiota and NAFLD: Pathogenetic Mechanisms, Microbiota Signatures, and Therapeutic Interventions. *Microorganisms* **2021**, *9*, 957. [CrossRef]
14. Jandhyala, S.M.; Talukdar, R.; Subramanyam, C.; Vuyyuru, H.; Sasikala, M.; Nageshwar Reddy, D. Role of the normal gut microbiota. *World J. Gastroenterol.* **2015**, *21*, 8787–8803. [CrossRef]
15. Wang, S.; Song, F.; Gu, H.; Shu, Z.; Wei, X.; Zhang, K.; Zhou, Y.; Jiang, L.; Wang, Z.; Li, J.; et al. Assess the diversity of gut microbiota among healthy adults for forensic application. *Microb. Cell Factories* **2022**, *21*, 46. [CrossRef]
16. Rinninella, E.; Raoul, P.; Cintoni, M.; Franceschi, F.; Miggiano, G.A.D.; Gasbarrini, A.; Mele, M.C. What is the Healthy Gut Microbiota Composition? A Changing Ecosystem across Age, Environment, Diet, and Diseases. *Microorganisms* **2019**, *7*, 14. [CrossRef]
17. Johnson, E.L.; Heaver, S.L.; Walters, W.A.; Ley, R.E. Microbiome and metabolic disease: Revisiting the bacterial phylum Bacteroidetes. *J. Mol. Med.* **2017**, *95*, 1–8. [CrossRef]
18. Mariat, D.; Firmesse, O.; Levenez, F.; Guimarães, V.; Sokol, H.; Doré, J.; Corthier, G.; Furet, J.P. Firmicutes/Bacteroidetes ratio of the human microbiota changes with age. *BMC Microbiol.* **2009**, *9*, 23. [CrossRef]
19. Sedighi, M.; Razavi, S.; Navab-Moghadam, F.; Khamseh, M.E.; Alaei-Shahmiri, F.; Mehrtash, A.; Amirmozafari, N. Comparison of gut microbiota in adult patients with type 2 diabetes and healthy individuals. *Microb. Pathog.* **2017**, *111*, 362–369. [CrossRef]
20. Magne, F.; Gotteland, M.; Gauthier, L.; Zazueta, A.; Pesoa, S.; Navarrete, P.; Balamurugan, R. Firmicutes/Bacteroidetes Ratio: A Relevant Marker of Gut Dysbiosis in Obese Patients? *Nutrients* **2020**, *12*, 1474. [CrossRef]
21. Grigor'eva, I.N. Gallstone Disease, Obesity and the Firmicutes/Bacteroidetes Ratio as a Possible Biomarker of Gut Dysbiosis. *J. Pers. Med.* **2020**, *11*, 13. [CrossRef]

22. Zhang, Y.; Yan, S.; Sheng, S.; Qin, Q.; Chen, J.; Li, W.; Li, T.; Gao, X.; Wang, L.; Ang, L.; et al. Comparison of gut microbiota in male MAFLD patients with varying liver stiffness. *Front. Cell. Infect. Microbiol.* **2022**, *12*, 873048. [CrossRef]
23. Yang, L.; Dai, Y.; He, H.; Liu, Z.; Liao, S.; Zhang, Y.; Liao, G.; An, Z. Integrative analysis of gut microbiota and fecal metabolites in metabolic associated fatty liver disease patients. *Front. Microbiol.* **2022**, *13*, 969757. [CrossRef]
24. Oh, J.H.; Lee, J.H.; Cho, M.S.; Kim, H.; Chun, J.; Lee, J.H.; Yoon, Y.; Kang, W. Characterization of Gut Microbiome in Korean Patients with Metabolic Associated Fatty Liver Disease. *Nutrients* **2021**, *13*, 1013. [CrossRef]
25. Yang, Q.; Zhang, L.; Li, Q.; Gu, M.; Qu, Q.; Yang, X.; Yi, Q.; Gu, K.; Kuang, L.; Hao, M.; et al. Characterization of microbiome and metabolite analyses in patients with metabolic associated fatty liver disease and type II diabetes mellitus. *BMC Microbiol.* **2022**, *22*, 105. [CrossRef]
26. Dorofeyev, A.; Rudenko, M.; Cheverda, T. State of The Gut Microbiota in Patients with Metabolic-Associated Fatty Liver Disease with Type 2 Diabetes Mellitus. *Proc. Shevchenko Sci. Soc. Med. Sci.* **2022**, *69*. [CrossRef]
27. Abenavoli, L.; Procopio, A.C.; Scarpellini, E.; Polimeni, N.; Aquila, I.; Larussa, T.; Boccuto, L.; Luzza, F. Gut microbiota and non-alcoholic fatty liver disease. *Minerva Gastroenterol. (Torino)* **2021**, *67*, 339–347. [CrossRef]
28. Abenavoli, L.; Giubilei, L.; Procopio, A.C.; Spagnuolo, R.; Luzza, F.; Boccuto, L.; Scarpellini, E. Gut Microbiota in Non-Alcoholic Fatty Liver Disease Patients with Inflammatory Bowel Diseases: A Complex Interplay. *Nutrients* **2022**, *14*, 5323. [CrossRef]
29. Li, H.; Guo, M.; An, Z.; Meng, J.; Jiang, J.; Song, J.; Wu, W. Prevalence and Risk Factors of Metabolic Associated Fatty Liver Disease in Xinxiang, China. *Int. J. Environ. Res. Public Health* **2020**, *17*, 1818. [CrossRef]
30. El Aidy, S.; Hooiveld, G.; Tremaroli, V.; Bäckhed, F.; Kleerebezem, M. The gut microbiota and mucosal homeostasis: Colonized at birth or at adulthood, does it matter? *Gut Microbes* **2013**, *4*, 118–124. [CrossRef]
31. Ma, N.; Guo, P.; Zhang, J.; He, T.; Kim, S.W.; Zhang, G.; Ma, X. Nutrients Mediate Intestinal Bacteria-Mucosal Immune Crosstalk. *Front. Immunol.* **2018**, *9*, 5. [CrossRef]
32. Ghosh, S.; Whitley, C.S.; Haribabu, B.; Jala, V.R. Regulation of Intestinal Barrier Function by Microbial Metabolites. *Cell. Mol. Gastroenterol. Hepatol.* **2021**, *11*, 1463–1482. [CrossRef]
33. Odenwald, M.A.; Choi, W.; Kuo, W.T.; Singh, G.; Sailer, A.; Wang, Y.; Shen, L.; Fanning, A.S.; Turner, J.R. The scaffolding protein ZO-1 coordinates actomyosin and epithelial apical specializations in vitro and in vivo. *J. Biol. Chem.* **2018**, *293*, 17317–17335. [CrossRef]
34. Rahman, K.; Desai, C.; Iyer, S.S.; Thorn, N.E.; Kumar, P.; Liu, Y.; Smith, T.; Neish, A.S.; Li, H.; Tan, S.; et al. Loss of Junctional Adhesion Molecule A Promotes Severe Steatohepatitis in Mice on a Diet High in Saturated Fat, Fructose, and Cholesterol. *Gastroenterology* **2016**, *151*, 733–746. [CrossRef]
35. Lukovac, S.; Belzer, C.; Pellis, L.; Keijser, B.J.; de Vos, W.M.; Montijn, R.C.; Roeselers, G. Differential modulation by Akkermansia muciniphila and Faecalibacterium prausnitzii of host peripheral lipid metabolism and histone acetylation in mouse gut organoids. *mBio* **2014**, *5*, e01438-14. [CrossRef]
36. Dao, M.C.; Everard, A.; Aron-Wisnewsky, J.; Sokolovska, N.; Prifti, E.; Verger, E.O.; Kayser, B.D.; Levenez, F.; Chilloux, J.; Hoyles, L.; et al. Akkermansia muciniphila and improved metabolic health during a dietary intervention in obesity: Relationship with gut microbiome richness and ecology. *Gut* **2016**, *65*, 426–436. [CrossRef]
37. Kobyliak, N.; Falalyeyeva, T.; Kyriachenko, Y.; Tseyslyer, Y.; Kovalchuk, O.; Hadiliia, O.; Eslami, M.; Yousefi, B.; Abenavoli, L.; Fagoonee, S.; et al. Akkermansia muciniphila as a novel powerful bacterial player in the treatment of metabolic disorders. *Minerva Endocrinol. (Torino)* **2022**, *47*, 242–252. [CrossRef]
38. Camilleri, M. Leaky gut: Mechanisms, measurement and clinical implications in humans. *Gut* **2019**, *68*, 1516–1526. [CrossRef]
39. Guerville, M.; Boudry, G. Gastrointestinal and hepatic mechanisms limiting entry and dissemination of lipopolysaccharide into the systemic circulation. *Am. J. Physiol. Gastrointest. Liver Physiol.* **2016**, *311*, G1–G15. [CrossRef]
40. Abu-Shanab, A.; Quigley, E.M. The role of the gut microbiota in nonalcoholic fatty liver disease. *Nat. Rev. Gastroenterol. Hepatol.* **2010**, *7*, 691–701. [CrossRef]
41. Abenavoli, L.; Scarpellini, E.; Colica, C.; Boccuto, L.; Salehi, B.; Sharifi-Rad, J.; Aiello, V.; Romano, B.; De Lorenzo, A.; Izzo, A.A.; et al. Gut Microbiota and Obesity: A Role for Probiotics. *Nutrients* **2019**, *11*, 2690. [CrossRef]
42. Portincasa, P.; Bonfrate, L.; Vacca, M.; De Angelis, M.; Farella, I.; Lanza, E.; Khalil, M.; Wang, D.Q.; Sperandio, M.; Di Ciaula, A. Gut Microbiota and Short Chain Fatty Acids: Implications in Glucose Homeostasis. *Int. J. Mol. Sci.* **2022**, *23*, 1105. [CrossRef]
43. Cani, P.D.; Van Hul, M.; Lefort, C.; Depommier, C.; Rastelli, M.; Everard, A. Microbial regulation of organismal energy homeostasis. *Nat. Metab.* **2019**, *1*, 34–46. [CrossRef]
44. Rahat-Rozenbloom, S.; Fernandes, J.; Gloor, G.B.; Wolever, T.M. Evidence for greater production of colonic short-chain fatty acids in overweight than lean humans. *Int. J. Obes.* **2014**, *38*, 1525–1531. [CrossRef]
45. Han, H.; Yi, B.; Zhong, R.; Wang, M.; Zhang, S.; Ma, J.; Yin, Y.; Yin, J.; Chen, L.; Zhang, H. From gut microbiota to host appetite: Gut microbiota-derived metabolites as key regulators. *Microbiome* **2021**, *9*, 162. [CrossRef]
46. Hill, J.W. Gene Expression and the Control of Food Intake by Hypothalamic POMC/CART Neurons. *Open Neuroendocrinol. J.* **2010**, *3*, 21–27.
47. Sato, T.; Nakamura, Y.; Shiimura, Y.; Ohgusu, H.; Kangawa, K.; Kojima, M. Structure, regulation and function of ghrelin. *J. Biochem.* **2012**, *151*, 119–128. [CrossRef]
48. Gil-Campos, M.; Aguilera, C.M.; Cañete, R.; Gil, A. Ghrelin: A hormone regulating food intake and energy homeostasis. *Br. J. Nutr.* **2006**, *96*, 201–226. [CrossRef]

49. Haugaard-Jónsson, L.M.; Hossain, M.A.; Daly, N.L.; Craik, D.J.; Wade, J.D.; Rosengren, K.J. Structure of human insulin-like peptide 5 and characterization of conserved hydrogen bonds and electrostatic interactions within the relaxin framework. *Biochem. J.* **2009**, *419*, 619–627. [CrossRef]
50. Ang, S.Y.; Hutchinson, D.S.; Patil, N.; Evans, B.A.; Bathgate, R.A.D.; Halls, M.L.; Hossain, M.A.; Summers, R.J.; Kocan, M. Signal transduction pathways activated by insulin-like peptide 5 at the relaxin family peptide RXFP4 receptor. *Br. J. Pharmacol.* **2017**, *174*, 1077–1089. [CrossRef]
51. Grosse, J.; Heffron, H.; Burling, K.; Akhter Hossain, M.; Habib, A.M.; Rogers, G.J.; Richards, P.; Larder, R.; Rimmington, D.; Adriaenssens, A.A.; et al. Insulin-like peptide 5 is an orexigenic gastrointestinal hormone. *Proc. Natl. Acad. Sci. USA* **2014**, *111*, 11133–11138. [CrossRef]
52. Zaykov, A.N.; Gelfanov, V.M.; Perez-Tilve, D.; Finan, B.; DiMarchi, R.D. Insulin-like peptide 5 fails to improve metabolism or body weight in obese mice. *Peptides* **2019**, *120*, 170116. [CrossRef]
53. Kim, K.N.; Yao, Y.; Ju, S.Y. Short Chain Fatty Acids and Fecal Microbiota Abundance in Humans with Obesity: A Systematic Review and Meta-Analysis. *Nutrients* **2019**, *11*, 2512. [CrossRef]
54. Martínez-Cuesta, M.C.; Del Campo, R.; Garriga-García, M.; Peláez, C.; Requena, T. Taxonomic Characterization and Short-Chain Fatty Acids Production of the Obese Microbiota. *Front. Cell. Infect. Microbiol.* **2021**, *11*, 598093. [CrossRef]
55. Kumar, R.; Mal, K.; Razaq, M.K.; Magsi, M.; Memon, M.K.; Memon, S.; Afroz, M.N.; Siddiqui, H.F.; Rizwan, A. Association of Leptin With Obesity and Insulin Resistance. *Cureus* **2020**, *12*, e12178. [CrossRef]
56. Al Maskari, M.Y.; Alnaqdy, A.A. Correlation between Serum Leptin Levels, Body Mass Index and Obesity in Omanis. *Sultan Qaboos Univ. Med. J.* **2006**, *6*, 27–31.
57. Wang, Y.; Wu, Q.; Zhou, Q.; Chen, Y.; Lei, X.; Chen, Y.; Chen, Q. Circulating acyl and des-acyl ghrelin levels in obese adults: A systematic review and meta-analysis. *Sci. Rep.* **2022**, *12*, 2679. [CrossRef]
58. Maier, S.; Wieland, A.; Cree-Green, M.; Nadeau, K.; Sullivan, S.; Lanaspa, M.A.; Johnson, R.J.; Jensen, T. Lean NAFLD: An underrecognized and challenging disorder in medicine. *Rev. Endocr. Metab. Disord.* **2021**, *22*, 351–366. [CrossRef]
59. Randeria, S.N.; Thomson, G.J.A.; Nell, T.A.; Roberts, T.; Pretorius, E. Inflammatory cytokines in type 2 diabetes mellitus as facilitators of hypercoagulation and abnormal clot formation. *Cardiovasc. Diabetol.* **2019**, *18*, 72. [CrossRef]
60. Wang, X.; Ota, N.; Manzanillo, P.; Kates, L.; Zavala-Solorio, J.; Eidenschenk, C.; Zhang, J.; Lesch, J.; Lee, W.P.; Ross, J.; et al. Interleukin-22 alleviates metabolic disorders and restores mucosal immunity in diabetes. *Nature* **2014**, *514*, 237–241. [CrossRef]
61. Ramakrishna, C.; Kujawski, M.; Chu, H.; Li, L.; Mazmanian, S.K.; Cantin, E.M. *Bacteroides fragilis* polysaccharide A induces IL-10 secreting B and T cells that prevent viral encephalitis. *Nat. Commun.* **2019**, *10*, 2153. [CrossRef]
62. Wu, S.; Zhang, Y.; Ma, J.; Liu, Y.; Li, W.; Wang, T.; Xu, X.; Wang, Y.; Cheng, K.; Zhuang, R. Interleukin-6 absence triggers intestinal microbiota dysbiosis and mucosal immunity in mice. *Cytokine* **2022**, *153*, 155841. [CrossRef]
63. Nunberg, M.; Werbner, N.; Neuman, H.; Bersudsky, M.; Braiman, A.; Ben-Shoshan, M.; Ben Izhak, M.; Louzoun, Y.; Apte, R.N.; Voronov, E.; et al. Interleukin 1α-Deficient Mice Have an Altered Gut Microbiota Leading to Protection from Dextran Sodium Sulfate-Induced Colitis. *mSystems* **2018**, *3*, e00213–e00217. [CrossRef]
64. Cunningham, A.L.; Stephens, J.W.; Harris, D.A. Gut microbiota influence in type 2 diabetes mellitus (T2DM). *Gut Pathog.* **2021**, *13*, 50. [CrossRef]
65. Foley, K.P.; Zlitni, S.; Duggan, B.M.; Barra, N.G.; Anhê, F.F.; Cavallari, J.F.; Henriksbo, B.D.; Chen, C.Y.; Huang, M.; Lau, T.C.; et al. Gut microbiota impairs insulin clearance in obese mice. *Mol. Metab.* **2020**, *42*, 101067. [CrossRef]
66. Mkumbuzi, L.; Mfengu, M.M.O.; Engwa, G.A.; Sewani-Rusike, C.R. Insulin Resistance is Associated with Gut Permeability Without the Direct Influence of Obesity in Young Adults. *Diabetes Metab. Syndr. Obes.* **2020**, *13*, 2997–3008. [CrossRef]
67. Sakurai, Y.; Kubota, N.; Yamauchi, T.; Kadowaki, T. Role of Insulin Resistance in MAFLD. *Int. J. Mol. Sci.* **2021**, *22*, 4156. [CrossRef]
68. Dongiovanni, P.; Meroni, M.; Longo, M.; Fargion, S.; Fracanzani, A.L. miRNA Signature in NAFLD: A Turning Point for a Non-Invasive Diagnosis. *Int. J. Mol. Sci.* **2018**, *19*, 3966. [CrossRef]
69. Donati, B.; Dongiovanni, P.; Romeo, S.; Meroni, M.; McCain, M.; Miele, L.; Petta, S.; Maier, S.; Rosso, C.; De Luca, L.; et al. MBOAT7 rs641738 variant and hepatocellular carcinoma in non-cirrhotic individuals. *Sci. Rep.* **2017**, *7*, 4492. [CrossRef]
70. Mu, T.; Peng, L.; Xie, X.; He, H.; Shao, Q.; Wang, X.; Zhang, Y. Single Nucleotide Polymorphism of Genes Associated with Metabolic Fatty Liver Disease. *J. Oncol.* **2022**, *2022*, 9282557. [CrossRef]
71. Liao, S.; An, K.; Liu, Z.; He, H.; An, Z.; Su, Q.; Li, S. Genetic variants associated with metabolic dysfunction-associated fatty liver disease in western China. *J. Clin. Lab. Anal.* **2022**, *36*, e24626. [CrossRef]
72. Nibali, L.; Henderson, B.; Sadiq, S.T.; Donos, N. Genetic dysbiosis: The role of microbial insults in chronic inflammatory diseases. *J. Oral. Microbiol.* **2014**, *6*, 22962. [CrossRef]
73. Li, D.; Wu, M. Pattern recognition receptors in health and diseases. *Signal. Transduct. Target. Ther.* **2021**, *6*, 291. [CrossRef]
74. Sobhani, I.; Tap, J.; Roudot-Thoraval, F.; Roperch, J.P.; Letulle, S.; Langella, P.; Corthier, G.; Tran Van Nhieu, J.; Furet, J.P. Microbial dysbiosis in colorectal cancer (CRC) patients. *PLoS ONE* **2011**, *6*, e16393. [CrossRef]
75. Iebba, V.; Totino, V.; Gagliardi, A.; Santangelo, F.; Cacciotti, F.; Trancassini, M.; Mancini, C.; Cicerone, C.; Corazziari, E.; Pantanella, F.; et al. Eubiosis and dysbiosis: The two sides of the microbiota. *New. Microbiol.* **2016**, *39*, 1–12.
76. Leeming, E.R.; Johnson, A.J.; Spector, T.D.; Le Roy, C.I. Effect of Diet on the Gut Microbiota: Rethinking Intervention Duration. *Nutrients* **2019**, *11*, 2862. [CrossRef]
77. Machado, M.V. What should we advise MAFLD patients to eat and drink? *Metab. Target Organ. Damage* **2021**, *1*, 9. [CrossRef]

78. Kurylowicz, A. The role of diet in the management of MAFLD-why does a new disease require a novel, individualized approach? *Hepatobiliary Surg. Nutr.* **2022**, *11*, 419–421. [CrossRef]
79. Italian Association for the Study of the Liver (AISF). AISF position paper on nonalcoholic fatty liver disease (NAFLD): Updates and future directions. *Dig. Liver Dis.* **2017**, *49*, 471–483. [CrossRef]
80. Abenavoli, L.; Boccuto, L.; Federico, A.; Dallio, M.; Loguercio, C.; Di Renzo, L.; De Lorenzo, A. Diet and Non-Alcoholic Fatty Liver Disease: The Mediterranean Way. *Int. J. Environ. Res. Public Health* **2019**, *16*, 3011. [CrossRef]
81. D'Innocenzo, S.; Biagi, C.; Lanari, M. Obesity and the Mediterranean Diet: A Review of Evidence of the Role and Sustainability of the Mediterranean Diet. *Nutrients* **2019**, *11*, 1306. [CrossRef]
82. Martín-Peláez, S.; Fito, M.; Castaner, O. Mediterranean Diet Effects on Type 2 Diabetes Prevention, Disease Progression, and Related Mechanisms. A Review. *Nutrients* **2020**, *12*, 2236. [CrossRef]
83. Slattery, M.L.; Lundgreen, A.; Wolff, R.K. Dietary influence on MAPK-signaling pathways and risk of colon and rectal cancer. *Nutr. Cancer* **2013**, *65*, 729–738. [CrossRef]
84. Khan, H.; Ullah, H.; Castilho, P.C.M.F.; Gomila, A.S.; D'Onofrio, G.; Filosa, R.; Wang, F.; Nabavi, S.M.; Daglia, M.; Silva, A.S.; et al. Targeting NF-κB signaling pathway in cancer by dietary polyphenols. *Crit. Rev. Food Sci. Nutr.* **2020**, *60*, 2790–2800. [CrossRef]
85. Gugliandolo, E.; Cordaro, M.; Siracusa, R.; D'Amico, R.; Peritore, A.F.; Genovese, T.; Impellizzeri, D.; Paola, R.D.; Crupi, R.; Cuzzocrea, S.; et al. Novel Combination of COX-2 Inhibitor and Antioxidant Therapy for Modulating Oxidative Stress Associated with Intestinal Ischemic Reperfusion Injury and Endotoxemia. *Antioxidants* **2020**, *9*, 930. [CrossRef]
86. Deledda, A.; Annunziata, G.; Tenore, G.C.; Palmas, V.; Manzin, A.; Velluzzi, F. Diet-Derived Antioxidants and Their Role in Inflammation, Obesity and Gut Microbiota Modulation. *Antioxidants* **2021**, *10*, 708. [CrossRef]
87. Zunica, E.R.M.; Heintz, E.C.; Axelrod, C.L.; Kirwan, J.P. Obesity Management in the Primary Prevention of Hepatocellular Carcinoma. *Cancers* **2022**, *14*, 4051. [CrossRef] [PubMed]
88. Hill, C.; Guarner, F.; Reid, G.; Gibson, G.R.; Merenstein, D.J.; Pot, B.; Morelli, L.; Canani, R.B.; Flint, H.J.; Salminen, S.; et al. Expert consensus document. The International Scientific Association for Probiotics and Prebiotics consensus statement on the scope and appropriate use of the term probiotic. *Nat. Rev. Gastroenterol. Hepatol.* **2014**, *11*, 506–514. [CrossRef]
89. Gibson, G.R.; Hutkins, R.; Sanders, M.E.; Prescott, S.L.; Reimer, R.A.; Salminen, S.J.; Scott, K.; Stanton, C.; Swanson, K.S.; Cani, P.D.; et al. Expert consensus document: The International Scientific Association for Probiotics and Prebiotics (ISAPP) consensus statement on the definition and scope of prebiotics. *Nat. Rev. Gastroenterol. Hepatol.* **2017**, *14*, 491–502. [CrossRef] [PubMed]
90. Salminen, S.; Collado, M.C.; Endo, A.; Hill, C.; Lebeer, S.; Quigley, E.M.M.; Sanders, M.E.; Shamir, R.; Swann, J.R.; Szajewska, H.; et al. The International Scientific Association of Probiotics and Prebiotics (ISAPP) consensus statement on the definition and scope of postbiotics. *Nat. Rev. Gastroenterol. Hepatol.* **2021**, *18*, 649–667. [CrossRef]
91. Kobyliak, N.; Abenavoli, L.; Mykhalchyshyn, G.; Kononenko, L.; Boccuto, L.; Kyriienko, D.; Dynnyk, O. A Multi-strain Probiotic Reduces the Fatty Liver Index, Cytokines and Aminotransferase levels in NAFLD Patients: Evidence from a Randomized Clinical Trial. *J. Gastrointest. Liver Dis.* **2018**, *27*, 41–49. [CrossRef] [PubMed]
92. Kobyliak, N.; Abenavoli, L.; Falalyeyeva, T.; Mykhalchyshyn, G.; Boccuto, L.; Kononenko, L.; Kyriienko, D.; Komisarenko, I.; Dynnyk, O. Beneficial effects of probiotic combination with omega-3 fatty acids in NAFLD: A randomized clinical study. *Minerva Med.* **2018**, *109*, 418–428. [CrossRef] [PubMed]
93. Kobyliak, N.; Abenavoli, L.; Falalyeyeva, T.; Beregova, T. Efficacy of Probiotics and Smectite in Rats with Non-Alcoholic Fatty Liver Disease. *Ann. Hepatol.* **2018**, *17*, 153–161. [CrossRef]
94. Nguyen, H.T.; Gu, M.; Werlinger, P.; Cho, J.H.; Cheng, J.; Suh, J.W. Lactobacillus sakei MJM60958 as a Potential Probiotic Alleviated Non-Alcoholic Fatty Liver Disease in Mice Fed a High-Fat Diet by Modulating Lipid Metabolism, Inflammation, and Gut Microbiota. *Int. J. Mol. Sci.* **2022**, *23*, 13436. [CrossRef]
95. Wang, Q.; Wang, Z.; Pang, B.; Zheng, H.; Cao, Z.; Feng, C.; Ma, W.; Wei, J. Probiotics for the improvement of metabolic profiles in patients with metabolic-associated fatty liver disease: A systematic review and meta-analysis of randomized controlled trials. *Front. Endocrinol. (Lausanne)* **2022**, *13*, 1014670. [CrossRef]
96. Wang, J.S.; Liu, J.C. Intestinal microbiota in the treatment of metabolically associated fatty liver disease. *World J. Clin. Cases* **2022**, *10*, 11240–11251. [CrossRef]
97. Lanthier, N.; Delzenne, N. Targeting the Gut Microbiome to Treat Metabolic Dysfunction-Associated Fatty Liver Disease: Ready for Prime Time? *Cells* **2022**, *11*, 2718. [CrossRef]

Disclaimer/Publisher's Note: The statements, opinions and data contained in all publications are solely those of the individual author(s) and contributor(s) and not of MDPI and/or the editor(s). MDPI and/or the editor(s) disclaim responsibility for any injury to people or property resulting from any ideas, methods, instructions or products referred to in the content.

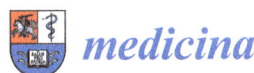

Review

Surgical Options for Peritoneal Surface Metastases from Digestive Malignancies—A Comprehensive Review

Mihai Adrian Eftimie [1,2], Gheorghe Potlog [1] and Sorin Tiberiu Alexandrescu [1,2,*]

1. Department of General Surgery, Fundeni Clinical Institute, 022328 Bucharest, Romania
2. Department of Surgery, Faculty of Medicine, Carol Davila University of Medicine and Pharmacy, 050474 Bucharest, Romania
* Correspondence: sorin.alexandrescu@umfcd.ro

Abstract: The peritoneum is a common site for the dissemination of digestive malignancies, particularly gastric, colorectal, appendix, or pancreatic cancer. Other tumors such as cholangiocarcinomas, digestive neuroendocrine tumors, or gastrointestinal stromal tumors (GIST) may also associate with peritoneal surface metastases (PSM). Peritoneal dissemination is proven to worsen the prognosis of these patients. Cytoreductive surgery (CRS), along with systemic chemotherapy, have been shown to constitute a survival benefit in selected patients with PSM. Furthermore, the association of CRS with hyperthermic intraperitoneal chemotherapy (HIPEC) seems to significantly improve the prognosis of patients with certain types of digestive malignancies associated with PSM. However, the benefit of CRS with HIPEC is still controversial, especially due to the significant morbidity associated with this procedure. According to the results of the PRODIGE 7 trial, CRS for PSM from colorectal cancer (CRC) achieved overall survival (OS) rates higher than 40 months, but the addition of oxaliplatin-based HIPEC failed to improve the long-term outcomes. Furthermore, the PROPHYLOCHIP and COLOPEC trials failed to demonstrate the effectiveness of oxaliplatin-based HIPEC for preventing peritoneal metastases development in high-risk patients operated for CRC. In this review, we discuss the limitations of these studies and the reasons why these results are not sufficient to refute this technique, until future well-designed trials evaluate the impact of different HIPEC regimens. In contrast, in pseudomyxoma peritonei, CRS plus HIPEC represents the gold standard therapy, which is able to achieve 10-year OS rates ranging between 70 and 80%. For patients with PSM from gastric carcinoma, CRS plus HIPEC achieved median OS rates higher than 40 months after complete cytoreduction in patients with a peritoneal cancer index (PCI) ≤6. However, the data have not yet been validated in randomized clinical trials. In this review, we discuss the controversies regarding the most efficient drugs that should be used for HIPEC and the duration of the procedure. We also discuss the current evidence and controversies related to the benefit of CRS (and HIPEC) in patients with PSM from other digestive malignancies. Although it is a palliative treatment, pressurized intraperitoneal aerosolized chemotherapy (PIPAC) significantly increases OS in patients with unresectable PSM from gastric cancer and represents a promising approach for patients with PSM from other digestive cancers.

Keywords: peritoneal surface metastases; digestive cancers; colorectal cancer; gastric cancer; appendix cancer; cytoreductive surgery (CRS); hyperthermic intraperitoneal chemotherapy (HIPEC); pressurized intraperitoneal aerosolized chemotherapy (PIPAC)

Citation: Eftimie, M.A.; Potlog, G.; Alexandrescu, S.T. Surgical Options for Peritoneal Surface Metastases from Digestive Malignancies—A Comprehensive Review. *Medicina* **2023**, *59*, 255. https://doi.org/10.3390/medicina59020255

Academic Editors: Ludovico Abenavoli and Marcello Candelli

Received: 30 December 2022
Revised: 25 January 2023
Accepted: 25 January 2023
Published: 28 January 2023

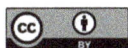

Copyright: © 2023 by the authors. Licensee MDPI, Basel, Switzerland. This article is an open access article distributed under the terms and conditions of the Creative Commons Attribution (CC BY) license (https:// creativecommons.org/licenses/by/ 4.0/).

1. Introduction

Although most guidelines recommend only palliative oncologic therapy for patients with peritoneal surface metastases (PSM) of digestive origin, the responsiveness of PSM to systemic therapy is significantly lower compared to other metastatic sites [1,2]. Peritoneal implants are believed to be the consequences of primary tumor cell detachment or dissemination during surgical procedure [3].

As a consequence of the low survival rates achieved by palliative systemic therapy, there has been increased interest in the complete surgical removal of peritoneal deposits. The first surgical resection of PSM was performed for ovarian cancer. Cytoreductive surgery (CRS), first performed in the 1980s, represents the complete (or near-complete) removal of macroscopic disease. CRS, accompanied by hyperthermic intraperitoneal chemotherapy (HIPEC), has emerged as an aggressive and efficient loco-regional therapy. In the 1990s, Sugarbaker described the surgical technique for peritonectomy and associated visceral resections [4]. During the same period, various investigators developed drug regimens and methods for HIPEC according to the primary tumor site [5–7]. For selected patients, this approach offered improved survival rates and even better quality of life. Other forms of intraperitoneal chemotherapy such as early postoperative intraperitoneal chemotherapy (EPIC—on days 1–5) and sequential intraperitoneal chemotherapy (SIPC) are less commonly used.

The most important prognostic factors related to the overall survival (OS) of patients treated by CRS +/− HIPEC are Sugarbaker's peritoneal cancer index (PCI), which quantifies the extent of the disease, and the completeness of the cytoreduction score (CC score), which evaluates the wholeness of the CRS. The impact of these parameters on OS rates depends on the site of the primary tumor and its histological type [8].

The completeness of the cytoreductive procedure has a direct impact on the survival of patients with PSM in most malignancies. Although the goal of CRS should be the achievement of a CC-0 score (no macroscopic residual tissue), at least in ovarian cancer, even a CC-1 score (persistent nodules less than 2.5 mm in largest diameter) seems to be associated with improved OS [9]. In order to achieve a CC-0/CC-1 score, a dedicated team involving surgeons, anesthesiologists, medical oncologists, and radiologists should evaluate the patient and subsequently perform the procedure, preferably in a high volume-center [10]. Preoperative chemotherapy seems to play an important role in the selection of patients who could really benefit from this aggressive procedure (CRS with or without HIPEC).

Even with optimal CRS, the majority of recurrences that occur are located intraperitoneally [9].

For patients with unresectable PSM, chemotherapy remains the gold standard treatment, even if its impact on survival is limited, ranging from 16.6 months for recurrent platinum-resistant ovarian cancer [11] to 16.3 months for colorectal carcinoma (CRC) [12], 10.7 months for gastric cancer [13], and less than 12 months for peritoneal mesothelioma [14]. For such patients, pressurized intraperitoneal aerosol chemotherapy (PIPAC) has been developed as a safe and well-tolerated palliative procedure that enhances the effect of chemotherapy (because of the physical properties of aerosol and pressure) and improves their OS [15].

With the increase in experience and the development of high-volume centers, the morbidity and mortality rates associated with these procedures has decreased, becoming similar to the respective rates of other major gastrointestinal surgeries [16]. A study conducted by Constance Houlze-Laroye [17] on 5562 patients, published in 2021, revealed that more than half of the postoperative deaths following CRS and HIPEC procedures were preventable.

Although the issue of CRS +/− HIPEC for PSM from specific malignancies has been addressed in other recent papers, there is a paucity of reviews that have presented, together, the latest evidence regarding the surgical options for all digestive carcinomas with peritoneal metastases. This paper aims to advance the field by informing current practice and by prompting clinicians to act and broaden the use of an aggressive surgical approach in patients with PSM from digestive carcinomas. Given the current evidence, concerted efforts should be made by general practitioners, gastroenterologists, oncologists, and surgeons to promote CRS with or without HIPEC in order to prolong the life-expectancy of these patients.

In this comprehensive review, the surgical approach of PSM is reported separately according to the primary site and/or histology. For each type of digestive malignancy, the patient selection protocols, specific approaches to CRS, HIPEC methodology and drug regimens, proper sequencing with other treatments, patient follow-up, and protocols used for recurrence are described and discussed. Furthermore, the paper reflects the most recent evidence regarding the prophylactic use of HIPEC in patients with colorectal or gastric carcinoma at high risk for developing PSM. We review the data critically, taking into account the limitations of the studies, and suggest future directions of research.

2. Paper Selection

We searched the PubMed database using the following terms: ((((((((((((peritoneal surface metastasis[Text Word]) OR (carcinomatosis[Text Word])) AND (colorectal cancer[Text Word])) OR (gastric carcinoma[Text Word])) OR (digestive malignancies[Text Word])) OR (biliary tract carcinoma[Text Word])) OR (pancreatic carcinoma[Text Word])) OR (gastrointestinal stromal tumors[Text Word])) OR (neuroendocrine tumors[Text Word])) OR (small bowel carcinoma[Text Word])) AND (cytoreductive surgery[Text Word])) OR (HIPEC[Text Word])) NOT (ovarian cancer[Text Word])) NOT (mesothelioma[Text Word]). The filters applied were: Clinical Trial, Meta-Analysis, Randomized Controlled Trial, Review, Systematic Review, from 1 January 2001 to 1 June 2022. The search generated 538 results. The abstracts of these results were evaluated by two authors (M.A.E. and G.P.), the relevant papers were extracted independently, and their full-text versions were assessed. Consensus for the relevance of a study was carried out by the third author (S.T.A.). We also evaluated the references of the relevant papers that were evaluated in order to identify additional articles that were not found during the initial search. Due to the heterogeneity of the studies, we report the results as a narrative review.

3. Surgical Options for PSM from Colorectal Carcinoma (CRC)

3.1. Epidemiology

CRC is the third most common type of cancer and generates the second most frequent cancer-related mortality globally. When diagnosed at an early stage, 70–80% of patients will benefit from a curative-intent surgical procedure, resulting in a 5-year survival rate of 72–93% for stages I–II [3].

For CRC, synchronous PSM is encountered in 6–7% of patients and almost half of them have peritoneal-only metastases [18]. Furthermore, the risk for metachronous PSM can be as high as 6% [19]. The literature reveals that an advanced T stage, the presence of positive lymph nodes, synchronous ovarian metastases, a poor differentiation of the primary tumor, a colonic versus a rectal origin, the R1/R2 resection of the primary tumor, the histologic type of mucinous or signet-ring adenocarcinoma, the perforation or stenosis of the primary tumor, and younger age are the most frequently reported risk factors for the development of metachronous PSM [19–21].

3.2. Treatment Options

Patients with PSM of colorectal origin have classically been treated only with systemic palliative oncologic therapy, and sometimes palliative surgery [3]. In patients who receive only palliative treatment, colorectal PSM is associated with a worse prognosis compared to non-peritoneal metastases (16.3 months for PSM vs. 19.1 months for liver-only metastases and 24.6 months for lung-only metastases [12,22].

In 2003, Verwaal et al. [23] published a Dutch phase 3 controlled trial comparing the OS rates achieved by CRS plus HIPEC vs. palliative surgery plus systemic chemotherapy in patients operated for bowel obstruction. They showed that the OS rates achieved by CRS plus HIPEC were significantly superior to those observed in patients treated with palliative surgery. Later on, many clinical protocols of CRS and HIPEC were evaluated in different high-volume centers to treat the patients with colorectal PSM. Thus, Elias D., Koga S., Quenet S. et al. [7,22,24,25] reported promising results for CRS and HIPEC when a macroscopically complete resection is performed (CC-0), with an average median OS of 40 months. In 2013, Goere D et al. [26] stated that, in specialized centers, CRS and HIPEC could even achieve a cure in one sixth of the patients who underwent a CC-0 resection, reporting 5-year disease free survival (DFS) rates of 16% in such patients. However, because all of these studies were retrospective, no definitive conclusions could be drawn, and most guidelines continued to recommend only palliative oncologic therapy in patients with PSM of colorectal origin, irrespective of the extent of peritoneal involvement.

To overcome this drawback, between February 2008 and January 2014, 265 patients were randomly assigned to CRS and HIPEC (133 patients) or to CRS alone (132 patients) in a randomized, open-label, phase 3 trial performed at 17 cancer centers in France (PRODIGE 7 trial). All patients were confirmed with CRC and PSM, had a PCI $\leq$ 25, a WHO performance status of 0 or 1, normal liver function, proper hematological function, and were eligible to receive chemotherapy for 6 months [27]. Any previous treatments were permitted, a 4-week wash-out period was indicated, and the main exclusion criteria were extraperitoneal metastases, previous HIPEC treatment, and grade 3 or worse peripheral neuropathy. For patients enrolled in the CRS plus HIPEC arm, the HIPEC technique was performed either in a closed or open abdomen manner, according to each center's approach. Systemic chemotherapy (400 mg/m^2 fluorouracil and 20 mg/m^2 folinic acid) was administered intravenously 20 min before HIPEC (bidirectional chemotherapy protocol) and intraperitoneal chemotherapy consisted of oxaliplatin at a dose of 460 mg/m^2 (for the open technique) or 360 mg/m^2 (for the closed abdomen technique). Oxaliplatin was delivered intraperitoneally in 2 L/m^2 of dextrose, heated at 43 °C, for 30 min. The follow-up was conducted one month after surgery, every 3 months for the first 3 years and every 6 months up to 5 years. The median OS was 41.7 months in the CRS plus HIPEC group and 41.2 months in the CRS alone group (p = 0.99). Although PRODIGE 7 did not reveal a survival benefit for the addition of HIPEC to CRS, this trial reported unexpectedly high OS rates in patients treated with CRS alone. These findings suggest that the completeness of CRS is the most important factor for survival in patients with PSM from CRCs, with similar observations already being reported by other authors in retrospective studies [23,24,28]. Furthermore, median relapse-free survival (RFS) between the two groups was not significantly different and 15% of patients in each group were considered cured at 5 years. According to the data of the PRODIGE 7 trial, CRS alone should be the cornerstone of therapeutic strategies with curative intent for colorectal peritoneal metastases [23], and the benefit of HIPEC is still debatable.

3.3. Prognostic Factors in Patients Treated with CRS +/− HIPEC

The only significant survival difference between the two study arms of the PRODIGE 7 trial was found in the subgroup of patients with a PCI between 11 and 15. In these patients, CRS and HIPEC were associated with significantly higher RFS rates than CRS alone, although the OS rates were similar among the two study arms. This might be the basis for further studies aiming to evaluate a potential survival benefit offered by CRS plus HIPEC vs. CRS alone in patients with more extensive PSM involvement.

Moreover, the cut-off value of the PCI associated with a significantly higher survival benefit after CRS + HIPEC has not been uniformly reported by different authors. Thus, Gustave Roussy's group revealed that the maximum survival benefit of CRS plus HIPEC was achieved in patients with a PCI $\leq$ 10. [26] The Consensus Guidelines from The American Society of Peritoneal Surface Malignancies on standardizing the delivery of hyperthermic intraperitoneal chemotherapy (HIPEC) in CRC patients in the United States, published in 2014 [29], state that CRS is particularly effective in patients with a low-volume peritoneal disease, suggesting that a PCI $\leq$ 12 and no evidence of systemic disease are the main prognostic factors for better survival. Yan TD [30] stated that patients with a PCI $\leq$ 13 had a better life expectancy. Authors such as Da Silva and Sugarbaker [31] set the limit of the PCI at 20. This value is also supported by data from Cavaliere et al. [32] and Van Sweringen et al. [33], whose data indicated that a PCI > 20 is associated with decreased survival rates, hence, they concluded that such patients should not be seen as candidates for CRS +/− HIPEC.

In and by itself, the PCI cannot predict unresectability for certain tumor locations [34]. Thus, some studies have suggested that the number of regions affected by PSM of colorectal origin and invasion of the small bowel in more than two different parts are independent prognostic factors for both unresectability and shorter survival [35,36]. A paper published by Elias D. et al. [37] in 2014 also revealed that the involvement of the lower ileum and a high PCI were negative prognostic factors for the efficacy of the multimodality treatment, while Verwaal et al. [23] demonstrated a clear decrease in the survival rates in patients with PSM involving six or more regions ($p < 0.0001$).

Alongside the CC score, the PCI, and the number of regions with PSM, other studies have suggested additional prognostic factors that were independently associated with OS and/or DFS in patients who underwent CRS +/− HIPEC for PSM of colorectal origin. However, the impact of these additional prognostic factors is still controversial, since most of the data are from relatively small retrospective studies. For example, Tonello M. et al. [38] found that operated patients with PSM of rectal origin had a worse prognosis than those with PSM of colonic origin. Hence, they proposed a more restrictive use of CRS and HIPEC in patients with PSM of rectal origin. The impact of the location of the primary tumor on OS in patients with PSM of colorectal origin was also assessed by Peron et al. [39] in a prospective study that included 796 patients undergoing complete CRS (CC-0) between January 2004 and January 2017 in 14 institutions from France (the BIG-RENAPE database) and two institutions from Canada. They revealed that the primary site had no impact on the long-term outcomes of patients with PSM undergoing a complete CRS. No impact on OS and DFS was encountered across all subgroups of patients. This study also found no impact of RAS and BRAF mutations on the outcomes after complete CRS. This evidence suggests that the side of the primary tumor should not represent an exclusion criterion for patients with PSM from colorectal origin that are amenable to CRS (with or without HIPEC). Similar results were reported by Massalou et al. [40], who found that the location of the primary tumor location as well as RAS and BRAF status had no significant impact on the OS or DFS. In their study, the only pathologic/molecular factors associated with worse OS after CRS + HIPEC were the signet ring and mucinous type of carcinoma, while the presence of microsatellite sequence stability (MSS) was associated with lower DFS rates. This study also found that BMI > 25 was associated with significantly lower OS and DFS rates.

3.4. Morbidity and Mortality after CRS +/− HIPEC

Higher BMI is also correlated with increased postoperative morbidity and mortality rates in colorectal procedures including CRS with or without HIPEC [41,42]. Regarding the 30-day mortality rates after CRS with/without HIPEC, most studies reported an average value of 2% [16,24,25,27]. In the PRODIGE 7 trial, there was no statistically significant difference ($p = 0.083$) concerning the frequency of grade 3 or worse adverse events at 30 days between the CRS alone group (32%) and the CRS + HIPEC group (42%) [23]. Similarly, Foster et al. [43] used the data from the American College of Surgeons National Surgical Quality Improvement Project database and found that CRS and HIPEC were associated with perioperative and 30-day postoperative morbidity and mortality rates similar to those of other oncological surgical procedures. However, the PRODIGE 7 trial showed a significantly increased 60-day rate of grade 3 or worse complication in the CRS plus oxaliplatin-based HIPEC group vs. the CRS alone group (26% vs. 15%, respectively; $p = 0.035$) [23]. This indicates that patients in the CRS + HIPEC group have a longer period of risk for developing complications, leading to a prolonged time to resumption of postoperative systemic chemotherapy. The lack of survival benefit and the significantly higher rate of grade 3 or worse adverse events at 60 days in the CRS + HIPEC group (vs. CRS alone group) seem to be reasonable arguments to refute the use of prophylactic HIPEC in patients with non-metastatic CRC at risk of developing PSM [27].

3.5. HIPEC Protocol

Although the PRODIGE 7 randomized controlled trial did not find any survival benefit from the association of HIPEC to CRS in patients with PSM of colorectal origin, its results were critically appraised by many authors including Paul H. Sugarbaker [44]. The major criticism of the PRODIGE 7 trial was related to the HIPEC protocol, concerning both the dose and the duration of chemotherapy.

In the PRODIGE 7 trial, the oxaliplatin-based HIPEC regimen was limited to 30 min. Kirstein MN [45] and Lemoine L [46] demonstrated that the response to local oxaliplatin was related to the duration of exposure. Furthermore, Levine EA et al. [47] used a HIPEC regimen lasting 120 min in their study, while Van Driel WJ [48] opted for a 90 min cisplatin-based HIPEC protocol for the treatment of ovarian cancer. Both reported increased overall survival rates with prolonged duration of HIPEC.

Regarding the cytotoxic agent used for HIPEC in the PRODIGE 7 trial, several concerns have been raised, because no standard regimen exists thus far. Hence, to increase the efficacy of intraoperative chemotherapy, many protocols have been put in place [49]. For example, the intensification of the HIPEC regimen with irinotecan has been explored in a previous study, but could not be associated with any survival benefit [25]. Furthermore, a cisplatin-based HIPEC protocol was associated with inferior long-term outcomes compared to an oxaliplatin-based regimen in an Italian multicentric study conducted by Cavaliere [32]. Thus, the most frequently used HIPEC regimens are based on oxaliplatin or mitomycin C. A Dutch series reported by Hompes et al. [50] as well as a large American retrospective study conducted by Prada-Villaverde [51] suggested no significant differences in the OS rates between the oxaliplatin-based and mytomicin C-based protocols. However, a single-center Australian study reported superior OS rates achieved by an oxaliplatin-based HIPEC regimen compared to the mytomicin C-based protocol [52]. The major criticism regarding the use of the oxaliplatin-based HIPEC protocol in the PRODIGE 7 trial is related to the extensive use of oxaliplatin in these patients before HIPEC. Previous studies [53,54] have suggested that the patients hard-treated with oxaliplatin could develop oxaliplatin resistance, resulting in decreased rates of response to a further oxaliplatin-based regimen. In the PRODIGE 7 trial, extensive oxaliplatin treatment before surgery might induce misleading results in the arm of patients treated with CRS + HIPEC, raising the question of whether a mitomycin-C based HIPEC regimen or an oxaliplatin-based HIPEC regimen prolonged to 120 min would be associated with higher survival rates in this arm.

3.6. Recurrent PSM

Despite the aggressive approach and curative intention, between 70% and 80% of patients with colorectal PSM treated by CRS (alone or combined with HIPEC) will develop recurrent disease [7,55]. This has led to the idea of iterative CRS and even HIPEC procedures. Several studies have suggested that in high-volume centers, the morbidity and mortality associated with these procedures are similar to those of the initial intervention [56]. This aggressive approach has led to a moderate increase in the median OS from 39 months to 42.9 months when compared to systemic treatment alone [3,56–58]. Although HIPEC has not been proven to be an independent risk factor for the development of postoperative complications [59], its benefit in the treatment of recurrent PSM from CRC needs further evaluation in prospective randomized controlled trials.

3.7. Prophylactic HIPEC in High-Risk Patients

Proactive strategies regarding high-risk patients with CRCs are still a matter of debate and no strong evidence supports their superiority versus proper surveillance. Authors such as Dominique Elias [60,61] and Serrano Del Moral [62] suggest that second-look surgery in conjunction with imagistic investigations, colonoscopies, and CEA level surveillance for high-risk patients can offer the early detection of PSM and precocious aggressive treatment. The promising results associated with prophylactic resection of target organs during the primary surgery (omentectomy, hepatic round ligament resection, appendicectomy, adnexectomy) [63] or prophylactic HIPEC administration at the time of the primary procedure for advanced tumors without PSM [64–66] represent the basis for some phase III randomized clinical trials evaluating the usefulness of such approaches (e.g., the ProphyloCHIP trial and COLOPEC trial). The PROPHYLOCHIP-PRODIGE 15 trial [67] evaluated the impact of second-look surgery and HIPEC vs. follow-up on 3-yr DFS of patients with resected CRC and high-risk of developing PSM (perforated primary tumor/peritoneal or ovarian metastases radically resected concomitant with CRC). The authors did not find a significant difference in the 3-yr DFS rates (44% vs. 53%, respectively; p value = 0.82). On the other hand, the COLOPEC trial [68] assessed the role of adjuvant HIPEC in preventing the occurrence of peritoneal metastases in patients with resected T4/perforated primary tumor, who received adjuvant systemic chemotherapy. There was no statistically significant difference in 18-months peritoneal DFS rates between patients treated with adjuvant systemic therapy only (76.2%) and those treated with adjuvant HIPEC and systemic therapy (80.9%; p value = 0.28). However, in both of these studies as well as in the PRODIGE 7 trial, the HIPEC protocol consisted in the administration of oxaliplatin only for 30 min. Although these trials have generated skepticism toward the usefulness of HIPEC, these results could be challenged by ongoing/future trials evaluating the different protocols of HIPEC. Until new HIPEC protocols are tested in well-designed comparative trials, this procedure should not be considered as an ineffective method [69].

Take home message: Complete CRS represents the cornerstone therapy in patients with PSM from colorectal carcinoma and a low PCI. The addition of HIPEC to complete CRS in such patients seems to have a limited benefit and this approach should be restricted to patients with a PCI > 10, operated in specialized centers, and preferably in the context of controlled trials. The current results cannot support the routine use of prophylactic HIPEC in patients operated for colorectal carcinoma with a high-risk for the development of PSM (T4/perforated primary).

4. Surgical Options for PSM from Gastric Carcinoma

4.1. Epidemiology

Gastric cancer is the third leading cause of cancer deaths worldwide and has the fifth highest incidence among solid cancers in adults. PSM from gastric adenocarcinoma is found in 17% of newly-diagnosed patients and is associated with a poor prognosis. Advanced stages such as stage III gastric adenocarcinomas can be associated in up to 40% of cases with PSM [70,71].

4.2. Treatment Modalities

According to the NCCN guidelines, the treatment options for patients with PSM from gastric carcinoma include palliative systemic therapy, supportive treatment, and surgery for complications [72]. Despite recent advances in oncologic therapy (e.g., trastuzumab in patients with HER-2/neu gene amplification, check-point inhibitors), the median overall survival of patients with PSM of gastric origin ranges from 8 to 10 months [73].

Due to the dismal prognosis associated with the current oncologic therapy, aggressive surgical approaches have been developed in the last two decades including CRS in combination with HIPEC as a potentially curative-intent therapy and PIPAC as a palliative therapy able to prolong survival in patients with unresectable PSM or high PCI. The CRS + HIPEC approach should be combined with neoadjuvant and adjuvant systemic therapy in order to better select patients and increase the DFS and OS rates.

The Japanese group of Yokemura suggested for the first time, in the 1990s, the feasibility and efficacy of CRS plus HIPEC for the treatment of PSM from gastric adenocarcinoma [74,75]. These findings were further supported by a European series reported by Glehen et al. [76]. In 2010, a large retrospective multicentric study from France (159 patients) added more evidence to the concept of CRS and HIPEC for the treatment of PSM of gastric origin. This study showed that complete CRS (CC-0 score) [77,78] was an independent predictor of prolonged OS. Thus, the median OS in patients who underwent CC-0 was

15 months, significantly higher than those achieved in the entire group of patients, irrespective of the completeness of cytoreduction (9.2 months). Furthermore, when complete CRS (CC-0) was achieved, the 5-year OS rate was 23%. In a large retrospective study with propensity score matching analysis, Glehen et al. [79] showed that incomplete CRS (CC-1) is associated with a 5-year OS rate of 6.2%, significantly lower than the 24.8% 5-year OS achieved by complete CRS (CC-0). Similarly, Coccolini et al. [80] found significantly higher 1- and 3-year OS rates in patients who underwent CC-0, compared to those achieved by CC-1. Both studies revealed that complete CRS (CC-0) was correlated with the initial tumor burden expressed by the value of the PCI. Similarly, Yonemura et al. evaluated 95 patients and found that CC-0 had been achieved in 91% of patients with a PCI $\leq$ 6, but only in 42% of the patients with a PCI $\geq$ 7. Furthermore, the OS rates were significantly higher in patients with PCI $\leq$ 6 compared to patients with a PCI > 6 [78]. The study of Cambay et al. [81] reported similar results. A more recent multicentric study from Italy, which included 91 patients with gastric carcinoma and synchronous PSM, reported median OS rates higher than 40 months in patients with a PCI $\leq$ 6 as well as in those who underwent complete cytoreduction [82]. Thus, the median OS after CC-0 was significantly higher compared to the OS of patients with incomplete resection (40.7 vs. 10.7 months, respectively; p value = 0.003). Moreover, in patients with a PCI > 6. the median OS was significantly lower than in patients with a PCI $\leq$ 6 (13.4 vs. 44.3 months, respectively; p value = 0.005) and the mortality was almost double [82].

4.3. Prognostic Factors in Patients Treated with CRS +/− HIPEC

Multiple retrospective studies from Italy, Spain, Germany, and Central-Eastern European countries have supported the observation that complete CRS (CC-0) and a low PCI are the main independent prognostic factors associated with better prognosis in this type of approach [82–85].

However, there is no universally-accepted cut-off value of the PCI to select patients with PSM of gastric origin for CRS plus HIPEC. Although most centers recommend such an aggressive surgical approach in patients with a PCI $\leq$ 6, some high-volume centers suggest that even in patients with a PCI between 7 and 12. there is a survival benefit from CRS + HIPEC [76,86,87].

Other negative prognostic factors such as signet ring cell histology, presence of lymph node metastasis, and lack of tumor regression after preoperative chemotherapy were revealed by these studies. A recent multicenter study by the "Italian Peritoneal Surface Malignancies Oncoteam—S.I.C.O." proved the beneficial effect of neoadjuvant chemotherapy on the long-term outcomes of patients eligible for CRS and HIPEC [82]. The same group highlighted a significant negative prognostic effect determined by positive peritoneal cytology [82,88].

However, the prognostic impact of signet ring cell histology on the long-term outcomes of patients treated by CRS plus HIPEC for PSM of gastric carcinoma is still debatable. In 2014, Konigsrainer et al. [89] hypothesized that for patients with PSM from gastric cancer with signet ring cell histology, CRS + HIPEC should not be considered due to the high recurrence rates. However, these authors did not support this hypothesis with evidence derived from a specific study. In 2019, Solomon et al. [90] revealed the negative impact of the signet ring cell histologic subtype on the OS of patients treated with CRS + HIPEC for PSM of various origins, but surprisingly, in PSM from gastric cancer, the OS was not significantly different between patients with signet ring cell pathology and those with other pathologic subtypes (p = 0.245). Similarly, a Spanish study published in 2018 found that the only prognostic factor that was independently associated with worse OS after CRS + HIPEC for PSM of gastric origin was perineural invasion (HR = 18.886, 95% CI: 1.104–323.123; p = 0.043), while the signet ring cell subtype did not significantly influence the OS [83].

Because most of these studies were retrospective and had a small sample-size, definitive conclusions on the real benefit of CRS + HIPEC for PSM of gastric origin cannot be drawn. The most reliable conclusions on this topic should probably be derived from the results of the CYTO-CHIP study, an observational study that included 277 patients from 19 French centers [79]. This is the largest study published thus far to assess the comparative results of CRS vs. CRS + HIPEC in patients with PSM from gastric carcinoma. Similar to the previously-mentioned studies, complete CRS (CC-0) was associated with significantly higher 5-year OS rates compared to CC-1 (24.8% vs. 6.2%, respectively; $p < 0.05$), and lower PCI was confirmed as an independent prognostic for better OS. The most important findings of this study are the significantly higher OS and DFS rates achieved by CRS + HIPEC compared to CRS alone, without significant increase in major morbidity and 90-day mortality. These results support the performance of CRS + HIPEC when CC-0 can be achieved in patients with limited PSM of gastric origin [79]. Furthermore, the study suggested that CRS + HIPEC performed in specialized centers was associated with morbidity rates similar to those reported after other aggressive surgical procedures [91].

The results of an ongoing phase III randomized controlled trial (PERISCOPE II), which compares the CRS + HIPEC vs. palliative systemic therapy in patients with gastric cancer and limited peritoneal dissemination or positive peritoneal cytology, will be able to improve the current knowledge on this topic, assuming or rejecting the current hypothesis about the usefulness of CRS + HIPEC [92].

4.4. Prophylactic HIPEC in High-Risk Patients

Gastric cancer is associated with a high risk for developing PSM. Around 50% of patients with potentially curable advanced gastric cancer die from recurrence in the peritoneum [93]. A total of 15 to 50% of patients with serosal involvement present peritoneal dissemination at the time of the initial surgical exploration [94].

A study by Seyfried et al. [95] on 1108 patients that were treated for gastric cancer with radical D2 gastrectomy revealed a 50% recurrence rate. Out of these patients, 15.5% developed metachronous PSM after a median time of 17.7 months. The major risk factors for PSM were found to be serosal involvement, the extent of nodal metastasis, and tumor pathology—signet ring cell and undifferentiated carcinoma.

Furthermore, the Japanese General Rules of Gastric Cancer Treatment divide PSM into two categories with the same prognosis [96,97]: (1) P0/Cy1—positive peritoneal wash cytology; (2) P1—macroscopic PSM.

Due to the high-risk of developing PSM in patients with such risk factors, some authors hypothesized that adjuvant HIPEC might be associated with decreased rates of recurrence and improved survival.

Jingxu Sun et al. [98] performed a meta-analysis on 280 studies analyzing the impact of adjuvant HIPEC on the prognosis of patients with serosal involvement from gastric cancer and found that HIPEC improved the long-term outcomes of these patients, with acceptable morbidity and mortality rates. Similarly, a 2019 study on 80 locally advanced gastric tumor patients (T stage ≥ 3) with no signs of PSM or systemic disease, conducted by Maneesh Kumarsing Beeharry [99], proved that the combination of radical gastrectomy with HIPEC has been associated with acceptable complication rates and improved the OS rates.

To evaluate these results in a European cohort of patients, a randomized multicenter phase III trial (GASTRICHIP) was initiated. This study aimed to evaluate the effects of HIPEC with oxaliplatin on patients with gastric cancer involving the serosa and/or lymph nodes and/or with positive peritoneal cytology, treated with perioperative systemic chemotherapy and D1-D2 curative gastrectomy [100].

Take home message: Current evidence supports the performance of CRS + HIPEC in carefully selected patients with a PCI ≤ 6, when CC-0 can be achieved in high-volume centers. Prophylactic HIPEC in patients with gastric carcinoma at high-risk of PSM development should not be routinely recommended until the results of ongoing trials are made available.

5. Surgical Options for PSM from Pseudomyxoma Peritonei (PMP)

Pseudomyxoma peritonei (PMP) is a rare peritoneal malignancy, most commonly originating from a perforated epithelial tumor of the appendix, also known as "Jelly Belly" and is characterized by the bulky accumulation of gelatinous tumor deposits in the peritoneal cavity.

CRS and HIPEC represent the gold standard treatment for PMP. The main factors that influence a patient's outcome are the histological type and the completeness of the cytoreduction. Thus, the peritoneal mucinous carcinomatosis (PMCA) histologic subtype is associated with significantly worse prognosis compared to the diffuse peritoneal adenomucinosis (DPAM) subtype or hybrid tumors [101]. For appendicular PMP, complete CRS (CC-0) combined with HIPEC was associated with 5- and 10-year OS rates of 85% and 75%, respectively [101,102]. The most frequently used HIPEC regimens are based on oxaliplatin or mitomycin C. However, Chua et al. found that HIPEC was significantly associated with an improved rate of PFS, but it had no significant impact on the OS rates. Thus, even though HIPEC may improve disease control, optimal cytoreduction seems to be the strongest predictor of long-term survival [101].

Some intraoperative findings such as the involvement of the hepatic hilum [34,103], the infiltration of the anterior pancreatic surface [104,105], the ureteric obstruction, or the need for complete gastric resection [106] can impede the achievement of complete CRS. In such instances, although incomplete CRS is known to be associated with significantly decreased OS rates compared with complete CRS, patients with appendiceal PMP seem to benefit from CC-1 resections (remaining nodules smaller than 2.5 mm) and even debulking surgical procedures [102]. The concept of "maximum tumor debulking" (MTD) has been accepted as an alternative to CC-0/CC-1 resection, when complete CRS is not possible or in patients who are not fit for complex surgery [107]. MTD usually involves a greater omentectomy, lower abdominal peritonectomies. and an extended right hemicolectomy, usually associated in women with bilateral oophorectomy [102]. Several studies have shown that MTD plus HIPEC is feasible (achieving low morbidity and mortality rates) and is associated with acceptable OS rates (5-year OS ranging between 24% and 46% after CC-2 or CC-3 resection, compared to 80% after CC-1 resection) [101,108–110].

Absolute contraindications to CRS and HIPEC in patients with PMP are extensive small bowel serosa involvement (at least 1.5 m of small bowel must remain after surgery) [111,112] and mesenteric retraction and infiltration.

Take-home message: In patients with PMP, complete CRS (CC-0) or near-complete CRS (CC-1) associated with HIPEC represents the gold standard therapy. The concept of "maximum tumor debulking" has been accepted in PMP as an alternative to CC-0/CC-1 resection, when complete CRS is not possible, or in patients who are not fit for complex surgery.

6. Surgical Options for PSM from Pancreatic Adenocarcinoma

PSM originating from pancreatic cancer are generally considered incurable and the only treatment option is palliative treatment. PSM is found in approximately 40% of patients, but free intraperitoneal tumor cells are detected in an additional one third of the cases without macroscopic PSM [113,114].

There is a lack of evidence regarding the possible benefits of CRS and HIPEC in patients with PSM from pancreatic cancer. Tentes et al. performed complete CRS or near-complete CRS with HIPEC in seven cases of PSM from pancreatic tail adenocarcinomas and four patients survived for more than 12 months without evidence of recurrence. They suggest that CRS with HIPEC may be considered as a treatment option for highly selected patients with pancreatic cancer and peritoneal metastases [115].

In addition, there is a series of patients with prophylactic use of HIPEC after R0 resection of pancreatic cancer, without peritoneal metastasis. Survival results achieved by this approach are among the highest reported in patients treated with curative intent for pancreatic adenocarcinoma [116]. However, Larentzakis et al. concluded that more controlled studies are needed to justify the use of HIPEC as a prophylactic therapy in resectable pancreatic adenocarcinoma, while CRS and HIPEC for the treatment of PSM of pancreatic origin seems to be useless (and possibly unsafe) at this level of evidence [117].

Take-home message: In patients with pancreatic adenocarcinoma, current evidence cannot support either the performance of CRS +/− HIPEC in the case of PSM, or the prophylactic use of HIPEC in high-risk patients, outside the controlled clinical trials.

7. Surgical Options for PSM from Biliary Tract Carcinoma

PSM from biliary carcinoma is associated with poor outcomes. The treatment for the majority of cases does not imply a surgical gesture and consists of palliative chemotherapy. Amblard et al. compared the impact on survival of CRS and HIPEC (34 cases) with palliative chemotherapy for patients with PSM from biliary carcinoma (25 cases) [118]. The median PCI in the surgical group was 9 (3–26). Macroscopically complete resection could be achieved in 25 patients (73%). Median OS and 3-year OS rate were 21.4 months and 30% in the CRS plus HIPEC group and 9.3 months and 10%, respectively, in the chemotherapy group. The authors concluded that CRS plus HIPEC could be considered for selected patients with a good performance status, low burden of disease, and PSM amenable to complete CRS [1].

Take home message: Currently, surgery for PSM from biliary carcinoma is controversial and future prospective/randomized controlled trials are needed before recommending such an aggressive approach, even in selected patients.

8. Surgical Options for PSM from Gastrointestinal Stromal Tumors (GISTs)

Gastrointestinal stromal tumors (GIST) are the most common mesenchymal neoplasms of the gastrointestinal tract. Surgery is the most effective treatment for resectable primary GIST without metastasis. Approximately 15–47% of patients present with overt metastatic disease with the most common sites of metastases being the liver, peritoneum, and omentum [119].

Surgical treatment for patients with metastatic gastrointestinal stromal tumors remains controversial. Prior to the introduction of systemic treatment with imatinib, outcomes for metastatic GIST were poor, median survival ranging between 10 and 20 months with 5-year OS rates lower than 10% [120]. With the introduction of imatinib in 2002, patient outcomes improved, with an acceptable systemic toxicity [121]. However, imatinib is not a curative treatment and needs to be associated with cytoreductive surgery to achieve better long-term outcomes.

Some retrospective studies [122,123] have reported that tumor size is an important factor in imatinib resistance. An et al. [124] reviewed 249 advanced GIST patients (102 patients with metastatic disease and 147 with multifocal disease relapse) and compared the outcomes achieved by CRS (more than 75% of the initial tumor bulk removed) vs. no CRS, prior to imatinib treatment. They found that CRS was not associated with better long-term outcomes. Their data suggest that cytoreductive surgery prior to imatinib treatment has no benefits for the outcome of the patient.

Thus, for most patients with metastatic GIST, imatinib is the first treatment option. The role of CRS in patients with metastatic GIST with variable responses to imatinib is still debated. Several studies have concluded that patients with disease response to tyrosine kinase inhibitor (TKI) treatment benefit more from CRS (R0/R1) than those with disease progression on TKIs [120,125–130]. Similarly, a multicenter retrospective study from Spain compared the long-term outcomes observed in two cohorts of patients (treated with CRS or without surgery) who achieved partial response (PR) or stable disease (SD) after initial imatinib treatment. This study reported lower median OS in the imatinib only group (59.9 months) compared to the imatinib and CRS group (87.6 months) [131].

CRS (R0/R1) for patients who respond to TKI should be considered no earlier than 6 months after starting the initial systemic therapy (in order to evaluate if they have PR or SD), but not later than 2 years after TKI initiation. TKI treatment should be resumed postoperatively [125,132,133].

The benefits of CRS for imatinib-resistant metastatic GIST are controversial. Several studies have shown that patients who undergo surgery for the focal progressive disease have a limited benefit [126]. However, for imatinib-resistant patients, sunitinib as a second-line therapy seems to be the most appropriate treatment option. The surgical management of patients with progressive metastatic GIST receiving sunitinib is even more controversial, although Yeh et al. [134] and Raut et al. [135] suggest that surgery is feasible and safe for highly selected patients with metastatic GIST who are receiving sunitinib.

Take-home message: CRS should be considered in patients with metastatic GIST whose disease responds to imatinib, with the goal of performing R0/R1 resection. However, debulking/palliative surgery should be limited to patients with complications due to PSM from GISTs (such as hemorrhage, pain or intestinal obstruction) [136]. According to most authors, the role of HIPEC for the treatment of PSM from GIST is still difficult to determine [137–139].

9. Surgical Options for PSM from Gastroenteropancreatic Neuroendocrine Tumors (GEP-NETs)

The incidence of PSM in patients with GEP-NETs is approximately 20%. Most of these metastases originate from primary tumors located in the midgut [140], especially in the ileum, and are often associated with other metastatic sites such as liver metastases, mesenteric lymph nodes, lung and bone metastases [141,142]. Hepatic involvement and tumor grade are the most important prognostic factors [143].

Complete CRS is the best option for patients with metastatic GEP-NETs and appears to improve patient outcomes [144–150]. Therefore, primary tumor resection should be performed during CRS [145,151]. All PCI levels were considered suitable for surgery if resectable [146]. Multivisceral resections and peritonectomy could be part of CRS, and in most cases, are associated with liver metastasis resection and/or radiofrequency ablation and the radiologic chemo-embolization of liver metastases [146,149].

Some studies have shown that a 90% decrease in tumor volume after CRS is associated with the best OS rates [150,152]. Recently, the cytoreduction level has been lowered to 70% of the initial tumor burden, according to several studies that have demonstrated a significant survival benefit for this level of cytoreduction [148,153,154].

The role of HIPEC remains undetermined in patients with PSM from GEP-NETs and a randomized study to evaluate the impact of HIPEC should be initiated [137,147,155].

Take-home message: Complete resection of PSM from GEP-NETs is recommended whenever possible. Patients whose PSM cannot be completely resected seem to achieve a significant survival benefit with debulking surgery, if at least 70% of the tumor burden can be removed. The potential benefit of HIPEC is still unknown.

10. Surgical Options for PSM from Small Bowel Adenocarcinoma

Small bowel cancer is a rare malignancy comprising less than 5% of all digestive cancers. Adenocarcinoma is a frequent subtype, accounting for 37% of all small bowel cancers [156]. Although surgical resection of the primary tumor is the mainstay of treatment management for localized disease, the recurrence rates remain as high as 40% [157]. Furthermore, approximately one third of patients present with stage IV disease [158]. One of the most frequent sites of metastatic involvement in patients with small bowel adenocarcinoma (SBA) is the peritoneal surface, especially in tumors arising from the jejunum and ileum. Other common metastatic sites include liver, lymph nodes, and lungs [159–162].

The prognosis of metastatic SBA is poor, with a 5-year survival rate of 15–33% and a median OS ranging from 12 to 20 months [156,163–165]. Six comparative studies showed a higher median OS in patients who received chemotherapy (12–16 months) versus patients who did not receive chemotherapy (2–8 months) [160,166].

PSM from SBA represents a therapeutic challenge. Several studies showed that CRS and HIPEC improved the outcomes for selected patients with PSM from SBA, achieving a median OS of 31–32 months [159]. The goal of CRS should be the achievement of CC-0.

Patients who received complete CRS (CC-0) had a median OS of 43 months, significantly higher than those achieved by CC-1, CC-2, or CC-3 [167].

The following significant prognostic variables associated with improved survival after CRS plus HIPEC were reported: resection of the primary tumor before CRS plus HIPEC, time interval shorter than 6 months between the detection of PSM and CRS plus HIPEC therapy, well-differentiated tumor, absence of lymph node metastasis, absence of extraperitoneal metastasis, normal value of CA 125 and CA 19-9, absence of ascites, a PCI $\leq$ 15, achievement of CC-0, absence of postoperative complications, and oxaliplatin-based regimen of HIPEC [160,162]. Oxaliplatin-based HIPEC showed a significant survival advantage over the mitomycin C-based HIPEC regimen [162].

Levine et al. suggest that earlier surgical intervention is likely to be more effective than those performed after extensive systemic chemotherapy [168,169]. The most frequently used regimens of systemic chemotherapy are FOLFIRI, FOLFOX, and CAPOX [167,170–172].

Take home message: Based on the available evidence, complete CRS (CC-0) plus HIPEC seems to be safe and more beneficial than systemic chemotherapy alone in selected patients with PSM from SBA. However, future larger studies are needed before routinely recommending this aggressive approach.

11. Pressurized Intraperitoneal Aerosolized Chemotherapy (PIPAC)

PIPAC, a palliative surgical technique designed to deliver chemotherapy (cisplatin, doxorubicin, oxaliplatin) into the peritoneum under pressure, has recently been added to the armamentarium of oncologists to address PSM in patients who are not eligible for CRS [173]. The first report of the successful application of PIPAC in three patients with PSM was published in 2014 [15], and since then, a small number of articles have described the effectiveness and safety of PIPAC for the treatment of PSM in patients with cancers of various origins, the most common being gastric cancer [174].

Systemic chemotherapy is the gold standard approach for unresectable PSM, even if its impact on survival is limited [175]. The expected median survival is estimated at 16.3 months for CRC [176] and 10.7 months for gastric cancer [13], while with PIPAC, the median survival in patients with PSM of gastric origin increases up to 15.4 months, according to the number of PIPAC procedures [177–179].

Alyami et al. [175] reported that complete CRS and HIPEC could be achieved after repeated PIPAC sessions in carefully selected patients with unresectable PSM at diagnosis. In their cohort, the median PCI was 16, all patients underwent systemic chemotherapy between PIPAC sessions, the median consecutive PIPAC procedure was 3 (1–8), and 14.4% of patients were eligible for a secondary CRS and HIPEC after being considered unresectable prior to PIPAC.

A study published by Girshally et al. [180] suggested that neoadjuvant PIPAC is feasible and can be considered before CRS/HIPEC in a select group of patients with PSM of gastric origin and small bowel involvement, in order to reduce the extent of CRS. In their cohort, 12 out of 21 patients had a low PCI (mean 5.8 ± 5.6) and the remaining nine patients had advanced peritoneal involvement (mean PCI 14.3 ± 5.3) at the initial laparoscopy. Repeated PIPAC (3–4 cycles per patient) led to radiological tumor regression in seven out of nine patients, while major histological regression was achieved in eight out of nine patients, allowing for the subsequent performance of CRS + HIPEC.

The PIPAC procedure for PSM from non-gastric cancers is controversial and there is a paucity of data related to the role of PIPAC in PSM of non-gastric origin. Di Giorgio et al. reported that PIPAC with cisplatin, doxorubicin, or oxaliplatin is safe and has antitumor activity against peritoneal metastases of pancreatic and biliary tract origin [181].

Take home message: PIPAC seems to be a valuable palliative approach in patients with unresectable PSM of gastric origin, and is able to significantly prolong the survival of these patients. For PSM from other digestive malignancies, PIPAC requires more prospective controlled trials to better define its role in the palliative treatment of such patients.

12. Conclusions

The aggressive surgical approach of PSM from digestive malignancies, consisting of CRS with or without HIPEC, has gained wider acceptance during the last decade, especially in patients with CRC or gastric carcinoma. This is the consequence of the evidence offered by high-quality randomized clinical trials and meta-analysis that revealed that CRS is the cornerstone therapy in patients with PSM from CRC, although the oxaliplatin-based HIPEC regimen failed to further improve the survival of these patients. Supplementary well-designed randomized trials testing new HIPEC regimens are needed before refuting this therapy. Similarly, in patients with PSM from gastric carcinoma, future randomized controlled trials are needed to confirm the favorable outcomes achieved by CRS with HIPEC in large retrospective studies and meta-analysis. While in PMP the role of CRS with HIPEC is well-established, for PSM from other digestive malignancies, further high-quality studies are needed before recommending this approach outside clinical trials.

Author Contributions: Conceptualization, S.T.A. and M.A.E.; Data curation, M.A.E. and G.P.; Methodology, S.T.A.; Formal analysis and investigation, M.A.E. and G.P.; Writing—original draft preparation, M.A.E. and G.P.; Writing—review and editing, S.T.A. and M.A.E.; Supervision, S.T.A. All authors have read and agreed to the published version of the manuscript.

Funding: This research received no external funding.

Institutional Review Board Statement: Not applicable because this manuscript is a review of the literature.

Informed Consent Statement: Not applicable because this manuscript is a review of the literature.

Data Availability Statement: Not applicable.

Conflicts of Interest: The authors declare no conflict of interest.

References

1. Neuwirth, M.G.; Alexander, H.R.; Karakousis, G.C. Then and now: Cytoreductive surgery with hyperthermic intraperitoneal chemotherapy (HIPEC), a historical perspective. *J. Gastrointest. Oncol.* **2016**, *7*, 18–28. [PubMed]
2. Thomassen, I.; van Gestel, Y.R.; Lemmens, V.E.; de Hingh, I.H. Incidence, prognosis, and treatment options for patients with synchronous peritoneal carcinomatosis and liver metastases from colorectal origin. *Dis. Colon Rectum* **2013**, *56*, 1373–1380. [CrossRef] [PubMed]
3. Sánchez-Hidalgo, J.M.; Rodríguez-Ortiz, L.; Arjona-Sánchez, Á.; Rufián-Peña, S.; Casado-Adam, Á.; Cosano-Álvarez, A.; Briceño-Delgado, J. Colorectal peritoneal metastases: Optimal management review. *World J. Gastroenterol.* **2019**, *25*, 3484–3502. [CrossRef]
4. Sugarbaker, P.H. Peritonectomy procedures. *Ann. Surg.* **1995**, *221*, 29–42. [CrossRef] [PubMed]
5. Gilly, F.N.; Beaujard, A.; Glehen, O.; Grandclement, E.; Caillot, J.L.; Francois, Y.; Sadeghi-Looyeh, B.; Gueugniaud, P.Y.; Garbit, F.; Benoit, M.; et al. Peritonectomy combined with intraperitoneal chemohyperthermia in abdominal cancer with peritoneal carcinomatosis: Phase I-II study. *Anticancer Res.* **1999**, *19*, 2317–2321.
6. Glehen, O.; Cotte, E.; Kusamura, S.; Deraco, M.; Baratti, D.; Passot, G.; Beaujard, A.-C.; Noel, G.F. Hyperthermic intraperitoneal chemotherapy: Nomenclature and modalities of perfusion. *J. Surg. Oncol.* **2008**, *98*, 242–246. [CrossRef]
7. Elias, D.; Antoun, S.; Goharin, A.; Otmany, A.E.; Puizillout, J.M.; Lasser, P. Research on the best chemohyperthermia technique of treatment of peritoneal carcinomatosis after complete resection. *Int. J. Surg. Investig.* **2000**, *1*, 431–439.
8. Jacquet, P.; Sugarbaker, P.H. Clinical research methodologies in diagnosis and staging of patients with peritoneal carcinomatosis. *Cancer Treat. Res.* **1996**, *82*, 359–374.
9. Somashekhar, S.P.; Ashwin, K.R.; Yethadka, R.; Zaveri, S.S.; Ahuja, V.K.; Rauthan, A.; Rohit, K.C. Impact of extent of parietal peritonectomy on oncological outcome after cytoreductive surgery and HIPEC. *Pleura Peritoneum* **2019**, *4*, 20190015. [CrossRef]
10. Chang, S.J.; Bristow, R.E.; Chi, D.S.; Cliby, W.A. Role of aggressive surgical cytoreduction in advanced ovarian cancer. *J. Gynecol. Oncol.* **2015**, *26*, 336–342. [CrossRef]
11. Pujade-Lauraine, E.; Hilpert, F.; Weber, B.; Reuss, A.; Poveda, A.; Kristensen, G.; Sorio, R.; Vergote, I.; Witteveen, P.; Bamias, A.; et al. Bevacizumab combined with chemotherapy for platinum-resistant recurrent ovarian cancer: The AURELIA open-label randomized phase III trial. *J. Clin. Oncol.* **2014**, *32*, 1302–1308. [CrossRef]
12. Rosa, F.; Galiandro, F.; Ricci, R.; Di Miceli, D.; Quero, G.; Fiorillo, C.; Cina, C.; Alfieri, S. Cytoreductive surgery and hyperthermic intraperitoneal chemotherapy (HIPEC) for colorectal peritoneal metastases: Analysis of short- and long-term outcomes. *Langenbeck's Arch. Surg.* **2021**, *406*, 2797–2805. [CrossRef]

13. Al-Batran, S.-E.; Homann, N.; Pauligk, C.; Illerhaus, G.; Martens, U.M.; Stoehlmacher, J.; Schmalenberg, H.; Luley, K.B.; Prasnikar, N.; Egger, M.; et al. Effect of Neoadjuvant Chemotherapy Followed by Surgical Resection on Survival in Patients With Limited Metastatic Gastric or Gastroesophageal Junction Cancer: The AIO-FLOT3 Trial. *JAMA Oncol.* **2017**, *3*, 1237–1244. [CrossRef]
14. Chua, T.C.; Yan, T.D.; Morris, D.L. Surgical biology for the clinician: Peritoneal mesothelioma: Current understanding and management. *Can. J. Surg.* **2009**, *52*, 59–64.
15. Solass, W.; Kerb, R.; Mürdter, T.; Giger-Pabst, U.; Strumberg, D.; Tempfer, C.; Zieren, J.; Schwab, M.; Reymond, M.A. Intraperitoneal chemotherapy of peritoneal carcinomatosis using pressurized aerosol as an alternative to liquid solution: First evidence for efficacy. *Ann. Surg. Oncol.* **2014**, *21*, 553–559. [CrossRef]
16. Chua, T.C.; Yan, T.D.; Saxena, A.; Morris, D.L. Should the treatment of peritoneal carcinomatosis by cytoreductive surgery and hyperthermic intraperitoneal chemotherapy still be regarded as a highly morbid procedure?: A systematic review of morbidity and mortality. *Ann. Surg.* **2009**, *249*, 900–907. [CrossRef]
17. Houlzé-Laroye, C.; Glehen, O.; Sgarbura, O.; Gayat, E.; Sourrouille, I.; Tuech, J.-J.; Delhorme, J.-B.; Dumont, F.; Ceribelli, C.; Amroun, K.; et al. Half of Postoperative Deaths After Cytoreductive Surgery and Hyperthermic Intraperitoneal Chemotherapy Could be Preventable: A French Root Cause Analysis on 5562 Patients. *Ann. Surg.* **2021**, *274*, 797–804. [CrossRef]
18. Alexandrescu, S.T.; Anastase, D.T.; Grigorie, R.T.; Zlate, C.A.; Andrei, S.; Costea, R.; Gramaticu, I.M.; Croitoru, A.E.; Popescu, I. Influence of the Primary Tumor Location on the Pattern of Synchronous Metastatic Spread in Patients with Stage IV Colorectal Carcinoma, According to the 8th Edition of the AJCC Staging System. *J. Gastrointestin Liver Dis.* **2020**, *29*, 561–568. [CrossRef]
19. Segelman, J.; Granath, F.; Holm, T.; Machado, M.; Mahteme, H.; Martling, A. Incidence, prevalence and risk factors for peritoneal carcinomatosis from colorectal cancer. *Br. J. Surg.* **2012**, *99*, 699–705. [CrossRef]
20. Quere, P.; Facy, O.; Manfredi, S.; Jooste, V.; Faivre, J.; Lepage, C.; Bouvier, A.-M. Epidemiology, Management, and Survival of Peritoneal Carcinomatosis from Colorectal Cancer: A Population-Based Study. *Dis. Colon Rectum* **2015**, *58*, 743–752. [CrossRef]
21. Honoré, C.; Goéré, D.; Souadka, A.; Dumont, F.; Elias, D. Definition of patients presenting a high risk of developing peritoneal carcinomatosis after curative surgery for colorectal cancer: A systematic review. *Ann. Surg. Oncol.* **2013**, *20*, 183–192. [CrossRef] [PubMed]
22. Koga, S.; Hamazoe, R.; Maeta, M.; Shimizu, N.; Kanayama, H.; Osaki, Y. Treatment of implanted peritoneal cancer in rats by continuous hyperthermic peritoneal perfusion in combination with an anticancer drug. *Cancer Res.* **1984**, *44*, 1840–1842. [PubMed]
23. Verwaal, V.J.; van Ruth, S.; de Bree, E.; van Sloothen, G.W.; van Tinteren, H.; Boot, H.; Zoetmulder, F.A.N. Randomized trial of cytoreduction and hyperthermic intraperitoneal chemotherapy versus systemic chemotherapy and palliative surgery in patients with peritoneal carcinomatosis of colorectal cancer. *J. Clin. Oncol.* **2003**, *21*, 3737–3743. [CrossRef] [PubMed]
24. Elias, D.; Gilly, F.; Boutitie, F.; Quénet, F.; Bereder, J.-M.; Mansvelt, B.; Lorimier, G.; Dubè, P.; Glehen, O. Peritoneal colorectal carcinomatosis treated with surgery and perioperative intraperitoneal chemotherapy: Retrospective analysis of 523 patients from a multicentric French study. *J. Clin. Oncol.* **2010**, *28*, 63–68. [CrossRef]
25. Quénet, F.; Goéré, D.; Mehta, S.S.; Roca, L.; Dumont, F.; Hessissen, M.; Saint-Aubert, B.; Elias, D. Results of two bi-institutional prospective studies using intraperitoneal oxaliplatin with or without irinotecan during HIPEC after cytoreductive surgery for colorectal carcinomatosis. *Ann. Surg.* **2011**, *254*, 294–301. [CrossRef]
26. Goéré, D.; Malka, D.; Tzanis, D.; Gava, V.; Boige, V.; Eveno, C.; Maggiori, L.; Dumont, F.; Ducreux, M.; Elias, D. Is there a possibility of a cure in patients with colorectal peritoneal carcinomatosis amenable to complete cytoreductive surgery and intraperitoneal chemotherapy? *Ann. Surg.* **2013**, *257*, 1065–1071. [CrossRef]
27. Quénet, F.; Elias, D.; Roca, L.; Goéré, D.; Ghouti, L.; Pocard, M.; Facy, O.; Arvieux, C.; Lorimier, G.; Pezet, D.; et al. Cytoreductive surgery plus hyperthermic intraperitoneal chemotherapy versus cytoreductive surgery alone for colorectal peritoneal metastases (PRODIGE 7): A multicentre, randomised, open-label, phase 3 trial. *Lancet Oncol.* **2021**, *22*, 256–266. [CrossRef]
28. Glehen, O.; Kwiatkowski, F.; Sugarbaker, P.H.; Elias, D.; Levine, E.A.; De Simone, M.; Barone, R.; Yonemura, Y.; Cavaliere, F.; Quenet, F.; et al. Cytoreductive surgery combined with perioperative intraperitoneal chemotherapy for the management of peritoneal carcinomatosis from colorectal cancer: A multi-institutional study. *J. Clin. Oncol.* **2004**, *22*, 3284–3292. [CrossRef]
29. Turaga, K.; Levine, E.; Barone, R.; Sticca, R.; Petrelli, N.; Lambert, L.; Nash, G.; Morse, M.; Adbel-Misih, R.; Alexander, H.R.; et al. Consensus guidelines from The American Society of Peritoneal Surface Malignancies on standardizing the delivery of hyperthermic intraperitoneal chemotherapy (HIPEC) in colorectal cancer patients in the United States. *Ann. Surg. Oncol.* **2014**, *21*, 1501–1505. [CrossRef]
30. Yan, T.D.; Chu, F.; Links, M.; Kam, P.C.; Glenn, D.; Morris, D.L. Cytoreductive surgery and perioperative intraperitoneal chemotherapy for peritoneal carcinomatosis from colorectal carcinoma: Non-mucinous tumour associated with an improved survival. *Eur. J. Surg. Oncol.* **2006**, *32*, 1119–1124. [CrossRef]
31. da Silva, R.G.; Sugarbaker, P.H. Analysis of prognostic factors in seventy patients having a complete cytoreduction plus perioperative intraperitoneal chemotherapy for carcinomatosis from colorectal cancer. *J. Am. Coll. Surg.* **2006**, *203*, 878–886. [CrossRef]
32. Cavaliere, F.; De Simone, M.; Virzì, S.; Deraco, M.; Rossi, C.R.; Garofalo, A.; Di Filippo, F.; Giannarelli, D.; Vaira, M.; Valle, M.; et al. Prognostic factors and oncologic outcome in 146 patients with colorectal peritoneal carcinomatosis treated with cytoreductive surgery combined with hyperthermic intraperitoneal chemotherapy: Italian multicenter study S.I.T.I.L.O. *Eur. J. Surg. Oncol.* **2011**, *37*, 148–154. [CrossRef]

33. Van Sweringen, H.L.; Hanseman, D.J.; Ahmad, S.A.; Edwards, M.J.; Sussman, J.J. Predictors of survival in patients with high-grade peritoneal metastases undergoing cytoreductive surgery and hyperthermic intraperitoneal chemotherapy. *Surgery* **2012**, *152*, 617–625. [CrossRef]
34. Cotte, E.; Passot, G.; Gilly, F.-N.; Glehen, O. Selection of patients and staging of peritoneal surface malignancies. *World J. Gastrointest. Oncol.* **2010**, *2*, 31–35. [CrossRef]
35. Yonemura, Y.; Canbay, E.; Ishibashi, H. Prognostic factors of peritoneal metastases from colorectal cancer following cytoreductive surgery and perioperative chemotherapy. *Sci. World J.* **2013**, *2013*, 978394. [CrossRef]
36. Benizri, E.I.; Bernard, J.-L.; Rahili, A.; Benchimol, D.; Bereder, J.-M. Small bowel involvement is a prognostic factor in colorectal carcinomatosis treated with complete cytoreductive surgery plus hyperthermic intraperitoneal chemotherapy. *World J. Surg. Oncol.* **2012**, *10*, 56–58. [CrossRef]
37. Elias, D.; Mariani, A.; Cloutier, A.-S.; Blot, F.; Goéré, D.; Dumont, F.; Honoré, C.; Billard, V.; Dartigues, P.; Ducreux, M. Modified selection criteria for complete cytoreductive surgery plus HIPEC based on peritoneal cancer index and small bowel involvement for peritoneal carcinomatosis of colorectal origin. *Eur. J. Surg. Oncol.* **2014**, *40*, 1467–1473. [CrossRef]
38. Tonello, M.; Ortega-Perez, G.; Alonso-Casado, O.; Torres-Mesa, P.; Guiñez, G.; Gonzalez-Moreno, S. Peritoneal carcinomatosis arising from rectal or colonic adenocarcinoma treated with cytoreductive surgery (CRS) hyperthermic intraperitoneal chemotherapy (HIPEC): Two different diseases. *Clin. Transl. Oncol.* **2018**, *20*, 1268–1273. [CrossRef]
39. Péron, J.; Mercier, F.; Tuech, J.-J.; Younan, R.; Sideris, L.; Gelli, M.; Dumont, F.; Le Roy, B.; Sgarbura, O.; Dico, R.L.; et al. The location of the primary colon cancer has no impact on outcomes in patients undergoing cytoreductive surgery for peritoneal metastasis. *Surgery* **2019**, *165*, 476–484. [CrossRef]
40. Massalou, D.; Benizri, E.; Chevallier, A.; Duranton-Tanneur, V.; Pedeutour, F.; Benchimol, D.; Bereder, J.-M. Peritoneal carcinomatosis of colorectal cancer: Novel clinical and molecular outcomes. *Am. J. Surg.* **2017**, *213*, 377–387. [CrossRef]
41. Bardou, M.; Rouland, A.; Martel, M.; Loffroy, R.; Barkun, A.N.; Chapelle, N. Review article: Obesity and colorectal cancer. *Aliment. Pharmacol. Ther.* **2022**, *56*, 407–418. [CrossRef] [PubMed]
42. Cohen, M.E.; Bilimoria, K.Y.; Ko, C.Y.; Richards, K.; Hall, B.L. Effect of subjective preoperative variables on risk-adjusted assessment of hospital morbidity and mortality. *Ann. Surg.* **2009**, *249*, 682–689. [CrossRef] [PubMed]
43. Foster, J.M.; Sleightholm, R.; Patel, A.; Shostrom, V.; Hall, B.; Neilsen, B.; Bartlett, D.; Smith, L. Morbidity and Mortality Rates Following Cytoreductive Surgery Combined with Hyperthermic Intraperitoneal Chemotherapy Compared with Other High-Risk Surgical Oncology Procedures. *JAMA Netw. Open* **2019**, *2*, e186847. [CrossRef] [PubMed]
44. Cashin, P.; Sugarbaker, P.H. Hyperthermic intraperitoneal chemotherapy (HIPEC) for colorectal and appendiceal peritoneal metastases: Lessons learned from PRODIGE 7. *J. Gastrointest Oncol.* **2021**, *12*, S120–S128. [CrossRef]
45. Kirstein, M.N.; Root, S.A.; Moore, M.M.; Wieman, K.M.; Williams, B.W.; Jacobson, P.A.; Marker, P.H.; Tuttle, T.M. Exposure-response relationships for oxaliplatin-treated colon cancer cells. *Anticancer Drugs* **2008**, *19*, 37–44. [CrossRef]
46. Lemoine, L.; Thijssen, E.; Carleer, R.; Geboers, K.; Sugarbaker, P.; van der Speeten, K. Body surface area-based vs concentration-based perioperative intraperitoneal chemotherapy after optimal cytoreductive surgery in colorectal peritoneal surface malignancy treatment: COBOX trial. *J. Surg. Oncol.* **2019**, *119*, 999–1010. [CrossRef]
47. Levine, E.A.; Stewart, J.H.; Shen, P.; Russell, G.B.; Loggie, B.L.; Votanopoulos, K.I. Intraperitoneal chemotherapy for peritoneal surface malignancy: Experience with 1000 patients. *J. Am. Coll. Surg.* **2014**, *218*, 573–585. [CrossRef]
48. van Driel, W.J.; Koole, S.N.; Sikorska, K.; van Leeuwen, J.H.S.; Schreuder, H.W.R.; Hermans, R.H.M.; de Hingh, I.H.J.T.; van der Velden, J.; Arts, H.J.; Massuger, L.F.A.G.; et al. Hyperthermic Intraperitoneal Chemotherapy in Ovarian Cancer. *N. Engl. J. Med.* **2018**, *378*, 230–240. [CrossRef]
49. Yurttas, C.; Hoffmann, G.; Tolios, A.; Haen, S.P.; Schwab, M.; Königsrainer, I.; Königsrainer, A.; Beckert, S.; Löffler, M.W. Systematic Review of Variations in Hyperthermic Intraperitoneal Chemotherapy (HIPEC) for Peritoneal Metastasis from Colorectal Cancer. *J. Clin. Med.* **2018**, *7*, 567. [CrossRef]
50. Hompes, D.; D'Hoore, A.; Wolthuis, A.; Fieuws, S.; Mirck, B.; Bruin, S.; Verwaal, V. The use of Oxaliplatin or Mitomycin C in HIPEC treatment for peritoneal carcinomatosis from colorectal cancer: A comparative study. *J. Surg. Oncol.* **2014**, *109*, 527–532. [CrossRef]
51. Prada-Villaverde, A.; Esquivel, J.; Lowy, A.M.; Markman, M.; Chua, T.; Pelz, J.; Baratti, D.; Baumgartner, J.M.; Berri, R.; Bretcha-Boix, P.; et al. The American Society of Peritoneal Surface Malignancies evaluation of HIPEC with Mitomycin C versus Oxaliplatin in 539 patients with colon cancer undergoing a complete cytoreductive surgery. *J. Surg. Oncol.* **2014**, *110*, 779–785. [CrossRef]
52. Leung, V.; Huo, Y.R.; Liauw, W.; Morris, D.L. Oxaliplatin versus Mitomycin C for HIPEC in colorectal cancer peritoneal carcinomatosis. *Eur. J. Surg. Oncol* **2017**, *43*, 144–149. [CrossRef]
53. Andreou, A.; Kopetz, S.; Maru, D.M.; Chen, S.S.; Zimmitti, G.; Brouquet, A.; Shindoh, J.; Curley, S.A.; Garrett, C.; Overman, M.J.; et al. Adjuvant chemotherapy with FOLFOX for primary colorectal cancer is associated with increased somatic gene mutations and inferior survival in patients undergoing hepatectomy for metachronous liver metastases. *Ann. Surg.* **2012**, *256*, 642–650. [CrossRef]
54. de Gramont, A.; Figer, A.; Seymour, M.; Homerin, M.; Hmissi, A.; Cassidy, J.; Boni, C.; Cortes-Funes, H.; Cervantes, A.; Freyer, G.; et al. Leucovorin and fluorouracil with or without oxaliplatin as first-line treatment in advanced colorectal cancer. *J. Clin. Oncol.* **2000**, *18*, 2938–2947. [CrossRef]

55. Powers, B.D.; Felder, S.; Veerapong, J.; Baumgartner, J.M.; Clarke, C.; Mogal, H.; Staley, C.A.; Maithel, S.K.; Patel, S.; Dhar, V.; et al. Repeat Cytoreductive Surgery and Hyperthermic Intraperitoneal Chemotherapy Is Not Associated with Prohibitive Complications: Results of a Multiinstitutional Retrospective Study. *Ann. Surg. Oncol.* **2020**, *27*, 4883–4891. [CrossRef]
56. Golse, N.; Bakrin, N.; Passot, G.; Mohamed, F.; Vaudoyer, D.; Gilly, F.-N.; Glehen, O.; Cotte, E. Iterative procedures combining cytoreductive surgery with hyperthermic intraperitoneal chemotherapy for peritoneal recurrence: Postoperative and long-term results. *J. Surg. Oncol.* **2012**, *106*, 197–203. [CrossRef]
57. Bijelic, L.; Yan, T.D.; Sugarbaker, P.H. Treatment failure following complete cytoreductive surgery and perioperative intraperitoneal chemotherapy for peritoneal dissemination from colorectal or appendiceal mucinous neoplasms. *J. Surg. Oncol.* **2008**, *98*, 295–299. [CrossRef]
58. Yap, D.R.Y.; Wong, J.S.M.; Tan, Q.X.; Tan, J.W.-S.; Chia, C.S.; Ong, C.-A.J. Effect of HIPEC on Peritoneal Recurrence in Peritoneal Metastasis Treated with Cytoreductive Surgery: A Systematic Review. *Front. Oncol.* **2021**, *11*, 795390. [CrossRef]
59. Newton, A.D.; Bartlett, E.K.; Karakousis, G.C. Cytoreductive surgery and hyperthermic intraperitoneal chemotherapy: A review of factors contributing to morbidity and mortality. *J. Gastrointest. Oncol.* **2016**, *7*, 99–111.
60. Elias, D.; Honoré, C.; Dumont, F.; Ducreux, M.; Boige, V.; Malka, D.; Burtin, P.; Dromain, C.; Goéré, D. Results of systematic second-look surgery plus HIPEC in asymptomatic patients presenting a high risk of developing colorectal peritoneal carcinomatosis. *Ann. Surg.* **2011**, *254*, 289–293. [CrossRef]
61. Elias, D.; Goéré, D.; Di Pietrantonio, D.; Boige, V.; Malka, D.; Kohneh-Shahri, N.; Dromain, C.; Ducreux, M. Results of systematic second-look surgery in patients at high risk of developing colorectal peritoneal carcinomatosis. *Ann. Surg.* **2008**, *247*, 445–450. [CrossRef] [PubMed]
62. Del Moral, Á.S.; Viejo, E.P.; Romero, I.M.; Caravaca, G.R.; Pérez, F.P. Systematic Second-Look Surgery Plus HIPEC in Patients without Evidence of Recurrence, at High Risk of Carcinomatosis after Colorectal Cancer Resection. *Cir. Esp.* **2018**, *96*, 96–101.
63. Sammartino, P.; Sibio, S.; Biacchi, D.; Cardi, M.; Mingazzini, P.; Rosati, M.S.; Cornali, T.; Sollazzo, B.; Atta, J.M.; Di Giorgio, A. Long-term results after proactive management for locoregional control in patients with colonic cancer at high risk of peritoneal metastases. *Int. J. Color. Dis.* **2014**, *29*, 1081–1089. [CrossRef] [PubMed]
64. Tentes, A.-A.K.; Kyziridis, D.; Kakolyris, S.; Pallas, N.; Zorbas, G.; Korakianitis, O.; Mavroudis, C.; Courcoutsakis, N.; Prasopoulos, P. Preliminary results of hyperthermic intraperitoneal intraoperative chemotherapy as an adjuvant in resectable pancreatic cancer. *Gastroenterol. Res. Pract.* **2012**, *2012*, 506571. [CrossRef]
65. Baratti, D.; Kusamura, S.; Iusco, D.; Gimondi, S.; Pietrantonio, F.; Milione, M.; Guaglio, M.; Bonomi, S.; Grassi, A.; Virzì, S.; et al. Hyperthermic Intraperitoneal Chemotherapy (HIPEC) at the Time of Primary Curative Surgery in Patients with Colorectal Cancer at High Risk for Metachronous Peritoneal Metastases. *Ann. Surg. Oncol.* **2017**, *24*, 167–175. [CrossRef]
66. Sloothaak, D.A.M.; Mirck, B.; Punt, C.J.A.; Bemelman, W.A.; van der Bilt, J.D.W.; D'Hoore, A.; Tanis, P.J. Intraperitoneal chemotherapy as adjuvant treatment to prevent peritoneal carcinomatosis of colorectal cancer origin: A systematic review. *Br. J. Cancer* **2014**, *111*, 1112–1121. [CrossRef]
67. Goéré, D.; Glehen, O.; Quenet, F.; Guilloit, J.M.; Bereder, J.M.; Lorimier, G.; Thibaudeau, E.; Ghouti, L.; Pinto, A.; Tuech, J.J.; et al. Second-look surgery plus hyperthermic intraperitoneal chemotherapy versus surveillance in patients at high risk of developing colorectal peritoneal metastases (PROPHYLOCHIP-PRODIGE 15): A randomised, phase 3 study. *Lancet Oncol.* **2020**, *21*, 1147–1154. [CrossRef]
68. Klaver, C.E.L.; Wisselink, D.D.; Punt, C.J.A.; Snaebjornsson, P.; Crezee, J.; Aalbers, A.G.J.; Brandt, A.; Bremers, A.J.A.; Fabry, H.F.J.; Ferenschild, F.; et al. Adjuvant hyperthermic intraperitoneal chemotherapy in patients with locally advanced colon cancer (COLOPEC): A multicentre, open-label, randomised trial. *Lancet Gastroenterol. Hepatol.* **2019**, *4*, 761–770. [CrossRef]
69. Sommariva, A.; Tonello, M.; Coccolini, F.; De Manzoni, G.; Delrio, P.; Pizzolato, E.; Gelmini, R.; Serra, F.; Rreka, E.; Pasqual, E.M.; et al. Colorectal Cancer with Peritoneal Metastases: The Impact of the Results of PROPHYLOCHIP, COLOPEC, and PRODIGE 7 Trials on Peritoneal Disease Management. *Cancers* **2022**, *15*, 165. [CrossRef]
70. Gretschel, S.; Siegel, R.; Estévez-Schwarz, L.; Hünerbein, M.; Schneider, U.; Schlag, P.M. Surgical strategies for gastric cancer with synchronous peritoneal carcinomatosis. *Br. J. Surg.* **2006**, *93*, 1530–1535. [CrossRef]
71. Roviello, F.; Caruso, S.; Neri, A.; Marrelli, D. Treatment and prevention of peritoneal carcinomatosis from gastric cancer by cytoreductive surgery and hyperthermic intraperitoneal chemotherapy: Overview and rationale. *Eur. J. Surg. Oncol.* **2013**, *39*, 1309–1316. [CrossRef]
72. Ajani, J.A.; Bentrem, D.J.; Besh, S.; D'Amico, T.A.; Das, P.; Denlinger, C.; Fakih, M.G.; Fuchs, C.S.; Gerdes, H.; Glasgow, R.E.; et al. Gastric cancer, version 2.2013: Featured updates to the NCCN Guidelines. *J. Natl. Compr. Cancer Netw.* **2013**, *11*, 531–546. [CrossRef]
73. Fuchs, C.S.; Shitara, K.; Di Bartolomeo, M.; Lonardi, S.; Al-Batran, S.-E.; Van Cutsem, E.; Ilson, D.H.; Alsina, M.; Chau, I.; Lacy, J.; et al. Ramucirumab with cisplatin and fluoropyrimidine as first-line therapy in patients with metastatic gastric or junctional adenocarcinoma (RAINFALL): A double-blind, randomised, placebo-controlled, phase 3 trial. *Lancet Oncol.* **2019**, *20*, 420–435. [CrossRef]
74. Fujimoto, S.; Takahashi, M.; Mutou, T.; Kobayashi, K.; Toyosawa, T.; Isawa, E.; Sumida, M.; Ohkubo, H. Improved mortality rate of gastric carcinoma patients with peritoneal carcinomatosis treated with intraperitoneal hyperthermic chemoperfusion combined with surgery. *Cancer* **1997**, *79*, 884–891. [CrossRef]

75. Yonemura, Y.; Fujimura, T.; Nishimura, G.; Falla, R.; Sawa, T.; Katayama, K.; Tsugawa, K.; Fushida, S.; Miyazaki, I.; Tanaka, M.; et al. Effects of intraoperative chemohyperthermia in patients with gastric cancer with peritoneal dissemination. *Surgery* **1996**, *119*, 437–444. [CrossRef]
76. Glehen, O.; Schreiber, V.; Cotte, E.; Sayag-Beaujard, A.C.; Osinsky, D.; Freyer, G.; Francois, Y.; Vignal, J.; Gilly, F.N. Cytoreductive surgery and intraperitoneal chemohyperthermia for peritoneal carcinomatosis arising from gastric cancer. *Arch. Surg.* **2004**, *139*, 20–26. [CrossRef]
77. Glehen, O.; Gilly, F.-N.; Arvieux, C.; Cotte, E.; Boutitie, F.; Mansvelt, B.; Bereder, J.-M.; Lorimier, G.; Quénet, F.; Elias, D.; et al. Peritoneal carcinomatosis from gastric cancer: A multi-institutional study of 159 patients treated by cytoreductive surgery combined with perioperative intraperitoneal chemotherapy. *Ann. Surg. Oncol.* **2010**, *17*, 2370–2377. [CrossRef]
78. Yonemura, Y.; Elnemr, A.; Endou, Y.; Hirano, M.; Mizumoto, A.; Takao, N.; Ichinose, M.; Miura, M.; Li, Y. Multidisciplinary therapy for treatment of patients with peritoneal carcinomatosis from gastric cancer. *World J. Gastrointest. Oncol.* **2010**, *2*, 85–97. [CrossRef]
79. Bonnot, P.-E.; Piessen, G.; Kepenekian, V.; Decullier, E.; Pocard, M.; Meunier, B.; Bereder, J.-M.; Abboud, K.; Marchal, F.; Quénet, F.; et al. Cytoreductive Surgery with or without Hyperthermic Intraperitoneal Chemotherapy for Gastric Cancer with Peritoneal Metastases (CYTO-CHIP study): A Propensity Score Analysis. *J. Clin. Oncol.* **2019**, *37*, 2028–2040. [CrossRef]
80. Coccolini, F.; Catena, F.; Glehen, O.; Yonemura, Y.; Sugarbaker, P.H.; Piso, P.; Montori, G.; Ansaloni, L. Complete versus incomplete cytoreduction in peritoneal carcinosis from gastric cancer, with consideration to PCI cut-off. Systematic review and meta-analysis. *Eur. J. Surg. Oncol.* **2015**, *41*, 911–919. [CrossRef]
81. Canbay, E.; Mizumoto, A.; Ichinose, M.; Ishibashi, H.; Sako, S.; Hirano, M.; Takao, N.; Yonemura, Y. Outcome data of patients with peritoneal carcinomatosis from gastric origin treated by a strategy of bidirectional chemotherapy prior to cytoreductive surgery and hyperthermic intraperitoneal chemotherapy in a single specialized center in Japan. *Ann. Surg. Oncol.* **2014**, *21*, 1147–1152. [CrossRef] [PubMed]
82. Marano, L.; Marrelli, D.; Sammartino, P.; Biacchi, D.; Graziosi, L.; Marino, E.; Coccolini, F.; Fugazzola, P.; Valle, M.; Federici, O.; et al. Cytoreductive Surgery and Hyperthermic Intraperitoneal Chemotherapy for Gastric Cancer with Synchronous Peritoneal Metastases: Multicenter Study of 'Italian Peritoneal Surface Malignancies Oncoteam-S.I.C.O. *Ann. Surg. Oncol.* **2021**, *28*, 9060–9070. [CrossRef] [PubMed]
83. Caro, C.R.; Manzanedo, I.; Pereira, F.; Carrion-Alvarez, L.; Serrano, Á.; Viejo, E.P. Cytoreductive surgery combined with hyperthermic intraperitoneal chemotherapy (HIPEC) in patients with gastric cancer and peritoneal carcinomatosis. *Eur. J. Surg. Oncol.* **2018**, *44*, 1805–1810. [CrossRef] [PubMed]
84. Yarema, R.; Mielko, J.; Fetsych, T.; Ohorchak, M.; Skorzewska, M.; Rawicz-Pruszyński, K.; Mashukov, A.; Maksimovsky, V.; Jastrzębski, T.; Polkowski, W.; et al. Hyperthermic intraperitoneal chemotherapy (HIPEC) in combined treatment of locally advanced and intraperitonealy disseminated gastric cancer: A retrospective cooperative Central-Eastern European study. *Cancer Med.* **2019**, *8*, 2877–2885. [CrossRef] [PubMed]
85. Rau, B.; Brandl, A.; Piso, P.; Pelz, J.; Busch, P.; Demtröder, C.; Schüle, S.; Schlitt, H.-J.; Roitman, M.; Tepel, J.; et al. Peritoneal metastasis in gastric cancer: Results from the German database. *Gastric Cancer* **2020**, *23*, 11–22. [CrossRef]
86. Rau, B.; Brandl, A.; Thuss-Patience, P.; Bergner, F.; Raue, W.; Arnold, A.; Horst, D.; Pratschke, J.; Biebl, M. The efficacy of treatment options for patients with gastric cancer and peritoneal metastasis. *Gastric Cancer* **2019**, *22*, 1226–1237. [CrossRef]
87. Glehen, O.; Gilly, F.N.; Boutitie, F.; Bereder, J.M.; Quénet, F.; Sideris, L.; Mansvelt, B.; Lorimier, G.; Msika, S.; Elias, D.; et al. Toward curative treatment of peritoneal carcinomatosis from nonovarian origin by cytoreductive surgery combined with perioperative intraperitoneal chemotherapy: A multi-institutional study of 1290 patients. *Cancer* **2010**, *116*, 5608–5618. [CrossRef]
88. Marano, L.; Marrelli, D.; Roviello, F. ASO Author Reflections: Gastric Cancer with Synchronous Peritoneal Disease—A Clinically Meaningful Survival after CRS and HIPEC in Selected Patients from Italian Peritoneal Surface Malignancies Oncoteam Network. *Ann. Surg. Oncol.* **2021**, *28*, 9071–9072. [CrossRef]
89. Königsrainer, I.; Horvath, P.; Struller, F.; Königsrainer, A.; Beckert, S. Initial clinical experience with cytoreductive surgery and hyperthermic intraperitoneal chemotherapy in signet-ring cell gastric cancer with peritoneal metastases. *J. Gastric Cancer* **2014**, *14*, 117–122. [CrossRef]
90. Solomon, D.; DeNicola, N.; Feingold, D.; Liu, P.H.; Aycart, S.; Golas, B.J.; Sarpel, U.; Labow, D.M.; Magge, D.R. Signet ring cell features with peritoneal carcinomatosis in patients undergoing cytoreductive surgery and hyperthermic intraperitoneal chemotherapy are associated with poor overall survival. *J. Surg. Oncol.* **2019**, *119*, 758–765. [CrossRef]
91. Hartwig, W.; Gluth, A.; Hinz, U.; Koliogiannis, D.; Strobel, O.; Hackert, T.; Werner, J.; Büchler, M.W. Outcomes after extended pancreatectomy in patients with borderline resectable and locally advanced pancreatic cancer. *Br. J. Surg.* **2016**, *103*, 1683–1694. [CrossRef]
92. Koemans, W.J.; van der Kaaij, R.T.; Boot, H.; Buffart, T.; Veenhof, A.A.F.A.; Hartemink, K.J.; Grootscholten, C.; Snaebjornsson, P.; Retel, V.P.; van Tinteren, H.; et al. Cytoreductive surgery and hyperthermic intraperitoneal chemotherapy versus palliative systemic chemotherapy in stomach cancer patients with peritoneal dissemination, the study protocol of a multicentre randomised controlled trial (PERISCOPE II). *BMC Cancer* **2019**, *19*, 420–428. [CrossRef]
93. Bieri, U.; Moch, H.; Dehler, S.; Korol, D.; Rohrmann, S. Changes in autopsy rates among cancer patients and their impact on cancer statistics from a public health point of view: A longitudinal study from 1980 to 2010 with data from Cancer Registry Zurich. *Virchows Arch.* **2015**, *466*, 637–643. [CrossRef]

94. Berretta, M.; Fisichella, R.; Borsatti, E.; Lleshi, A.; Ioffredo, S.; Meneguzzo, N.; Canzonieri, V.; Di Grazia, A.; Cannizzaro, R.; Tirelli, U.; et al. Feasibility of intraperitoneal Trastuzumab treatment in a patient with peritoneal carcinomatosis from gastric cancer. *Eur. Rev. Med. Pharmacol. Sci.* **2014**, *18*, 689–692.
95. Seyfried, F.; von Rahden, B.H.; Miras, A.D.; Gasser, M.; Maeder, U.; Kunzmann, V.; Germer, C.-T.; Pelz, J.; Kerscher, A.G. Incidence, time course and independent risk factors for metachronous peritoneal carcinomatosis of gastric origin-a longitudinal experience from a prospectively collected database of 1108 patients. *BMC Cancer* **2015**, *15*, 73. [CrossRef]
96. Bando, E.; Yonemura, Y.; Takeshita, Y.; Taniguchi, K.; Yasui, T.; Yoshimitsu, Y.; Fushida, S.; Fujimura, T.; Nishimura, G.; Miwa, K. Intraoperative lavage for cytological examination in 1,297 patients with gastric carcinoma. *Am. J. Surg.* **1999**, *178*, 256–262. [CrossRef]
97. Nio, Y.; Tsubono, M.; Kawabata, K.; Masai, Y.; Hayashi, H.; Meyer, C.; Inoue, K.; Tobe, T. Comparison of survival curves of gastric cancer patients after surgery according to the UICC stage classification and the General Rules for Gastric Cancer Study by the Japanese Research Society for gastric cancer. *Ann. Surg.* **1993**, *218*, 47–53. [CrossRef]
98. Sun, J.; Song, Y.; Wang, Z.; Gao, P.; Chen, X.; Xu, Y.; Liang, J.; Xu, H. Benefits of hyperthermic intraperitoneal chemotherapy for patients with serosal invasion in gastric cancer: A meta-analysis of the randomized controlled trials. *BMC Cancer* **2012**, *12*, 526. [CrossRef]
99. Beeharry, M.K.; Zhu, Z.-L.; Liu, W.-T.; Yao, X.-X.; Yan, M.; Zhu, Z.-G. Correction to: Prophylactic HIPEC with radical D2 gastrectomy improves survival and peritoneal recurrence rates for locally advanced gastric cancer: Personal experience from a randomized case control study. *BMC Cancer* **2019**, *19*, 1256. [CrossRef]
100. Glehen, O.; Passot, G.; Villeneuve, L.; Vaudoyer, D.; Bin-Dorel, S.; Boschetti, G.; Piaton, E.; Garofalo, A. GASTRICHIP: D2 resection and hyperthermic intraperitoneal chemotherapy in locally advanced gastric carcinoma: A randomized and multicenter phase III study. *BMC Cancer* **2014**, *14*, 183. [CrossRef]
101. Chua, T.C.; Moran, B.J.; Sugarbaker, P.H.; Levine, E.A.; Glehen, O.; Gilly, F.N.; Baratti, D.; Deraco, M.; Elias, D.; Sardi, A.; et al. Early- and long-term outcome data of patients with pseudomyxoma peritonei from appendiceal origin treated by a strategy of cytoreductive surgery and hyperthermic intraperitoneal chemotherapy. *J. Clin. Oncol.* **2012**, *30*, 2449–2456. [CrossRef] [PubMed]
102. Govaerts, K.; Lurvink, R.J.; De Hingh, I.H.J.T.; Van der Speeten, K.; Villeneuve, L.; Kusamura, S.; Kepenekian, V.; Deraco, M.; Glehen, O.; Moran, B.J.; et al. Appendiceal tumours and pseudomyxoma peritonei: Literature review with PSOGI/EURACAN clinical practice guidelines for diagnosis and treatment. *Eur. J. Surg. Oncol.* **2011**, *47*, 11–35. [CrossRef] [PubMed]
103. Esquivel, J.; Elias, D.; Baratti, D.; Kusamura, S.; Deraco, M. Consensus statement on the loco regional treatment of colorectal cancer with peritoneal dissemination. *J. Surg. Oncol.* **2008**, *98*, 263–267. [CrossRef] [PubMed]
104. Downs-Canner, S.; Ding, Y.; Magge, D.R.; Jones, H.; Ramalingam, L.; Zureikat, A.; Holtzman, M.; Ahrendt, S.; Pingpank, J.; Zeh, H.J.; et al. A comparative analysis of postoperative pancreatic fistulas after surgery with and without hyperthermic intraperitoneal chemoperfusion. *Ann. Surg. Oncol.* **2015**, *22*, 1651–1657. [CrossRef]
105. Doud, A.N.; Randle, R.W.; Clark, C.J.; Levine, E.A.; Swett, K.R.; Shen, P.; Stewart, J.H.; Votanopoulos, K.I. Impact of distal pancreatectomy on outcomes of peritoneal surface disease treated with cytoreductive surgery and hyperthermic intraperitoneal chemotherapy. *Ann. Surg. Oncol.* **2015**, *22*, 1645–1650. [CrossRef]
106. Di Fabio, F.; Mehta, A.; Chandrakumaran, K.; Mohamed, F.; Cecil, T.; Moran, B. Advanced Pseudomyxoma Peritonei Requiring Gastrectomy to Achieve Complete Cytoreduction Results in Good Long-Term Oncologic Outcomes. *Ann. Surg. Oncol.* **2016**, *23*, 4316–4321. [CrossRef]
107. Moran, B.J.; Tzivanakis, A. The concept of 'Obstruction-Free Survival' as an outcome measure in advanced colorectal cancer management. *Pleura Peritoneum* **2018**, *3*, 20180101. [CrossRef]
108. Yan, T.D.; Deraco, M.; Baratti, D.; Kusamura, S.; Elias, D.; Glehen, O.; Gilly, F.N.; Levine, E.A.; Shen, P.; Mohamed, F.; et al. Cytoreductive surgery and hyperthermic intraperitoneal chemotherapy for malignant peritoneal mesothelioma: Multi-institutional experience. *J. Clin. Oncol.* **2009**, *27*, 6237–6242. [CrossRef]
109. Delhorme, J.-B.; Elias, D.; Varatharajah, S.; Benhaim, L.; Dumont, F.; Honoré, C.; Goéré, D. Can a Benefit be Expected from Surgical Debulking of Unresectable Pseudomyxoma Peritonei? *Ann. Surg. Oncol.* **2016**, *23*, 1618–1624. [CrossRef]
110. Glehen, O.; Mohamed, F.; Sugarbaker, P.H. Incomplete cytoreduction in 174 patients with peritoneal carcinomatosis from appendiceal malignancy. *Ann. Surg.* **2004**, *240*, 278–285. [CrossRef]
111. Low, R.N.; Barone, R.M.; Gurney, J.M.; Muller, W.D. Mucinous appendiceal neoplasms: Preoperative MR staging and classification compared with surgical and histopathologic findings. *Am. J. Roentgenol.* **2008**, *190*, 656–665. [CrossRef]
112. Elias, D.; Benizri, E.; Vernerey, D.; Eldweny, H.; Dipietrantonio, D.; Pocard, M. Preoperative criteria of incomplete resectability of peritoneal carcinomatosis from non-appendiceal colorectal carcinoma. *Gastroenterol. Clin. Biol.* **2005**, *29*, 1010–1013. [CrossRef]
113. Heeckt, P.; Safi, F.; Binder, T.; Büchler, M. Free intraperitoneal tumors cells in pancreatic cancer-significance for clinical course and therapy. *Der Chir.* **1992**, *63*, 563–567.
114. Tani, M.; Kawai, M.; Terasawa, H.; Ina, S.; Hirono, S.; Shimamoto, T.; Miyazawa, M.; Uchiyama, K.; Yamaue, H. Prognostic factors for long-term survival in patients with locally invasive pancreatic cancer. *J. Hepatobiliary Pancreat. Surg.* **2007**, *14*, 545–550. [CrossRef]
115. Tentes, A.-A.; Pallas, N.; Karamveri, C.; Kyziridis, D.; Hristakis, C. Cytoreduction and HIPEC for peritoneal carcinomatosis of pancreatic cancer. *J. BUON* **2018**, *23*, 482–487.

116. Tentes, A.-A.; Stamou, K.; Pallas, N.; Karamveri, C.; Kyziridis, D.; Hristakis, C. The effect of hyperthermic intraoperative intraperitoneal chemotherapy (HIPEC) as an adjuvant in patients with resectable pancreatic cancer. *Int. J. Hyperth.* **2016**, *32*, 895–899. [CrossRef]
117. Larentzakis, A.; Anagnostou, E.; Georgiou, K.; Vrakopoulou, G.-Z.; Zografos, C.G.; Zografos, G.C.; Toutouzas, K.G. Place of hyperthermic intraperitoneal chemotherapy in the armament against pancreatic adenocarcinoma: A survival, mortality and morbidity systematic review. *Oncol. Lett.* **2021**, *21*, 246. [CrossRef]
118. Amblard, I.; Mercier, F.; Bartlett, D.L.; Ahrendt, S.A.; Lee, K.W.; Zeh, H.J.; Levine, E.A.; Baratti, D.; Deraco, M.; Piso, P.; et al. Cytoreductive surgery and HIPEC improve survival compared to palliative chemotherapy for biliary carcinoma with peritoneal metastasis: A multi-institutional cohort from PSOGI and BIG RENAPE groups. *Eur. J. Surg. Oncol.* **2018**, *44*, 1378–1383. [CrossRef]
119. Quek, R.; George, S. Gastrointestinal stromal tumor: A clinical overview. *Hematol. Oncol. Clin. N. Am.* **2009**, *23*, 69–78. [CrossRef]
120. Tielen, R.; Verhoef, C.; van Coevorden, F.; Gelderblom, H.; Sleijfer, S.; Hartgrink, H.H.; Bonenkamp, J.J.; van der Graaf, W.T.; de Wilt, J.H.W. Surgery after treatment with imatinib and/or sunitinib in patients with metastasized gastrointestinal stromal tumors: Is it worthwhile? *World J. Surg. Oncol.* **2012**, *10*, 111. [CrossRef]
121. Keung, E.Z.; Fairweather, M.; Raut, C.P. The Role of Surgery in Metastatic Gastrointestinal Stromal Tumors. *Curr. Treat Options Oncol.* **2016**, *17*, 8–12. [CrossRef]
122. Van Glabbeke, M.; Verweij, J.; Casali, P.G.; Le Cesne, A.; Hohenberger, P.; Ray-Coquard, I.; Schlemmer, M.; van Oosterom, A.T.; Goldstein, D.; Sciot, R.; et al. Initial and late resistance to imatinib in advanced gastrointestinal stromal tumors are predicted by different prognostic factors: A European Organisation for Research and Treatment of Cancer-Italian Sarcoma Group-Australasian Gastrointestinal Trials Group study. *J. Clin. Oncol.* **2005**, *23*, 5795–5804.
123. GSTMA Group. Comparison of two doses of imatinib for the treatment of unresectable or metastatic gastrointestinal stromal tumors: A meta-analysis of 1640 patients. *J. Clin. Oncol.* **2010**, *28*, 1247–1253. [CrossRef] [PubMed]
124. An, H.J.; Ryu, M.-H.; Ryoo, B.-Y.; Sohn, B.S.; Kim, K.-H.; Oh, S.T.; Yu, C.S.; Yook, J.H.; Kim, B.S.; Kang, Y.-K. The effects of surgical cytoreduction prior to imatinib therapy on the prognosis of patients with advanced GIST. *Ann. Surg. Oncol.* **2013**, *20*, 4212–4218. [CrossRef] [PubMed]
125. Bonvalot, S.; Eldweny, H.; Péchoux, C.L.; Vanel, D.; Terrier, P.; Cavalcanti, A.; Robert, C.; Lassau, N.; Cesne, A.L. Impact of surgery on advanced gastrointestinal stromal tumors (GIST) in the imatinib era. *Ann. Surg. Oncol.* **2006**, *13*, 1596–1603. [CrossRef]
126. Raut, C.P.; Posner, M.; Desai, J.; Morgan, J.A.; George, S.; Zahrieh, D.; Fletcher, C.D.M.; Demetri, G.D.; Bertagnolli, M.M. Surgical management of advanced gastrointestinal stromal tumors after treatment with targeted systemic therapy using kinase inhibitors. *J. Clin. Oncol.* **2006**, *24*, 2325–2331. [CrossRef] [PubMed]
127. Andtbacka, R.H.I.; Ng, C.S.; Scaife, C.L.; Cormier, J.N.; Hunt, K.K.; Pisters, P.W.T.; Pollock, R.E.; Benjamin, R.S.; Burgess, M.A.; Chen, L.L.; et al. Surgical resection of gastrointestinal stromal tumors after treatment with imatinib. *Ann. Surg. Oncol.* **2007**, *14*, 14–24. [CrossRef]
128. DeMatteo, R.P.; Maki, R.G.; Singer, S.; Gonen, M.; Brennan, M.F.; Antonescu, C.R. Results of tyrosine kinase inhibitor therapy followed by surgical resection for metastatic gastrointestinal stromal tumor. *Ann. Surg.* **2007**, *245*, 347–352. [CrossRef]
129. Gronchi, A.; Fiore, M.; Miselli, F.; Lagonigro, M.S.; Coco, P.; Messina, A.; Pilotti, S.; Casali, P.G. Surgery of residual disease following molecular-targeted therapy with imatinib mesylate in advanced/metastatic GIST. *Ann. Surg.* **2007**, *245*, 341–346. [CrossRef]
130. Bischof, D.A.; Kim, Y.; Blazer, D.G.; Behman, R.; Karanicolas, P.J.; Law, C.H.; Quereshy, F.A.; Maithel, S.K.; Gamblin, T.C.; Bauer, T.W.; et al. Surgical management of advanced gastrointestinal stromal tumors: An international multi-institutional analysis of 158 patients. *J. Am. Coll. Surg.* **2014**, *219*, 439–449. [CrossRef]
131. Rubió-Casadevall, J.; Martinez-Trufero, J.; Garcia-Albeniz, X.; Calabuig, S.; Lopez-Pousa, A.; Del Muro, J.G.; Fra, J.; Redondo, A.; Lainez, N.; Poveda, A.; et al. Role of surgery in patients with recurrent, metastatic, or unresectable locally advanced gastrointestinal stromal tumors sensitive to imatinib: A retrospective analysis of the Spanish Group for Research on Sarcoma (GEIS). *Ann. Surg. Oncol.* **2015**, *22*, 2948–2957. [CrossRef]
132. Mussi, C.; Ronellenfitsch, U.; Jakob, J.; Tamborini, E.; Reichardt, P.; Casali, P.G.; Fiore, M.; Hohenberger, P.; Gronchi, A. Post-imatinib surgery in advanced/metastatic GIST: Is it worthwhile in all patients? *Ann. Oncol.* **2010**, *21*, 403–408. [CrossRef]
133. Sym, S.J.; Ryu, M.-H.; Lee, J.-L.; Chang, H.M.; Kim, T.-W.; Kim, H.C.; Kim, K.-H.; Yook, J.H.; Kim, B.S.; Kang, Y.-K. Surgical intervention following imatinib treatment in patients with advanced gastrointestinal stromal tumors (GISTs). *J. Surg. Oncol.* **2008**, *98*, 27–33. [CrossRef]
134. Yeh, C.-N.; Wang, S.-Y.; Tsai, C.-Y.; Chen, Y.-Y.; Liu, C.-T.; Chiang, K.-C.; Chen, T.-W.; Liu, Y.-Y.; Yeh, T.-S. Surgical management of patients with progressing metastatic gastrointestinal stromal tumors receiving sunitinib treatment: A prospective cohort study. *Int. J. Surg.* **2017**, *39*, 30–36. [CrossRef]
135. Raut, C.P.; Wang, Q.; Manola, J.; Morgan, J.A.; George, S.; Wagner, A.J.; Butrynski, J.E.; Fletcher, C.D.M.; Demetri, G.D.; Bertagnolli, M.M. Cytoreductive surgery in patients with metastatic gastrointestinal stromal tumor treated with sunitinib malate. *Ann. Surg. Oncol.* **2010**, *17*, 407–415. [CrossRef]
136. Zhang, X.H.; He, Y.L. Significance of surgical treatment for recurrent and metastatic gastrointestinal stromal tumors. *Chin. J. Gastrointest. Surg.* **2020**, *23*, 840–844.

137. Goéré, D.; Passot, G.; Gelli, M.; Levine, E.A.; Bartlett, D.L.; Sugarbaker, P.H.; Glehen, O. Complete cytoreductive surgery plus HIPEC for peritoneal metastases from unusual cancer sites of origin: Results from a worldwide analysis issue of the Peritoneal Surface Oncology Group International (PSOGI). *Int. J. Hyperth.* **2017**, *33*, 520–527. [CrossRef]
138. Bonvalot, S.; Cavalcanti, A.; Le Péchoux, C.; Terrier, P.; Vanel, D.; Blay, J.Y.; Le Cesne, A.; Elias, D. Randomized trial of cytoreduction followed by intraperitoneal chemotherapy versus cytoreduction alone in patients with peritoneal sarcomatosis. *Eur. J. Surg. Oncol.* **2005**, *31*, 917–923. [CrossRef]
139. Baratti, D.; Pennacchioli, E.; Kusamura, S.; Fiore, M.; Balestra, M.R.; Colombo, C.; Mingrone, E.; Gronchi, A.; Deraco, M. Peritoneal sarcomatosis: Is there a subset of patients who may benefit from cytoreductive surgery and hyperthermic intraperitoneal chemotherapy? *Ann. Surg. Oncol.* **2010**, *17*, 3220–3228. [CrossRef]
140. Kianmanesh, R.; Ruszniewski, P.; Rindi, G.; Kwekkeboom, D.; Pape, U.-F.; Kulke, M.; Garcia, I.S.; Scoazec, J.-Y.; Nilsson, O.; Fazio, N.; et al. ENETS consensus guidelines for the management of peritoneal carcinomatosis from neuroendocrine tumors. *Neuroendocrinology* **2010**, *91*, 333–340. [CrossRef]
141. de Mestier, L.; Lardière-Deguelte, S.; Brixi, H.; O'Toole, D.; Ruszniewski, P.; Cadiot, G.; Kianmanesh, R. Updating the surgical management of peritoneal carcinomatosis in patients with neuroendocrine tumors. *Neuroendocrinology* **2015**, *101*, 105–111. [CrossRef] [PubMed]
142. Ejaz, A.; Reames, B.N.; Maithel, S.; Poultsides, G.A.; Bauer, T.W.; Fields, R.C.; Weiss, M.; Marques, H.P.; Aldrighetti, L.; Pawlik, T.M. The impact of extrahepatic disease among patients undergoing liver-directed therapy for neuroendocrine liver metastasis. *J. Surg. Oncol.* **2017**, *116*, 841–847. [CrossRef] [PubMed]
143. Tomassetti, P.; Campana, D.; Piscitelli, L.; Casadei, R.; Nori, F.; Brocchi, E.; Santini, D.; Pezzilli, R.; Corinaldesi, R. Endocrine tumors of the ileum: Factors correlated with survival. *Neuroendocrinology* **2006**, *83*, 380–386. [CrossRef] [PubMed]
144. Group, C.C.W. The Chicago Consensus on peritoneal surface malignancies: Management of neuroendocrine tumors. *Cancer* **2020**, *126*, 2561–2565.
145. Group, C.C.W. The Chicago Consensus on Peritoneal Surface Malignancies: Management of Neuroendocrine Tumors. *Ann. Surg. Oncol.* **2020**, *27*, 1788–1792.
146. Benhaim, L.; Faron, M.; Hadoux, J.; Gelli, M.; Sourrouille, I.; Burtin, P.; Honoré, C.; Malka, D.; Leboulleux, S.; Ducreux, M.; et al. Long-Term Results after Surgical Resection of Peritoneal Metastasis from Neuroendocrine Tumors. *Neuroendocrinology* **2021**, *111*, 599–608. [CrossRef]
147. Elias, D.; David, A.; Sourrouille, I.; Honoré, C.; Goéré, D.; Dumont, F.; Stoclin, A.; Baudin, E. Neuroendocrine carcinomas: Optimal surgery of peritoneal metastases (and associated intra-abdominal metastases). *Surgery* **2014**, *155*, 5–12. [CrossRef]
148. Wonn, S.M.; Limbach, K.E.; Pommier, S.J.; Ratzlaff, A.N.; Leon, E.J.; McCully, B.H.; Pommier, R.F. Outcomes of cytoreductive operations for peritoneal carcinomatosis with or without liver cytoreduction in patients with small bowel neuroendocrine tumors. *Surgery* **2021**, *169*, 168–174. [CrossRef]
149. Chan, D.L.; Dixon, M.; Law, C.H.L.; Koujanian, S.; Beyfuss, K.A.; Singh, S.; Myrehaug, S.; Hallet, J. Outcomes of Cytoreductive Surgery for Metastatic Low-Grade Neuroendocrine Tumors in the Setting of Extrahepatic Metastases. *Ann. Surg. Oncol.* **2018**, *25*, 1768–1774. [CrossRef]
150. Sarmiento, J.M.; Heywood, G.; Rubin, J.; Ilstrup, D.M.; Nagorney, D.M.; Que, F.G. Surgical treatment of neuroendocrine metastases to the liver: A plea for resection to increase survival. *J. Am. Coll. Surg.* **2003**, *197*, 29–37. [CrossRef]
151. Wind, G.G. *Applied Laparoscopic Anatomy: Abdomen and Pelvis*, 1st ed.; Lippincott Williams & Wilkins: Baltimore, MD, USA, 1997.
152. McEntee, G.P.; Nagorney, D.M.; Kvols, L.K.; Moertel, C.G.; Grant, C.S. Cytoreductive hepatic surgery for neuroendocrine tumors. *Surgery* **1990**, *108*, 1091–1096.
153. Woltering, E.A.; Voros, B.A.; Beyer, D.T.; Wang, Y.-Z.; Thiagarajan, R.; Ryan, P.; Wright, A.; Ramirez, R.A.; Ricks, M.J.; Boudreaux, J.P. Aggressive Surgical Approach to the Management of Neuroendocrine Tumors: A Report of 1000 Surgical Cytoreductions by a Single Institution. *J. Am. Coll. Surg.* **2017**, *224*, 434–447. [CrossRef]
154. Maxwell, J.E.; Sherman, S.K.; O'Dorisio, T.M.; Bellizzi, A.M.; Howe, J.R. Liver-directed surgery of neuroendocrine metastases: What is the optimal strategy? *Surgery* **2016**, *159*, 320–335. [CrossRef]
155. Bhatt, A. *Management of Peritoneal Metastases-Cytoreductive Surgery, HIPEC and beyond*; Springer: Berlin/Heidelberg, Germany, 2018.
156. Bilimoria, K.Y.; Bentrem, D.J.; Wayne, J.D.; Ko, C.Y.; Bennett, C.L.; Talamonti, M.S. Small bowel cancer in the United States: Changes in epidemiology, treatment, and survival over the last 20 years. *Ann. Surg.* **2009**, *249*, 63–71. [CrossRef]
157. Talamonti, M.S.; Goetz, L.H.; Rao, S.; Joehl, R.J. Primary cancers of the small bowel: Analysis of prognostic factors and results of surgical management. *Arch. Surg.* **2002**, *137*, 564–571. [CrossRef]
158. Overman, M.J.; Hu, C.-Y.; Kopetz, S.; Abbruzzese, J.L.; Wolff, R.A.; Chang, G.J. A population-based comparison of adenocarcinoma of the large and small intestine: Insights into a rare disease. *Ann. Surg. Oncol.* **2012**, *19*, 1439–1445. [CrossRef]
159. Legué, L.M.; Simkens, G.A.; Creemers, G.-J.M.; Lemmens, V.E.P.P.; de Hingh, I.H.J.T. Synchronous peritoneal metastases of small bowel adenocarcinoma: Insights into an underexposed clinical phenomenon. *Eur. J. Cancer* **2017**, *87*, 84–91. [CrossRef]
160. Dabaja, B.S.; Suki, D.; Pro, B.; Bonnen, M.; Ajani, J. Adenocarcinoma of the small bowel: Presentation, prognostic factors, and outcome of 217 patients. *Cancer* **2004**, *101*, 518–526. [CrossRef]
161. Legué, L.M.; Bernards, N.; Gerritse, S.L.; van Oudheusden, T.R.; de Hingh, I.H.J.T.; Creemers, G.-J.M.; Tije, A.J.T.; Lemmens, V.E.P.P. Trends in incidence, treatment and survival of small bowel adenocarcinomas between 1999 and 2013: A population-based study in The Netherlands. *Acta Oncol.* **2016**, *55*, 1183–1189. [CrossRef]

162. Liu, Y.; Ishibashi, H.; Takeshita, K.; Mizumoto, A.; Hirano, M.; Sako, S.; Takegawa, S.; Takao, N.; Ichinose, M.; Yonemura, Y. Cytoreductive Surgery and Hyperthermic Intraperitoneal Chemotherapy for Peritoneal Dissemination from Small Bowel Malignancy: Results from a Single Specialized Center. *Ann. Surg. Oncol.* **2016**, *23*, 1625–1631. [CrossRef]
163. Howe, J.R.; Karnell, L.H.; Menck, H.R.; Scott-Conner, C. The American College of Surgeons Commission on Cancer and the American Cancer Society. Adenocarcinoma of the small bowel: Review of the National Cancer Data Base, 1985–1995. *Cancer* **1999**, *86*, 2693–2706. [CrossRef]
164. Frost, D.B.; Mercado, P.D.; Tyrell, J.S. Small bowel cancer: A 30-year review. *Ann. Surg. Oncol.* **1994**, *1*, 290–295. [CrossRef]
165. Aparicio, T.; Zaanan, A.; Svrcek, M.; Laurent-Puig, P.; Carrere, N.; Manfredi, S.; Locher, C.; Afchain, P. Small bowel adenocarcinoma: Epidemiology, risk factors, diagnosis and treatment. *Dig. Liver Dis.* **2014**, *46*, 97–104. [CrossRef] [PubMed]
166. Halfdanarson, T.R.; McWilliams, R.R.; Donohue, J.H.; Quevedo, J.F. A single-institution experience with 491 cases of small bowel adenocarcinoma. *Am. J. Surg* **2010**, *199*, 797–803. [CrossRef] [PubMed]
167. Liu, Y.; Yonemura, Y.; Levine, E.A.; Glehen, O.; Goéré, D.; Elias, D.; Morris, D.L.; Sugarbaker, P.H.; Tuech, J.J.; Cashin, P.; et al. Cytoreductive Surgery Plus Hyperthermic Intraperitoneal Chemotherapy for Peritoneal Metastases From a Small Bowel Adenocarcinoma: Multi-Institutional Experience. *Ann. Surg. Oncol.* **2018**, *25*, 1184–1192. [CrossRef]
168. Tsushima, T.; Taguri, M.; Honma, Y.; Takahashi, H.; Ueda, S.; Nishina, T.; Kawai, H.; Kato, S.; Suenaga, M.; Tamura, F.; et al. Multicenter retrospective study of 132 patients with unresectable small bowel adenocarcinoma treated with chemotherapy. *Oncologist* **2012**, *17*, 1163–1170. [CrossRef]
169. Sun, Y.; Shen, P.; Stewart, J.H.; Russell, G.B.; Levine, E.A. Cytoreductive surgery and hyperthermic intraperitoneal chemotherapy for peritoneal carcinomatosis from small bowel adenocarcinoma. *Am. Surg.* **2013**, *79*, 644–648. [CrossRef]
170. Khan, K.; Peckitt, C.; Sclafani, F.; Watkins, D.; Rao, S.; Starling, N.; Jain, V.; Trivedi, S.; Stanway, S.; Cunningham, D.; et al. Prognostic factors and treatment outcomes in patients with Small Bowel Adenocarcinoma (SBA): The Royal Marsden Hospital (RMH) experience. *BMC Cancer* **2015**, *15*, 15. [CrossRef]
171. Overman, M.J.; Hu, C.-Y.; Wolff, R.A.; Chang, G.J. Prognostic value of lymph node evaluation in small bowel adenocarcinoma: Analysis of the surveillance, epidemiology, and end results database. *Cancer* **2010**, *116*, 5374–5382. [CrossRef]
172. Zaanan, A.; Costes, L.; Gauthier, M.; Malka, D.; Locher, C.; Mitry, E.; Tougeron, D.; Lecomte, T.; Gornet, J.-M.; Sobhani, I.; et al. Chemotherapy of advanced small-bowel adenocarcinoma: A multicenter AGEO study. *Ann. Oncol.* **2010**, *21*, 1786–1793. [CrossRef]
173. Alberto, M.; Brandl, A.; Garg, P.K.; Gül-Klein, S.; Dahlmann, M.; Stein, U.; Rau, B. Pressurized intraperitoneal aerosol chemotherapy and its effect on gastric-cancer-derived peritoneal metastases: An overview. *Clin. Exp. Metastasis* **2019**, *36*, 1–14. [CrossRef]
174. Garg, P.K.; Jara, M.; Alberto, M.; Rau, B. The role of Pressurized IntraPeritoneal Aerosol Chemotherapy in the management of gastric cancer: A systematic review. *Pleura Peritoneum* **2019**, *4*, 20180127. [CrossRef]
175. Alyami, M.; Mercier, F.; Siebert, M.; Bonnot, P.-E.; Laplace, N.; Villeneuve, L.; Passot, G.; Glehen, O.; Bakrin, N.; Kepenekian, V. Unresectable peritoneal metastasis treated by pressurized intraperitoneal aerosol chemotherapy (PIPAC) leading to cytoreductive surgery and hyperthermic intraperitoneal chemotherapy. *Eur. J. Surg. Oncol.* **2021**, *47*, 128–133. [CrossRef]
176. Franko, J.; Shi, Q.; Meyers, J.P.; Maughan, T.S.; Adams, R.A.; Seymour, M.T.; Saltz, L.; Punt, C.J.A.; Koopman, M.; Tournigand, C.; et al. Prognosis of patients with peritoneal metastatic colorectal cancer given systemic therapy: An analysis of individual patient data from prospective randomised trials from the Analysis and Research in Cancers of the Digestive System (ARCAD) database. *Lancet Oncol.* **2016**, *17*, 1709–1719. [CrossRef]
177. Khomyakov, V.; Ryabov, A.; Ivanov, A.; Bolotina, L.; Utkina, A.; Volchenko, N.; Kaprin, A. Bidirectional chemotherapy in gastric cancer with peritoneal metastasis combining intravenous XELOX with intraperitoneal chemotherapy with low-dose cisplatin and Doxorubicin administered as a pressurized aerosol: An open-label, Phase-2 study (PIPAC-GA2). *Pleura Peritoneum* **2016**, *1*, 159–166. [CrossRef]
178. Nadiradze, G.; Giger-Pabst, U.; Zieren, J.; Strumberg, D.; Solass, W.; Reymond, M.A. Pressurized Intraperitoneal Aerosol Chemotherapy (PIPAC) with Low-Dose Cisplatin and Doxorubicin in Gastric Peritoneal Metastasis. *J. Gastrointest. Surg.* **2015**, *20*, 367–373. [CrossRef]
179. Di Giorgio, A.; Schena, C.A.; El Halabieh, M.A.; Abatini, C.; Vita, E.; Strippoli, A.; Inzani, F.; Rodolfino, E.; Romanò, B.; Pacelli, F.; et al. Systemic chemotherapy and pressurized intraperitoneal aerosol chemotherapy (PIPAC): A bidirectional approach for gastric cancer peritoneal metastasis. *Surg. Oncol.* **2020**, *34*, 270–275. [CrossRef]
180. Girshally, R.; Demtröder, C.; Albayrak, N.; Zieren, J.; Tempfer, C.; Reymond, M.A. Pressurized intraperitoneal aerosol chemotherapy (PIPAC) as a neoadjuvant therapy before cytoreductive surgery and hyperthermic intraperitoneal chemotherapy. *World J. Surg. Oncol.* **2016**, *14*, 253. [CrossRef]
181. Di Giorgio, A.; Sgarbura, O.; Rotolo, S.; Schena, C.A.; Bagalà, C.; Inzani, F.; Russo, A.; Chiantera, V.; Pacelli, F. Pressurized intraperitoneal aerosol chemotherapy with cisplatin and doxorubicin or oxaliplatin for peritoneal metastasis from pancreatic adenocarcinoma and cholangiocarcinoma. *Ther. Adv. Med. Oncol.* **2020**, *12*, 1758835920940887. [CrossRef]

Disclaimer/Publisher's Note: The statements, opinions and data contained in all publications are solely those of the individual author(s) and contributor(s) and not of MDPI and/or the editor(s). MDPI and/or the editor(s) disclaim responsibility for any injury to people or property resulting from any ideas, methods, instructions or products referred to in the content.

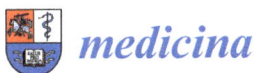

Review

International Consensus on Definition of Mild-to-Moderate Ulcerative Colitis Disease Activity in Adult Patients

Bénédicte Caron [1], Vipul Jairath [2,3], Ferdinando D'Amico [4,5], Sameer Al Awadhi [6], Axel Dignass [7], Ailsa L. Hart [8], Taku Kobayashi [9], Paulo Gustavo Kotze [10], Fernando Magro [11,12,13], Britta Siegmund [14,15], Kristine Paridaens [16], Silvio Danese [4,*] and Laurent Peyrin-Biroulet [1]

1. Department of Gastroenterology and Inserm NGERE U1256, Nancy University Hospital, University of Lorraine, 54500 Vandoeuvre-lès-Nancy, France
2. Department of Medicine, Western University, London, ON N6A 3K7, Canada
3. Department of Epidemiology and Biostatistics, Western University, London, ON N6A 3K7, Canada
4. Gastroenterology and Endoscopy, IRCCS Ospedale San Raffaele and University Vita-Salute San Raffaele, 20132 Milan, Italy
5. Department of Biomedical Sciences, Humanitas University, Pieve Emanuele, 20090 Milan, Italy
6. Gastroenterology Division, Rashid Hospital, Dubai Health Authority, Dubai 003206, United Arab Emirates
7. Department of Medicine I, Agaplesion Markus Hospital, Goethe-University, 60431 Frankfurt am Main, Germany
8. Inflammatory Bowel Disease Unit, St. Mark's Hospital, Harrow HA1 3UJ, UK
9. Center for Advanced IBD Research and Treatment, Kitasato University Kitasato Institute Hospital, Tokyo 108-8642, Japan
10. IBD Outpatient Clinics, Colorectal Surgery Unit, Pontificia Universidade Católica do Paraná (PUCPR), Curitiba 80215-901, Brazil
11. Unit of Pharmacology and Therapeutics, Department of Biomedicine, Faculty of Medicine, University of Porto, 4200319 Porto, Portugal
12. Department of Clinical Pharmacology, São João University Hospital Center (CHUSJ), 4200319 Porto, Portugal
13. Center for Health Technology and Services Research (CINTESIS), 4200319 Porto, Portugal
14. Charité–Universitätsmedizin Berlin, Corporate Member of Freie Universität Berlin, Humboldt-Universität zu Berlin and Berlin Institute of Health, 10117 Berlin, Germany
15. Department of Gastroenterology, Rheumatology and Infectious Disease, Campus Benjamin Franklin, 10117 Berlin, Germany
16. Ferring International Center S.A. Ch. De la Vergognausaz 50, 1162 Saint-Prex, Switzerland
* Correspondence: sdanese@hotmail.com

Abstract: *Background and Objectives*: At present, there is no consensus definition of mild-to-moderate disease activity in patients with ulcerative colitis. The objective of the present study was to establish a reliable definition of mild-to-moderate disease activity in adult patients with ulcerative colitis. *Materials and Methods*: Twelve physicians from around the world participated in a virtual consensus meeting on 26 September 2022. All the physicians had expertise in the diagnosis and treatment of inflammatory bowel disease. After a systematic review of the literature and expert opinion, a modified version of the RAND/University of California, Los Angeles appropriateness method was applied. A total of 49 statements were identified and then anonymously rated (on a 9-point scale) as being appropriate (scores of 7 to 9), uncertain (4 to 6) or inappropriate (1 to 3). The survey results were reviewed and amended before a second round of voting. *Results*: Symptom and endoscopic-based measurements are of prime importance for assessing mild-to-moderate ulcerative colitis activity in clinical trials. The experts considered that clinical activity should be assessed in terms of stool frequency, rectal bleeding and fecal urgency, whereas endoscopic activity should be evaluated with regard to the vascular pattern, bleeding, erosions and ulcers. Fecal calprotectin was considered to be a suitable disease activity marker in mild-to-moderate ulcerative colitis. Lastly, mild-to-moderate ulcerative colitis should not have more than a small impact on the patient's daily activities. *Conclusions*: The present recommendations constitute a standardized framework for defining mild-to-moderate disease activity in clinical trials in the field of ulcerative colitis.

Keywords: ulcerative colitis; mild; moderate; definition; activity

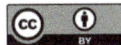

1. Introduction

In terms of severity, ulcerative colitis (UC) is typically classified as being "mild-to-moderate" or "moderate-to-severe" [1]. However, a great variety of definition of "mild-to-moderate" disease activity in UC can be found in the medical literature and in clinical practice [1]. Several metrics have been developed to monitor and standardize the assessment of clinical activity in UC; these include the Simple Colitis Clinical Activity Index (SCCAI), the Mayo Clinic Score (MCS), the Ulcerative Colitis Disease Activity Index (UC-DAI) and the Truelove and Witts criteria for severe disease [2–7]. Nevertheless, there is no consensus on the definition of mild-to-moderate disease activity in UC [1,8,9].

Sedano et al. have systematically reviewed definitions of mild-to-moderate UC found in protocols listed at clinicaltrials.gov (accessed on 10 October 2022) [10]. The MCS was the most frequently used score, while the UCDAI was detected in a small proportion of trials (13.1%) [10]. Twenty different MCS cut-offs have been used to define mild-to-moderate active UC: The minimum cut-off ranged from 1 to 6, and the maximum cut-off ranged from 4 to 11 [10]. However, the MCS and UCDAI have some limitations because they include the subjective Physician Global Assessment (PGA) sub-score [11]. Most regulatory authorities recommend excluding the PGA sub-score in order to reduce subjectivity and thus focus on the patient's self-reported symptoms and objective endoscopic findings [11].

Sedano et al.'s review emphasized that the definitions of mild-to-moderate UC vary markedly from one clinical trial to another. The lack of a consensus on the definition of mild-to-moderate UC means that the clinical trial data are heterogeneous and non-reproducible. We therefore lack a standardized definition of mild-to-moderate UC disease activity in patients eligible for inclusion in clinical trials; this constitutes a key unmet need in the field of inflammatory bowel disease (IBD).

In the present study, we first comprehensively reviewed the literature on (i) definitions of mild-to-moderate active UC and (ii) factors that were predictive of a treatment response in randomized controlled trials (RCTs) of 5-aminosalicylic acid (5-ASA) and/or budesonide Multi Matrix®. Secondly, we formed an international expert panel and conducted a multiple-round survey. The objective was to establish a robust definition of mild-to-moderate UC disease activity for use in clinical trials with adult patients.

2. Materials and Methods

Firstly, we systematically reviewed the definitions of mild-to-moderate active UC used in 39 RCTs of 5-ASA and/or budesonide Multi Matrix® [12]. Six different indexes were used to define mild-to-moderate active UC in these trials—emphasizing the high degree of heterogeneity in the literature [12]. Most RCTs used the UCDAI [12]. Four different UCDAI cut-offs were used to define mild-to-moderate active UC. The most common UCDAI cut-offs (reported in more than half of the included RCTs) were ≥ 4 and ≤ 10, with a sigmoidoscopy score of ≥ 1 and a PGA score ≤ 2 [12].

Secondly, we used the modified RAND/University of California, Los Angeles (UCLA) appropriateness method by incorporating a Delphi panel approach with iterative rounds of voting and discussion [13]. This approach combined the best available evidence with expert opinion, in order to (i) assess the face validity and the feasibility of items identified in the systematic review and (ii) generate a robust definition of mild-to-moderate disease activity in UC [12,13].

There were two rounds of voting. Two of the authors (VJ and BC) prepared 49 preliminary statements based on the needs identified in the systematic review. The list of statements was then disseminated online. The expert panel members anonymously rated each item for appropriateness on a 9-point scale (ranging from 1 = inappropriate to 5 = uncertain and 9 = highly appropriate). As specified in the RAND/University of California Los Angeles (UCLA) manual, each statement was classified (according to the panel's median rating and extent of disagreement) as inappropriate (a median score of 1 to 3.5, with no disagreement); uncertain (a median score of 3.5 to 6.5 with no disagreement or a median score of any value with disagreement); or appropriate (a median score of 6.5 to 9, with no disagreement). Disagreement for a given statement was defined as six or more votes in the lowest three-point region (i.e., 1–3) and six or more votes in the highest three-point region (i.e., 6–9).

The first-round survey results were reviewed, discussed and amended during a videoconference that took place on 26 September 2022. The latter included 12 physicians from nine different countries (Brazil, Canada, France, Germany, Italy, Japan, Portugal, the United Arab Emirates and the United Kingdom); all had significant expertise in the field of IBD. The videoconference's objective was to identify areas of disagreement on item appropriateness and the rationale for answers. The survey was then revised as a function of the panel's discussions in order to clarify statements prior to a second round of voting. This second round occurred only if no agreement was achieved during the first round, and the appropriateness of statements was scored in the same way. If no agreement was found, the statement in question was excluded. All the experts helped to write the manuscript and approved the final version for publication.

3. Results

The results of our systematic review of the literature (39 RCTs) have been published elsewhere; they emphasized the great variety of definitions of mild-to-moderate UC applied to the inclusion of patients in RCTs [12].

3.1. Item Generation and the Survey

The previously published results of the systematic review were used to support the survey statements. Items were grouped according to the following topics: symptom-based disease activity assessments, endoscopy-based disease activity assessments, histology-based disease activity assessments, biomarker-based disease activity assessments, composite disease activity scales, societal guideline-based definitions of mild-to-moderate UC and quality of life/disability-based definitions of mild-to-moderate UC. The first survey consisted of 49 items. The virtual panel for the final survey comprised 12 voting members. Overall, 29 (59.2%) items were considered to be appropriate. Three (6.1%) items were discussed, voted on and approved after the second round of voting. The statements on which the experts agreed are summarized in Table 1. Statements that were excluded are shown in Supplementary data Table S1.

Table 1. Approved statements for definition of mild-to-moderate ulcerative colitis for inclusion in clinical trials.

Proposed Statements	Median Panel Score
Symptom measurements are important to define mild-to-moderate ulcerative colitis.	8
The symptom-based items of the UCDAI should be used to assess mild-to-moderate ulcerative colitis disease activity	7
The symptom-based items of the MCS should be used to assess mild-to-moderate ulcerative colitis disease activity.	8
Stool frequency should be used to assess mild-to-moderate ulcerative colitis disease activity.	8
MCS stool frequency score of 2 is appropriate for defining mild-to-moderate ulcerative colitis disease activity	7
Rectal bleeding should be used to assess mild-to-moderate ulcerative colitis disease activity.	8

Table 1. *Cont.*

Proposed Statements	Median Panel Score
MCS rectal bleeding score of 1 is appropriate for defining mild-to-moderate ulcerative colitis disease activity.	8
The presence of fecal urgency should be used to assess mild-to-moderate ulcerative colitis disease activity.	8
Fecal urgency should be defined according to a global rating scale	7
Endoscopic measurements are important to define mild-to-moderate ulcerative colitis.	9
The endoscopic-based items of the MCS should be used to assess mild-to-moderate ulcerative colitis disease activity.	8
The endoscopic-based items of the MMCS should be used to assess mild-to-moderate ulcerative colitis disease activity.	7
The endoscopic-based items of the UCEIS should be used to assess mild-to-moderate ulcerative colitis disease activity.	7
Mucosal appearance should be used to assess mild-to-moderate ulcerative colitis disease activity.	7
MES score of 1 for mucosal appearance based on the MCS is appropriate for defining mild-to-moderate ulcerative colitis disease activity.	8
Vascular pattern should be used to assess mild-to-moderate ulcerative colitis disease activity	7
Patchy obliteration of vascular pattern based on the UCEIS is appropriate for defining mild-to-moderate ulcerative colitis disease activity.	7
Bleeding should be used to assess mild-to-moderate ulcerative colitis disease activity.	8
Mucosal bleeding based on the UCEIS is appropriate for defining mild-to-moderate ulcerative colitis disease activity.	7
Erosions and ulcers should be used to assess mild-to-moderate ulcerative colitis disease activity.	7
The presence of erosions based on the UCEIS are appropriate for defining mild-to-moderate ulcerative colitis disease activity.	7
Biomarker measurements are important to define mild-to-moderate ulcerative colitis.	7
The fecal calprotectin level is an appropriate marker for classifying disease activity in mild-to-moderate ulcerative colitis.	8
MCS score of at least 4 including an endoscopic sub-score of at least 2 and a rectal bleeding sub-score of at least 1 should be used to define mild-to-moderate ulcerative colitis disease activity.	7
Quality of life-based measurements are important to define mild-to-moderate ulcerative colitis.	7
Disability based measurements are important to define mild-to-moderate ulcerative colitis.	7
Fatigue measurements are important to define mild-to-moderate ulcerative colitis.	7
Work productivity measurements are important to define mild-to-moderate ulcerative colitis.	7
Mild-to-moderate ulcerative colitis should be defined as disease that does not have a significant impact on daily activities.	7

UCDAI: ulcerative colitis disease activity index; MCS: Mayo clinic score; MMCS: modified Mayo clinic score; UCEIS: Ucerative Colitis Endoscopic Index of Severity; MES: Mayo endoscopic score.

3.2. Symptom Based Disease Activity Assessments

The panel decided that measurements of symptoms were important for defining mild-to-moderate UC. The Clinical Activity Index (CAI), the Disease Activity Index (DAI), the UCDAI and the MCS have been used in clinical trials. The panel considered that the UCDAI or the MCS should be used to assess mild-to-moderate UC disease activity. However, the panel did not recommend the use of these scores in clinical practice. The clinical items deemed to be appropriate for disease assessment included stool frequency and rectal bleeding, which are symptom-based items of the UCDAI and the MCS. For the MCS, a stool frequency score of 2 and a rectal bleeding score of 1 were deemed to be appropriate for defining mild-to-moderate UC disease activity. The presence of fecal urgency should be used to assess mild-to-moderate UC, on a global rating scale. The presence of UC-related fever ruled out mild-to-moderate disease activity.

3.3. Endoscopy-Based Disease Activity Assessments

Endoscopic measurements were judged to be important for defining mild-to-moderate UC. The MCS, the Modified MCS (MMCS) or the Ulcerative Colitis Endoscopic Index of Severity (UCEIS) should be used to assess mild-to-moderate UC disease activity. Endoscopic items deemed to be appropriate for disease measurement included the appearance of the mucosa, the vascular pattern, bleeding and erosion/ulcers. When evaluating UC activity endoscopically, the panel determined that a Mayo Endoscopic Sub-score (MES) of 1 is appropriate for mild-to-moderate disease. For each UCEIS item, the panel determined that the patchy obliteration of vascular patterns, mucosal bleeding and the presence of erosions were appropriate for defining mild-to-moderate UC disease activity.

3.4. Histology-Based Disease Activity Assessments

The panel did not agree on histology-based measurements, and so, these should not be included in the definition of mild-to-moderate UC. There is a lack of robust evidence concerning the putative association between the histological grade and disease activity.

3.5. Biomarker-Based Disease Activity Assessments

The panel considered that biomarker-based measurements were important for defining mild-to-moderate UC. Fecal calprotectin was considered to be an appropriate marker for classifying disease activity in mild-to-moderate UC. However, the panel could not agree on whether a minimum fecal calprotectin cut-off should be applied to inpatients with mild-to-moderate disease. Furthermore, there was uncertainty as to whether CRP levels are an appropriate marker for classifying disease activity in mild-to-moderate UC as CRP can be correlated with disease severity.

3.6. Composite Disease Activity Scales

The panel agreed that an MCS score of at least 4 (including an endoscopic sub-score of at least 2 and a rectal bleeding sub-score of at least 1) should be used to define mild-to-moderate UC disease activity. The experts emphasized that an MCS score cut-off had not been fully validated in the assessment of UC disease activity.

3.7. Quality of Life/Disability-Based Definitions of Mild-to-Moderate UC

The panel agreed that quality of life, disability, fatigue and work productivity measurements were important when defining mild-to-moderate UC; the latter should not have more than a small impact on daily activities.

4. Discussion

For RCTs in patients with UC, the lack of a commonly accepted definition of mild-to-moderate disease activity means that the data are heterogeneous and poorly replicable. This can have a negative impact in clinical practice via the undertreatment or overtreatment of patients. Our international panel of experts suggested a consensus list of items that should be included in the definition of mild-to-moderate disease activity in adult patients screened for inclusion in UC clinical trials (Table 2).

Using a modified RAND/UCLA method, a consensus was reached for 29 statements. The expert panel members came from different countries/continents and diverse practice settings. However, not all countries with expertise in the field of IBD were represented in this panel of experts. The consensus statements were considered for use in future RCTs in patients with UC.

Table 2. Proposal for a definition of mild to moderate ulcerative colitis for clinical trials.

Mayo Clinic score of at least 4 including:
▪ Endoscopic sub-score of at least 2
▪ Rectal bleeding sub-score of at least 1
▪ No significant impact on the patient's daily activities

The panel members emphasized the need to combine clinic and endoscopic evaluations when seeking to define mild-to-moderate UC. They agreed that fecal urgency, stool frequency and rectal bleeding are appropriate in the assessment of mild-to-moderate UC disease activity. Fecal urgency is one of the common and most disabling symptoms that patients with UC experience [14–17]. Although fecal urgency is a key symptom for defining severity of disease activity in clinical practice and has a particularly distressing impact on patients, it is not included in the tools currently used to define IBD severity [18]. The Urgency Numeric Rating Scale (NRS), a validated score to evaluate severity of fecal urgency in adult patients with UC, could be used for a more appropriate and extensive evaluation and categorization of disease activity [19].

The panel members agreed that it is appropriate to use the endoscopic-based items of the UCEIS and the MCS to assess mild-to-moderate UC disease activity: vascular pattern, bleeding, erosions and ulcers. Several composite disease activity scales were considered by the panel. An MCS score of at least 4 (including an endoscopic sub-score of at least 2 and a rectal bleeding sub-score of at least 1) was voted as being appropriate; this decision is consistent with the results of a recent study [10]. Sedano et al. defined mild-to-moderate active UC on the basis of a MCS of 4 to 9 and an MES ≥ 2 combined with a Rectal Bleeding Sub-score (RBS) ≥ 1, and a Stool Frequency Sub-score ≥ 1 or MES ≥ 1 and a Geboes score > 2.0 or Robarts Histopathology Index (RHI) ≥ 10 and/or fecal calprotectin > 250 µg/g [10]. In our consensus, there was no agreement on the use of histological measurements to define mild-to-moderate UC. The panel members determined that fecal calprotectin is an appropriate marker for classifying disease activity in mild-to-moderate UC. However, an optimal fecal calprotectin cut-off has not yet been determined [20]. Calprotectin levels are not correlated with disease activity and can be affected by disease extension and blood in the stool samples. Significant intraindividual variations are seen.

In line with the guidelines issued by regulatory authorities, the panel considered that it was inappropriate to use the subjective PGA sub-score to assess disease activity [11]. The PGA sub-score is not derived directly from the patient and cannot adequately determine whether or not major symptoms are relieved [11].

UC can have a major impact on a patient's life [21]. The panel agreed that mild-to-moderate UC should be defined as disease that does not have more than a small impact on the patient's daily activities.

The present study provided a consensus definition of mild-to-moderate disease activity in UC. The definition could be used as an inclusion criterion in RCTs in the field of UC. With the ultimate goal of improving patient care and quality of life, there is a constant need for therapeutic trials in patients with mild-to-moderate UC. The results of our initiative will lead to higher-quality clinical studies in mild-to-moderate UC and will facilitate comparison of the latter's results.

Supplementary Materials: The following supporting information can be downloaded at: https://www.mdpi.com/article/10.3390/medicina59010183/s1, Supplementary Table S1: Statements excluded.

Author Contributions: L.P.-B., S.D. and V.J. conceived the study. B.C. wrote the article and created tables. B.C., V.J., F.D., S.A.A., A.D., A.L.H., T.K., P.G.K., F.M., B.S., K.P., S.D. and L.P.-B. critically reviewed the content of the paper. All authors discussed the statements and approved the final manuscript. All authors have read and agreed to the published version of the manuscript.

Funding: This research was funded by Ferring Pharmaceuticals.

Institutional Review Board Statement: Not applicable.

Informed Consent Statement: Not applicable.

Data Availability Statement: The data underlying this article are available in the article and in its online Supplementary Materials.

Conflicts of Interest: B.C. reports lecture and/or consulting fees from Abbvie, Amgen, Celltrion, Ferring, Galapagos, Janssen, Takeda. V.J. reports consulting/advisory board fees from AbbVie, Alimentiv Inc (formerly Robarts Clinical Trials), Arena pharmaceuticals, Asahi Kasei Pharma, Asieris, Bristol Myers Squibb, Celltrion, Eli Lilly, Ferring, Flagship Pioneering, Fresenius Kabi, Galapagos, GlaxoSmithKline, Genentech, Gilead, Janssen, Merck, Mylan, Pandion, Pendopharm, Pfizer, Protagonist, Reistone Biopharma, Roche, Sandoz, Second Genome, Takeda, Teva, Topivert, Vividion; speaker's fees from, Abbvie, Ferring, Galapagos, Janssen Pfizer Shire, Takeda, Fresenius Kabi. F D'Amico has served as a speaker for Janssen, Galapagos, Sandoz, and Omega Pharma. S Al Awadhi reports no conflict of interest. A Dignass received fees for participation in clinical trials and review activities (ie, data monitoring boards, statistical analysis, and end point committees) from AbbVie, Celgene/Bristol Myers Squibb, Falk Foundation, Gilead, Janssen, and Pfizer; received consultancy fees from AbbVie, Amgen, Biogen, Boehringer Ingelheim, Celgene/Bristol Myers Squibb, Eli Lilly, Falk, Ferring, Fresenius Kabi, Galapagos, Gilead, Janssen, MSD, Pfizer, Pharmacosmos, Roche/Genentech, Sandoz/Hexal, Takeda, Tillotts, and Vifor; and received payment for lectures, including service on speaker bureaus, from AbbVie, Eli Lilly, Falk Foundation, Ferring, Gilead/Galapagos, Janssen, MSD, Pfizer, Takeda, Tillotts, and Vifor; received payment for development of educational presentations from Ferring and Tillotts. A L Hart has served as a speaker, consultant, and advisory board member for AbbVie, AstraZeneca, BMS, Celltrion, Ferring, Galapagos, Genentech, Janssen, Johnson and Johnson, Takeda, MSD, Pfizer, Roche, Pharmacosmos. T Kobayashi has served as a speaker, a consultant or an advisory board member for AbbVie, Activaid, Astellas, Alfresa Pharma, Bristol Myers Squibb, Celltrion, Covidien, EA Pharma, Eli Lilly, Ferring Pharmaceuticals, Gilead Sciences, Janssen, JIMRO, JMDC, Kissei, Kyorin Pharmaceutical, Mitsubishi Tanabe Pharma, Mochida Pharmaceutical, Nippon Kayaku, Pfizer, Takeda Pharmaceutical, Thermo Scientific and Zeria Pharmaceutical, and has received research funding from AbbVie, Alfresa Pharma, EA Pharma, Kyorin Pharmaceutical, Mochida Pharmaceutical, Nippon Kayaku, Otsuka Holdings, Sekisui Medical, Thermo Fisher Scientific and Zeria Pharmaceutical. P G Kotze has served as a speaker and consultant for Abbvie, Janssen, Pfizer and Takeda. He also received scientific grants from Pfizer and Takeda. F Magro severd as speaker for: Abbvie, Arena, Biogen, Bristol-Myers Squibb, Falk, Ferring, Hospira, Janssen, Laboratórios Vitoria, Pfizer, Lilly, Merck Sharp & Dohme, Sandoz, Takeda, UCB, Vifor. B Siegmund has served as consultant for Abbvie, Arena, BMS, Boehringer, Celgene, Falk, Galapagos, Janssen, Lilly, Pfizer, PredictImmune and Takeda and received speaker's fees from Abbvie, BMS, CED Service GmbH, Falk, Ferring, Janssen, Novartis, Pfizer, Takeda, grants from Pfizer [served as representative of the Charité]. K Paridaens is an employee of Ferring Pharmaceuticals. S Danese has served as a speaker, consultant, and advisory board member for Schering-Plough, AbbVie, Actelion, Alphawasserman, AstraZeneca, Cellerix, Cosmo Pharmaceuticals, Ferring, Genentech, Grunenthal, Johnson and Johnson, Millenium Takeda, MSD, Nikkiso Europe GmbH, Novo Nordisk, Nycomed, Pfizer, Pharmacosmos, UCB Pharma and Vifor. L Peyrin-Biroulet reports personal fees from Galapagos, AbbVie, Janssen, Genentech, Ferring, Tillots, Celltrion, Takeda, Pfizer, Index Pharmaceuticals, Sandoz, Celgene, Biogen, Samsung Bioepis, Inotrem, Allergan, MSD, Roche, Arena, Gilead, Amgen, BMS, Vifor, Norgine, Mylan, Lilly, Fresenius Kabi, OSE Immunotherapeutics, Enthera, Theravance, Pandion Therapeutics, Gossamer Bio, Viatris, Thermo Fisher; grants from Abbvie, MSD, Takeda, Fresenius Kabi; stock options: CTMA.

References

1. Ko, C.W.; Singh, S.; Feuerstein, J.D.; Falck-Ytter, C.; Falck-Ytter, Y.; Cross, R.K.; Crockett, S.; Flamm, S.; Inadomi, J.; Muniraj, T.; et al. AGA Clinical Practice Guidelines on the Management of Mild-to-Moderate Ulcerative Colitis. *Gastroenterology* **2019**, *156*, 748–764. [CrossRef] [PubMed]
2. Walsh, A.J.; Bryant, R.V.; Travis, S.P.L. Current best practice for disease activity assessment in IBD. *Nat. Rev. Gastroenterol. Hepatol.* **2016**, *13*, 567–579. [CrossRef] [PubMed]
3. Walmsley, R.S.; Ayres, R.C.; Pounder, R.E.; Allan, R.N. A simple clinical colitis activity index. *Gut* **1998**, *43*, 29–32. [CrossRef] [PubMed]
4. Schroeder, K.W.; Tremaine, W.J.; Ilstrup, D.M. Coated oral 5-aminosalicylic acid therapy for mildly to moderately active ulcerative colitis. A randomized study. *New Engl. J. Med.* **1987**, *317*, 1625–1629. [CrossRef] [PubMed]

5. Sandborn, W.J.; Sands, B.E.; Wolf, D.C.; Valentine, J.F.; Safdi, M.; Katz, S.; Isaacs, K.L.; Wruble, L.D.; Katz, J.; Present, D.H.; et al. Repifermin (keratinocyte growth factor-2) for the treatment of active ulcerative colitis: A randomized, double-blind, placebo-controlled, dose-escalation trial. *Aliment. Pharmacol. Ther.* **2003**, *17*, 1355–1364. [CrossRef] [PubMed]
6. Truelove, S.C.; Witts, L.J. Cortisone in ulcerative colitis; final report on a therapeutic trial. *Br. Med. J.* **1955**, *2*, 1041–1048. [CrossRef] [PubMed]
7. D'Haens, G.; Sandborn, W.J.; Feagan, B.G.; Geboes, K.; Hanauer, S.B.; Irvine, E.J.; Lémann, M.; Marteau, P.; Rutgeerts, P.; Schölmerich, J.; et al. A Review of Activity Indices and Efficacy End Points for Clinical Trials of Medical Therapy in Adults with Ulcerative Colitis. *Gastroenterology* **2007**, *132*, 763–786. [CrossRef] [PubMed]
8. Raine, T.; Bonovas, S.; Burisch, J.; Kucharzik, T.; Adamina, M.; Annese, V.; Bachmann, O.; Bettenworth, D.; Chaparro, M.; Czuber-Dochan, W.; et al. ECCO Guidelines on Therapeutics in Ulcerative Colitis: Medical Treatment. *J. Crohns Colitis* **2022**, *16*, 2–17. [CrossRef] [PubMed]
9. Lamb, C.A.; Kennedy, N.A.; Raine, T.; Hendy, P.A.; Smith, P.J.; Limdi, J.K.; Hayee, B.; Lomer, M.C.E.; Parkes, G.C.; Selinger, C.; et al. British Society of Gastroenterology consensus guidelines on the management of inflammatory bowel disease in adults. *Gut* **2019**, *68*, s1–s106. [CrossRef] [PubMed]
10. Sedano, R.; Jairath, V.; Ma, C.; Hanzel, J.; Shackelton, L.M.; McFarlane, S.; D'Haens, G.R.; Sandborn, W.J.; Feagan, B.G. Design of Clinical Trials for Mild to Moderate Ulcerative Colitis. *Gastroenterology* **2022**, *162*, 1005–1018. [CrossRef] [PubMed]
11. Ulcerative Colitis: Clinical Trial Endpoints Guidance for Industry. U.S. Food and Drug Administration. 2020. Available online: https://www.fda.gov/regulatory-information/search-fda-guidance-documents/ulcerative-colitis-clinical-trial-endpoints-guidance-industry (accessed on 1 September 2022).
12. Caron, B.; Jairath, V.; D'Amico, F.; Paridaens, K.; Magro, F.; Danese, S.; Peyrin-Biroulet, L. Definition of mild to moderate ulcerative colitis in clinical trials: A systematic literature review. *United Eur. Gastroenterol. J.* **2022**, *10*, 854–867. [CrossRef] [PubMed]
13. Fitch, K.; Bernstein, S.J.; Aguilar, M.D.; Burnand, B.; LaCalleet, J.R.; Lazaro, P.; van het Loo, M.; McDonnell, J.; Vader, J.; Kahan, J.P. The RAND/UCLA Appropriateness Method User's Manual. 2021. Available online: https://www.rand.org/pubs/monograph_reports/MR1269.html (accessed on 1 September 2022).
14. Petryszyn, P.W.; Paradowski, L. Stool patterns and symptoms of disordered anorectal function in patients with inflammatory bowel diseases. *Adv. Clin. Exp. Med.* **2018**, *27*, 813–818. [CrossRef] [PubMed]
15. Newton, L.; Randall, J.A.; Hunter, T.; Keith, S.; Symonds, T.; Secrest, R.J.; Komocsar, W.J.; Curtis, S.E.; Abetz-Webb, L.; Kappelman, M.; et al. A qualitative study exploring the health-related quality of life and symptomatic experiences of adults and adolescents with ulcerative colitis. *J. Patient Rep. Outcomes* **2019**, *3*, 66. [CrossRef] [PubMed]
16. Dulai, P.S.; Jairath, V.; Khanna, R.; Ma, C.; McCarrier, K.P.; Martin, M.L.; Parker, C.E.; Morris, J.; Feagan, B.G.; Sandborn, W.J. Development of the symptoms and impacts questionnaire for Crohn's disease and ulcerative colitis. *Aliment. Pharmacol. Ther.* **2020**, *51*, 1047–1066. [CrossRef] [PubMed]
17. Snisky, J.A.; Barnes, E.L.; Zhang, X.; Long, M.D. Urgency and its association with quality of life and clinical outcomes in ulcerative colitis patients. *Am. J. Gastroenterol.* **2022**, *117*, 769–776. [CrossRef] [PubMed]
18. Joyce, J.C.; Waljee, A.K.; Khan, T.; A Wren, P.; Dave, M.; Zimmermann, E.M.; Wang, S.; Zhu, J.; Higgins, P. Identification of symptom domains in ulcerative colitis that occur frequently during flares and are responsive to changes in disease activity. *Health Qual Life Outcomes* **2008**, *6*, 69. [CrossRef] [PubMed]
19. Dubinsky, M.C.; Irving, P.M.; Panaccione, R.; Naegeli, A.N.; Potts-Bleakman, A.; Arora, V.; Shan, M.; Travis, S. Incorporating patient experience into drug development for ulcerative colitis: Development of the Urgency Numeric Rating Scale, a patient-reported outcome measure to assess bowel urgency in adults. *J. Patient-Reported Outcomes* **2022**, *6*, 31. [CrossRef] [PubMed]
20. D'Amico, F.; Bonovas, S.; Danese, S.; Peyrin-Biroulet, L. Review article: Faecal calprotectin and histologic remission in ulcerative colitis. *Aliment. Pharmacol. Ther.* **2020**, *51*, 689–698. [CrossRef] [PubMed]
21. Le Berre, C.; Ananthakrishnan, A.N.; Danese, S.; Singh, S.; Peyrin-Biroulet, L. Ulcerative Colitis and Crohn's Disease Have Similar Burden and Goals for Treatment. *Clin. Gastroenterol. Hepatol.* **2020**, *18*, 14–23. [CrossRef] [PubMed]

Disclaimer/Publisher's Note: The statements, opinions and data contained in all publications are solely those of the individual author(s) and contributor(s) and not of MDPI and/or the editor(s). MDPI and/or the editor(s) disclaim responsibility for any injury to people or property resulting from any ideas, methods, instructions or products referred to in the content.

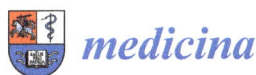

Case Report

Complex Refractory Esophageal Stricture Due to Chronic Gasoline Ingestion: A Case Report

Henry Sutanto [1,2] and Amie Vidyani [1,2,3,*]

[1] Department of Internal Medicine, Faculty of Medicine, Universitas Airlangga, Surabaya 60132, Indonesia; henry1988md@gmail.com
[2] Department of Internal Medicine, Dr. Soetomo General Academic Hospital, Surabaya 60286, Indonesia
[3] Division of Gastroenterology and Hepatology, Department of Internal Medicine, Faculty of Medicine, Universitas Airlangga, Surabaya 60132, Indonesia
* Correspondence: amie.vidyani@fk.unair.ac.id

Abstract: Esophageal stricture is a narrowing of the esophageal lumen which is often characterized by impaired swallowing or dysphagia. It can be induced by inflammation, fibrosis or neoplasia which damages the mucosa and/or submucosa of the esophagus. Corrosive substance ingestion is one of the major causes of esophageal stricture, particularly in children and young adults. For instance, accidental ingestion or attempted suicide with corrosive household products is not uncommon. Gasoline is a liquid mixture of aliphatic hydrocarbons derived from the fractional distillation of petroleum, which is then combined with additives such as isooctane and aromatic hydrocarbons (e.g., toluene and benzene). Gasoline also contains several other additives including ethanol, methanol and formaldehyde, which make it a corrosive agent. Interestingly, to the best of our knowledge, the incidence of esophageal stricture caused by chronic gasoline ingestion has not been reported. In this paper, we report the case of a patient with dysphagia due to complex esophageal stricture due to chronic gasoline ingestion who underwent a series of esophago-gastro-duodenoscopy (EGD) procedures and repeated esophageal dilation.

Keywords: esophageal stricture; gasoline ingestion; corrosive; gastroenterology; dilation of esophagus; upper gastrointestinal endoscopy; Savary-Gilliard bougie; controlled radial expansion balloon

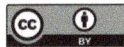

1. Introduction

Esophageal stricture is a narrowing of the esophageal lumen which is often characterized by impaired swallowing or dysphagia [1,2]. It can be caused by inflammation, fibrosis or neoplasia which causes damage to the mucosa and/or submucosa of the esophagus. The incidence of esophageal stricture has not been widely reported in previous studies. One study reported an incidence of esophageal stricture of 1.1 per 10,000 person-years, which increased with age [1,3]. Peptic stricture is the most common type of esophageal stricture (accounting for 70–80% of cases of esophageal stricture in adults) and is commonly caused by gastroesophageal reflux disease (GERD). Ingestion of corrosive substances is also a major cause of esophageal stricture, especially in children and young adults. Accidental ingestion or attempted suicide by ingestion of corrosive household products is not uncommon. According to data from the American Association of Poison Control Centers (AAPCC), exposure to corrosive substances is one of the five most common causes of poisoning in adults and children under the age of five [4], and the resulting damage can range from mild injury to extensive esophageal necrosis [5]. In addition to these two main causes, esophageal stricture can also be induced by eosinophilic esophagitis, drug-induced esophagitis (e.g., due to non-steroidal anti-inflammatory drugs/NSAIDs, potassium chloride [KCl] tablets and tetracycline antibiotics), radiation injuries, iatrogenic strictures, anastomotic strictures, chemotherapy, temperature injuries and even infections.

In addition, esophageal strictures can also be due to malignancy in the esophagus, such as esophageal adenocarcinoma, squamous cell carcinoma or lung malignancy metastases [1].

Corrosive substances are defined as materials that can attack and destroy living tissue, organic compounds and metals through chemical reactions. The more acidic or alkaline a substance is, the more effective it is as a corrosive agent. Some examples of corrosive substances are hydrochloric acid (HCl), sulfuric acid (H_2SO_4), nitric acid, chromic acid, acetic acid, ammonium hydroxide (NH_4OH), potassium hydroxide (KOH), sodium hydroxide (NaOH) and sodium hypochlorite (NaClO). Gasoline is a liquid mixture of aliphatic hydrocarbons derived from fractional distillation of petroleum, which is combined with additives such as isooctane and aromatic hydrocarbons (e.g., toluene and benzene). Gasoline also contains several other additives including ethanol, methanol, formaldehyde, xylene, 1,3-butadiene, methyl tert-butyl ether (MTBE), and hexane [6]. As previously reported, acute ingestion of toluene can cause irritation, corrosion and injury to the gastrointestinal tract, which manifests as abdominal pain, nausea, vomiting and vomiting of blood [7]. In addition, the ethanol content in gasoline may increase the ability of gasoline to absorb water and will make gasoline corrosive [8]. Interestingly, the incidence of esophageal stricture caused by chronic gasoline ingestion has not been reported. In this paper, we report the case of a patient with dysphagia due to complex esophageal stricture due to chronic gasoline ingestion who underwent a series of esophago-gastro-duodenoscopy (EGD) procedures and repeated esophageal dilation.

2. The Case Description

A 50-year-old woman came to the emergency room (ER) at the Dr. Soetomo General Academic Hospital in Surabaya, Indonesia with a chief complaint of vomiting every time she ate and drank. Vomiting was experienced by the patient a few seconds after eating or drinking without being preceded by nausea. The vomit contained food or drink consumed seconds before. This complaint was experienced by the patient 3 weeks before coming to the ER. The patient also had difficulty swallowing which had gotten worse 5 months before the ER visit. When she was in the emergency room, the patient complained of not being able to consume any liquids, including water. The patient admitted that she had lost more than 20 kg in the last 5 months. The patient defecated approximately once every 2–3 days. The patient's urination was normal. Any history of fever, cough, runny nose, pain when swallowing, tightness and the appearance of a lump in the body, especially in the neck, was denied. History of a burning sensation in the chest that rose to the throat and gastric acid reflux, especially when lying down or sleeping at night, was denied. There was a history of hypertension, and the patient claimed not to have diabetes mellitus, heart disease or other chronic diseases.

The patient had previously been examined at Sidoarjo General Hospital 1 month before coming to the ER and had undergone an upper gastrointestinal endoscopy or EGD. The findings showed that in the lower third of the esophagus, the mucosa was bizarre and appeared ulcerated, the lumen was narrow with a hard consistency that bled easily, and the scope could not pass through the lumen (Figure 1). The EGD results concluded that the patient had a tumor in the lower third of the esophagus leading to malignancy. A tissue biopsy was performed during the EGD and the results of histopathological examination of the esophageal tissue revealed tissue without a lining epithelium with dense inflammatory cells that were predominately neutrophils, histiocytes, plasma cells and a number of eosinophils, with many small blood vessels lined with reactive endothelium. In addition, small foci of squamous epithelial fragments with similar inflammatory cell infiltration were seen. However, no malignancy was found in the histopathological examination of the tissue preparations, and the conclusion was chronic suppurative inflammation. On this basis, the patient was then referred to the Dr. Soetomo General Academic Hospital for esophageal dilation.

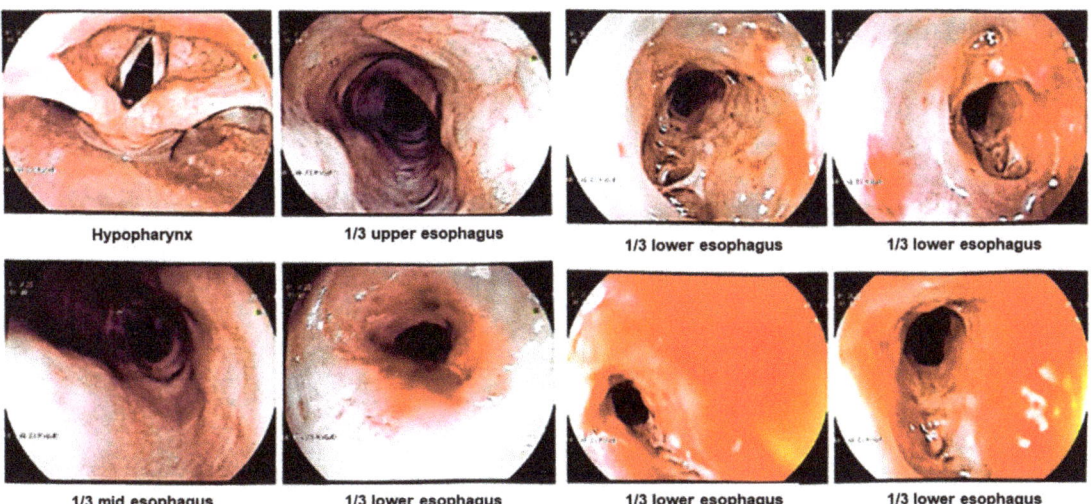

Figure 1. The narrowed and easily bled esophageal lumen was documented during the EGD at Sidoarjo General Hospital.

At the initial physical examination, the patient was found to be moderately ill with *compos mentis* alertness. Her blood pressure was 119/84 mmHg, her pulse rate was 75 beats per minute and her respiratory rate was 18 beats per minute and she had a body temperature of 36.5 °C. The patient's weight was 50 kg and her height was 160 cm. Her body mass index (BMI) was 19.5 kg/m^2 and the patient gave the impression of adequate nutrition. On head examination, the conjunctiva was not anemic, the sclera was not icteric, and the pupil was isochorous. Normal tonsils were observed and no sore throat was evident. In the neck area, no dilated veins were found; the trachea was centrally located, no increase in jugular venous pressure was found. The chest appeared symmetrical, in a static and dynamic state, with normal left and right lung fremitus, no crackles or wheezing was heard. On cardiac examination, the *ictus cordis* was not visible or palpable; on percussion, the left border of the heart was at the fourth intercostal space 1 cm lateral to the left mid-clavicular line and the right border of the heart was at the fourth intercostal space of the right sternal line. The first and second heart sounds were within the normal limits, and no murmurs or galops were heard. On abdominal examination, inspection found a flat abdomen; on auscultation, bowel sounds were within the normal limits; on palpation, there was epigastric tenderness, there was no enlargement of the liver or spleen, no lump was palpable, and there was no kidney ballottement. On percussion, there was a tympanic sound throughout the abdominal field. Extremities were warm and no limb edema was observed.

Laboratory examinations in the ER revealed a hemoglobin concentration (Hb) of 11.7 g/dL, hematocrit (HCT) concentration of 35.1%, mean corpuscular volume (MCV) of 83 fL, mean corpuscular hemoglobin (MCH) of 27.7 pg, mean corpuscular hemoglobin concentration (MCHC) of 33.3 g/dL, leukocyte count of 5670/μL with neutrophils 42.1% and lymphocytes 47.4%, and platelet count of 257,000/μL. The random blood glucose (RBG) was 82 mg/dL, blood urea nitrogen (BUN) was 4.0 mg/dL, serum creatinine was 0.6 mg/dL, serum glutamic oxaloacetic transaminase (SGOT) was 57 U/L, serum glutamic pyruvic transaminase (SGPT) was 37 U/L, serum albumin was 2.88 g/dL, direct bilirubin was 0.25 mg/dL, sodium was 150 mmol/L, potassium was 2.3 mmol/L and chloride was 116 mmol/L. Examination of the hemostasis panel showed an activated partial thromboplastin time (APTT) of 24.5 s and a partial thromboplastin time (PPT) of 15.7 s. Arterial blood gas analysis with free air showed pH 7.44, pCO$_2$ 43, pO$_2$ 104, HCO$_3$ 29.2 with a base excess (BE) of 5.0 and oxygen saturation (SO$_2$) of 98%. Additionally, HbsAg, antihepatitis C virus (HCV), and anti-human immunodeficiency virus (HIV) rapid test results were non-reactive. A chest X-ray (CXR) performed in the ER showed traces of pulmonary inflammation without abnormalities in the heart and no visualized metastatic processes in the lungs and bones.

Based on the medical history, physical examination and supporting examinations mentioned above, the patient was diagnosed with dysphagia due to a suspected esophageal tumor with hypokalemia and hypoalbuminemia. The patient was scheduled to be hospitalized and to receive an intravenous fluid drip (IVFD) containing Triofusin500®:WidaKN2®:Kalbamin® 1:1:1 with a total of 1500 mL administered every 24 h. She was also scheduled to receive an intravenous injection of 30 mg of lansoprazole every 12 h, an injection of 10 mg of metoclopramide every 8 h and 15 mL of KCl syrup every 8 h. To meet the nutritional needs of the patient, a 150 mL milk diet was also administered every 4 h (containing a total energy of 1200 kcal/day). The patient was then scheduled to have another EGD for further evaluation and confirmation of previous EGD results from Sidoarjo General Hospital, as well as a re-reading of tissue preparations in the form of paraffin blocks from Sidoarjo General Hospital.

3. The Disease Course and Treatment Progression

3.1. Treatment Day-2

The patient continued to complain of swallowing difficulty and vomiting whenever she tried to drink milk. Because there was no food or drink that could be administered orally and parenteral nutrition through peripheral veins was inadequate to support the patient's nutritional needs, it was decided to install a central venous catheter (CVC). The CVC on the right clavicle was inserted in the ER and from then on, the patient was completely fasted and received total parenteral nutrition (TPN) in the form of Clinimix®:Aminofluid® 1:1 in a total amount of 1500 mL every 24 h via the first port and KCl premix 50 meq in 500 mL of 0.9% NaCl every 24 h via the second port. Other intravenous drugs were continued, but the KCl syrup was discontinued due to the patient's dysphagia.

3.2. Treatment Day-4

On the fourth day of treatment, the patient underwent a cardiac examination and evaluation of the cardiac risk index (CRI) to prepare for the EGD. The electrocardiographic (ECG) examination revealed a sinus rhythm of 79 beats/minute with normal frontal and horizontal axes, as well as a T-wave inversion in V1–V4. The cardiology peer assessment concluded that the heart condition was stable with good functional capacity. The patient was then classified into CRI class I with a 3.9% risk of death, myocardial infarction or cardiac arrest within 30 days. However, the T-wave inversion that appeared on the ECG could have been due to hypokalemia. On this basis, hypokalemia correctional therapy was escalated from KCl premix 50 meq in 500 mL 0.9% NaCl every 24 h to KCl premix 50 meq in 500 mL 0.9% NaCl every 8 h via CVC.

3.3. Treatment Day-5

The evaluation of serum electrolytes showed improvement with serum sodium 138 mmol/L, potassium 4.7 mmol/L and chloride 113 mmol/L, and the serum albumin was 2.64 g/dL. To improve the patient's hypoalbuminemia, the TPN in the first port of the CVC was modified to Clinimix®:Aminofluid®:Kalbamin® 1:1:1 per 24 h and because the hypokalemia had been corrected, the administration of KCl premix was terminated on the fifth day of treatment.

3.4. Treatment Day-9

The patient underwent an EGD procedure on the ninth day of treatment. The results (Figure 2) showed that a 12 mm endoscope could enter the esophagus through the oral cavity and reach as far as 25 cm before resistance was felt. Then, the endoscope was replaced with a smaller (6 mm) scope which was able to enter the esophagus as far as the narrowing site. A narrowing of the esophageal lumen with the thickening of the mucosa was seen, and this matched the appearance of a corrosive stricture. Subsequently, the narrowing was dilated using a 9 mm Savary bougie slowly for one minute, and minimal bleeding was seen in the stricture location. Thereafter, a 6 mm scope could enter the gastric cavity. Minimal bleeding was observed. Because the endoscopic appearance matched that of a corrosive stricture, the patient was confronted by the operator and admitted that she had worked as a retail gasoline seller and often inhaled and swallowed gasoline little by little when selling. On this basis, the patient was diagnosed with esophageal stricture due to ingestion of a corrosive substance (gasoline) and was advised to undergo a second esophageal dilation a week later.

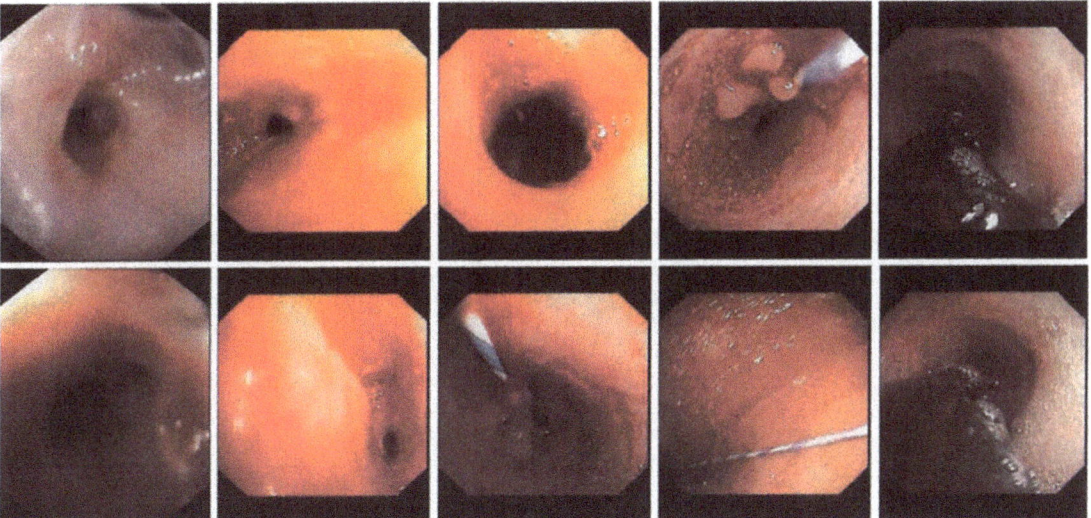

Figure 2. The first round of EGD performed at the Dr. Soetomo General Academic hospital showing a narrowing of esophageal lumen, which is consistent with the appearance of a corrosive stricture.

3.5. Treatment Day-10

After the first esophageal dilation on the ninth day of treatment, the patient felt that the barrier to swallowing in her throat was greatly reduced. The patient claimed to be able to drink water and milk without vomiting. From the physical examination, the general condition of the patient seemed adequate, with compos mentis alertness and a GCS of E4V5M6. The examination of vital signs showed a blood pressure of 114/77 mmHg, pulse rate of 85 times/min, respiratory rate of 18 times/min, body temperature of 36.5 °C and a 99% oxygen saturation with room air. A CBC on the tenth day of treatment showed Hb 9.8 g/dL, HCT 29.9%, MCV 83.1 fL, MCH 27.2 pg, MCHC 32.8 g/dL, leukocyte count 4130/μL with 55.0% neutrophils and 30.0% lymphocytes, and a platelet count of 189,000/μL. The clinical chemistry examination obtained BUN 15.9 mg/dL, serum creatinine 0.5 mg/dL, uric acid 1.8 mg/dL, SGOT 16.1 U/L, SGPT 10 U/L, serum albumin 3.19 g/dL, total bilirubin 0.40 mg/dL, direct bilirubin 0.20 mg/dL, sodium 129 mmol/L, potassium 3.6 mmol/L and chloride 104 mmol/L. The results of the patient's hemostasis panel examination were as follows: APTT 25.7 s and PPT 13.9 s. Arterial blood gas analysis with free air showed pH 7.32, pCO_2 44, pO_2 99, HCO_3 22.7 with BE −3.4 and SO_2 97%.

The re-assessment of histopathological preparations (i.e., paraffin block) from Sidoarjo General Hospital showed pieces of tissue without lining epithelium. In the stroma, a dense layer of inflammatory cells, lymphocytes, histiocytes, plasma cells, neutrophils and eosinophils were seen. Among them, there was a proliferation of blood vessels lined with a layer of endothelium. Taken together, this picture suggested chronic inflammation.

3.6. Treatment Day-11

The results of thoracolumbar axial reformatted coronal and sagittal slices on multislice computed tomography (MSCT), with and without contrast, showed diffuse, symmetrical thickening of the esophageal lumen by about +/−4.5 cm at the height of thoracic vertebrae bodies (VTh) 7 to 9, which narrowed the esophageal lumen and caused dilation of its proximal esophageal lumen. A cyst (14 HU) with dimensions of +/−1.4 × 1.6 cm in the left adrenal gland was seen. The liver was observed to be of normal size and density, with no intrahepatic bile duct (IHBD)/extrahepatic bile duct (EHBD) dilation. The portal vein/hepatica appeared normal, and no masses/nodules were seen. The GB was of normal size and density, and no masses/stones/cysts were seen. The pancreas was of normal size and parenchyma density, and no masses/cysts were seen. The spleen was of normal size and parenchyma density, and no masses/cysts were seen. The right and left kidneys were of normal size and normal parenchymal density with no ectasia of the pelvicalyceal system. Cysts (20 HU) with dimensions of +/−0.7 × 1.1 cm were seen in the lower pole of the right kidney and +/−0.9 × 0.8 cm in the lower pole of the left kidney. No extraluminal free fluid density was seen in the right and left abdominal cavity or pleural cavity. There was a lymph node in the right upper paratracheal region with a size of +/−0.8 cm. No visible osteolytic/osteoblastic process was observed. Double curve scoliosis was seen, with convexity of the thoracic vertebrae to the right and lumbar to the left. Osteophytes of the thoracic and lumbar vertebral bodies were visible. The patient appeared to have had a CVC attached with a distal tip in the right atrium. There was an appearance of fibrosis accompanied by dilation of the cylindrical type of bronchus in the apical segment of the superior lobe of the right lung. Based on these findings, it was concluded that there was diffuse, symmetrical thickening of the esophageal lumen by +/−4.5 cm as high in the body as VTh 7 to 9 which narrowed the esophageal lumen and caused dilation proximally (Figure 3). These findings indicated esophageal stricture, a left adrenal cyst, a bilateral kidney cyst, former lung inflammation, bronchiectasis, dextroscoliosis thoracalis and levoscoliosis thoracalis, as well as thoracolumbar spondylosis.

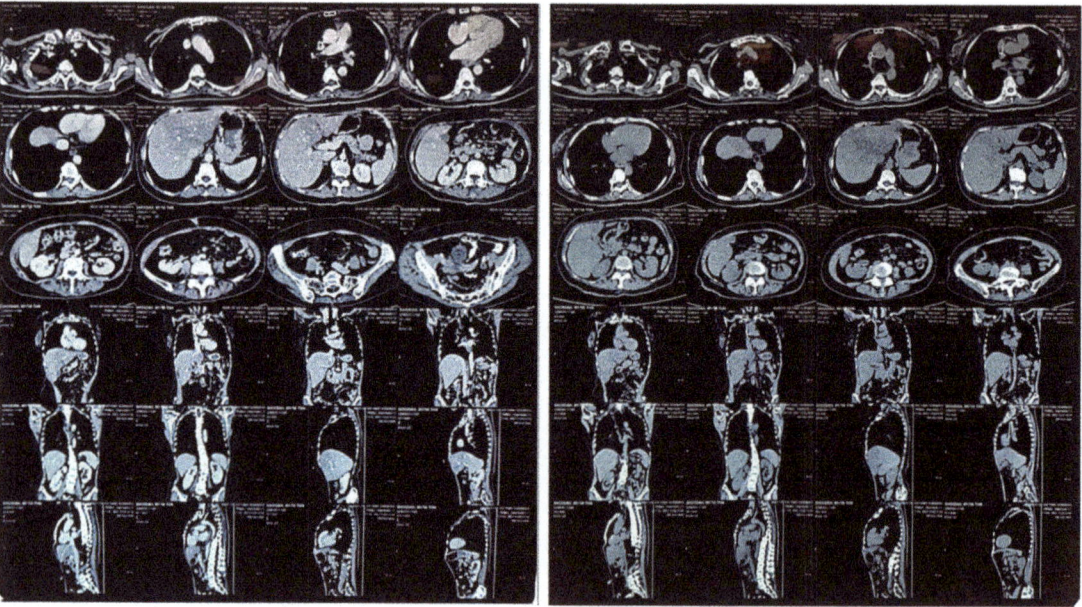

Figure 3. The thoracolumbar MSCT also revealed narrowing of esophageal lumen by about +/−4.5 cm.

3.7. Treatment Day-14

The patient underwent a second EGD and esophageal dilation. The patient had no complaints and was able to drink water and milk without vomiting. From the physical examination, the general condition of the patient seemed adequate. The results of the examination of vital signs showed a blood pressure of 125/73 mmHg, pulse rate of 104 times/min, respiratory rate of 18 times/min, body temperature of 36.5 °C and a 99% oxygen saturation with room air.

Laboratory test results on the 12th day of treatment (2 days before the procedure) showed Hb 9.4 g/dL, HCT 28.4%, MCV 85.8 fL, MCH 28.4 pg, MCHC 33.1 g/dL, leukocyte count 3680/μL with 42.4% neutrophils and 39.7% lymphocytes, and platelet count 197,000/μL, and the clinical chemistry examination obtained BUN 15.3 mg/dL, serum creatinine 0.5 mg/dL, SGOT 20.8 U/L, SGPT 14 U/L, serum albumin 3.17 g/dL, sodium 130 mmol/dL. l, potassium 3.8 mmol/L and chloride 101 mmol/L.

The second EGD report (Figure 4) showed that the scope entered the oral cavity (with scope 1.2) and a narrowing was seen at the insertion of 30 cm from the incisor. Subsequently, dilation was carried out using an 11 mm Savary-Gilliard. After dilation, scope 1.2 could not enter. Scope 0.6 entered from the oral cavity, erosion and bleeding were seen in the dilated area, and a polypoid mass was seen at 35 cm insertion (near the esophagogastric junction). Then, a biopsy was performed on the mass. In the gastric mucosa, no abnormalities were seen, and no erosions/ulcers/masses were seen, whereas in the duodenum, the D1 and D2 villi were intact, and the mucosa was not visible. From the results of the EGD, it was concluded that there was a stricture of the lower third of the esophagus that had been dilated with an 11 mm Savary-Gilliard and a distal esophageal polypoid mass. The patient was scheduled for a third EGD and dilation within 2 weeks.

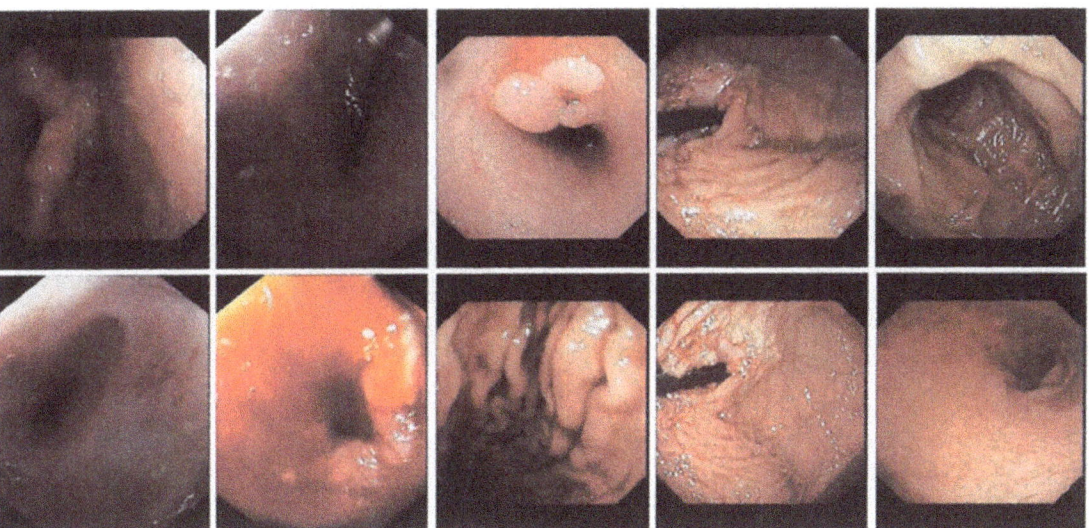

Figure 4. The second round of EGD performed at the Dr. Soetomo General Academic hospital.

3.8. The Third EGD and Dilation (2 Weeks after the Second EGD)

After the second dilation, the patient was discharged and received further treatment at the gastroenterology outpatient clinic at the Dr. Soetomo General Academic Hospital. The patient informed that she could eat soft foods (e.g., porridge) and drink without choking or vomiting. The results of the esophageal tissue biopsy taken during the second EGD showed pieces of polypoid-shaped tissue covered with squamous epithelium, which appeared to be intact. In the stroma, lymphocytes, histiocytes, plasma cells and a few eosinophils were seen. No dysplasia was seen; no intestinal metaplasia was seen. There was no specific process or signs of malignancy. Based on these findings, it can be concluded that there was non-specific chronic esophagitis.

Two weeks after the second EGD, the patient returned for the third EGD (Figure 5) and obtained the following results: the scope could go through the oral cavity up to D2. In the esophagus, there was a narrowing of the esophageal lumen starting 25–30 cm from the incisors. Dilation was carried out using 1ATM/2ATM/3ATM CRE balloons for 1 min each. Post dilation, mucosal break was visible, and no active bleeding was seen. There were two polyps in the distal esophagus. On the gastric cardia, a mass resembling granulation tissue was seen (the red dot in Figure 5), and a biopsy was performed. The fundus and body of the stomach showed no abnormalities. In the gastric antrum, an ulcer was seen with granulation tissue and cicatricial tissue, and a biopsy was performed. Normal pyloric ostium was observed. In the duodenum, the D1 and D2 villi were intact. Based on these findings, it was concluded that there was an esophageal stricture due to corrosive injury that had been dilated, as well as esophageal polyps, masses (granulation impressions) on the cardia and ulcers on the gastric antrum. Proton pump inhibitors and mucoprotectors were advised, as well as a high-protein coarse porridge diet and the patient was scheduled for another round of esophageal dilation within 2 weeks after the third EGD.

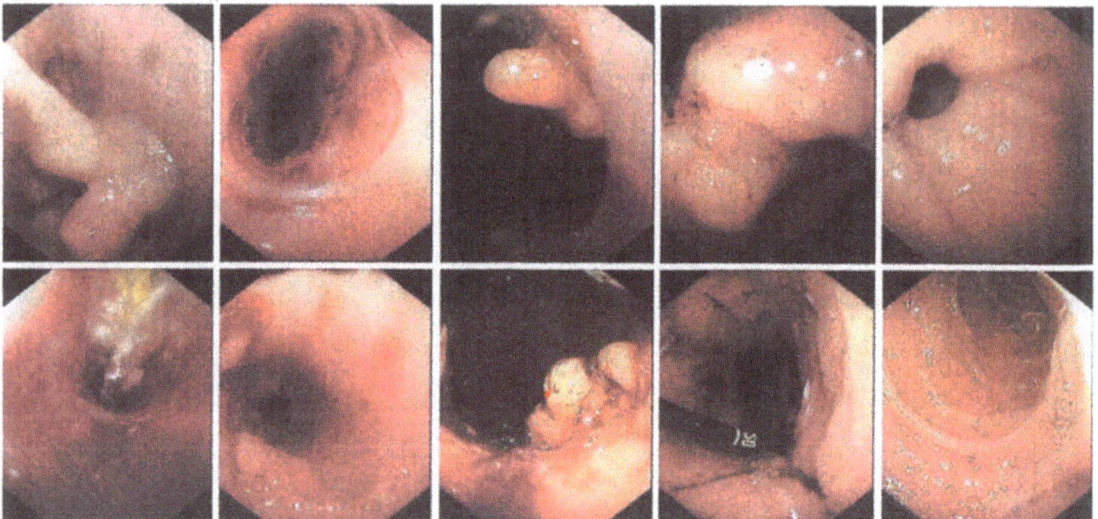

Figure 5. The third round of EGD performed at the Dr. Soetomo General Academic hospital.

3.9. The Fourth EGD and Dilation (2 Weeks after the Third EGD)

After the third EGD, the patient had no further swallowing issue. The results of the histopathological examination of gastric tissue taken during the third EGD revealed pieces of gastric mucosal tissue covered with glands with shortened (eroded) gastric pits. In the lamina propria, lymphocyte inflammatory cells and 1–2 plasma cells could be seen. Locally, glandular foci were covered with epithelium with hyperchromatic nuclei. The submucosal layer was composed of fibrous connective tissue with proliferation of muscle tissue accompanied by infiltration of lymphocyte cells. There were no signs of malignancy in any tissues, which indicated the presence of granulation tissue accompanied by reactive bleeding in the gastric mucosal epithelium.

During the fourth EGD session, the scope entered through the oral cavity at a 25 cm insertion. Thereafter, an esophageal stricture was detected and could not be passed by a 12 mm scope. The insertion of a 0.035 guidewire and dilation using an 8 mm balloon for

2 min were performed, followed by 12 mm balloon dilation for 2 min. Mucosal tears were visible. The lumen could not be passed by a 12 mm scope (Figure 6). In this patient, it was concluded that there was a complex esophageal stricture, which had been dilated with 8 mm and 12 mm balloons. The patient was advised to eat refined porridge and undergo another round of esophageal dilation within 1 week.

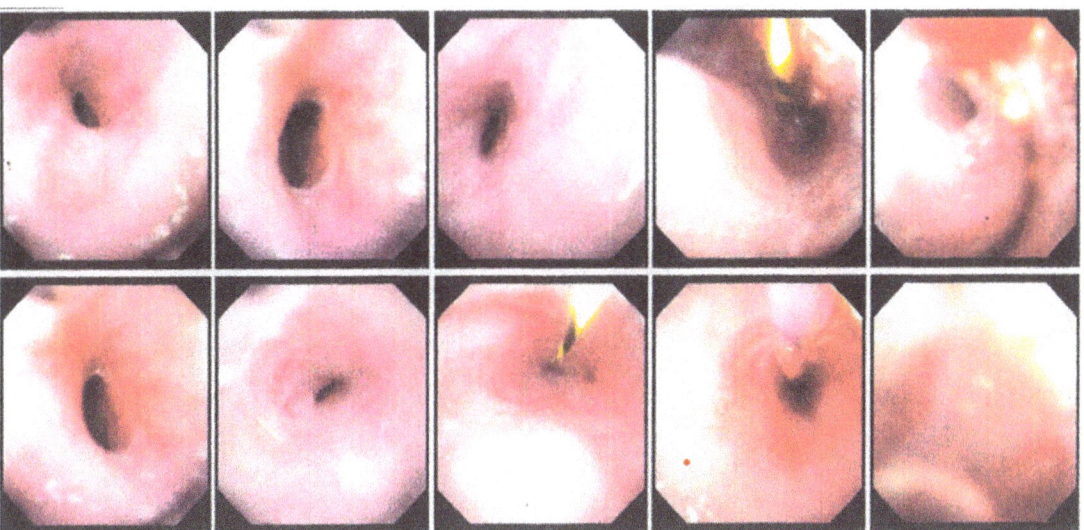

Figure 6. The fourth round of EGD performed at the Dr. Soetomo General Academic hospital.

4. Discussion

Severe corrosive injury can induce upper gastrointestinal stricture typically three weeks post ingestion. Barium contrast swallow or contrast fluoroscopy and EGD are important initial examinations to determine further management strategies for upper gastrointestinal stricture [1,9]. Contrast fluoroscopy is only performed in patients who develop complex strictures or when endoscopy is not optimal due to excessive narrowing of the lumen, whereas EGD is more commonly recommended because it provides overall information about the anatomy of the esophagus and not only establishes the diagnosis of stricture, but also allows for mucosal biopsies and can provide an opportunity for therapeutic dilation of strictures when indicated [1]. In addition, CT scanning is also important to exclude suspected esophageal perforation due to corrosive materials that are caustic, or for strictures that are suspected to be related to esophageal malignancy (for staging purposes) [1]. This was consistent with the case presented above, where EGD was the chosen diagnostic tool employed to identify the esophageal stricture, followed by esophageal dilation as the main treatment modality.

Pathophysiologically, corrosive injury activates an inflammatory response in the affected gastrointestinal tract, followed by thrombosis of the arterioles and venules leading to ischemic necrosis. Then, fibroblasts are recruited and the reparation of the damaged mucosa begins thereafter. The stricture usually develops in the third week and the formation is complete several months after exposure. From the third week onwards, scar tissue retraction leads to stricture formation and shortening of the gastrointestinal tract. At this point, the lower esophageal sphincter pressure decreases and allows gastroesophageal reflux to occur. As a result, repeated exposure to gastric acid will accelerate the formation of strictures [9]. This was consistent with the case above because in the histopathological examination of the biopsy sample of the esophageal tissue, inflammatory cells were predominantly neutrophils, histiocytes, plasma cells and a number of eosinophils, with many small blood vessels lined with reactive endothelium, which was identical to the picture of chronic inflammation. In addition, during endoscopy, the mucosa was fragile and bled easily, reflecting the fragility of the esophageal wall exposed to corrosive materials. Clinically, the patient also had complaints of epigastric pain and vomiting every time she ate/drank, so it is likely that gastric acid reflux into the esophagus will further accelerate the development of esophageal strictures.

Management of esophageal strictures includes prevention and management of the causes of strictures, for example, in esophageal strictures caused by corrosive substances, prevention of repeated exposure to corrosive substances must be carried out. Then, dilation of the esophageal stricture can be performed to restore the patency of the narrowed esophageal lumen. Dilation using an endoscopic bougie and a balloon is the key to managing esophageal strictures [9]. The bougie-type or mechanical pusher-type dilators usually come in different sizes and are made of different materials, such as rubber. Maloney's bougie can be passed freely without using a guidewire. Meanwhile, the Savary-Gilliard bougie has a guidewire to help it travel through the upper gastrointestinal tract. The balloon-type dilator has a way of working where the expansion of the balloon will produce a radial force that can widen the lumen [1]. Mercury-weighted rubber bougies (e.g., Maloney dilators) are commonly used for mild-to-moderate degrees of simple esophageal strictures, whereas balloon dilators (hydrostatic and pneumatic) and wire-guided polyvinyl bougies are standard modalities for more complex esophageal strictures (Table 1). A study conducted in the United States involving 348 esophageal dilation procedures over 4 years compared the performance of three methods of esophageal stricture dilation: Maloney, Savary-Gilliard and balloon (hydrostatic and pneumatic types). As a result, four incidents of esophageal perforation were reported with the use of Maloney's bougie without fluoroscopic guidance and all of them occurred in complex esophageal strictures, whereas no incidents of perforation were reported with the use of the Savary-Gilliard dilator or balloon [10]. Of note, endoscopic-associated iatrogenic perforation is a major cause of esophageal perforation, accounting for more than half of all reported cases of esophageal perforation [11].

Table 1. Differences between simple and complex esophageal strictures.

	Simple Stricture	Complex Stricture
Endoscopy scope access	Yes	No (usually)
Size	Short (<2 cm)	Long (>2 cm)
Focal	Yes	No
Angulation/irregularity	No	Yes
Cause	Peptic, Shatzki's ring, anastomosis, pill-induced	Caustic ingestion, malignancy, photodynamic therapy, radiation
Recommended dilation method	Balloon or rigid dilator	Rigid dilator
Fluoroscopy	Rarely needed	Recommended
Frequency of dilation	1–3 (commonly)	≥ 3
Recurrence risk	Low	High

In this case, esophageal dilation with a Savary-Gilliard bougie was used in the first and second EGD, and a controlled radial expansion (CRE) endoscopic balloon was used in the third and fourth EGD. The patient's stricture can be classified as a complex stricture because after four dilation sessions, patency of the esophagus has not been achieved (the lumen still cannot be passed by the 12 mm scope) and additional episodes of EGD and dilation are still needed.

A previous study mentioned the superiority of the Savary-Gilliard bougie over the Maloney, arguing that the Savary-Gilliard bougie provides greater assurance that the dilator will follow the contour of the esophageal lumen, thereby reducing the risk of perforation. In addition, wire-guided dilators offer a potential effect of radial and longitudinal dilation, depending on whether additional alternating movements are made after the initial static radial dilation. When using a Savary-Gilliard bougie, fluoroscopic assistance is recommended to monitor the guidewire position, which should be targeted at least 30 cm below the lowest point of the stricture. Usually, the distal end is positioned in the gastric antrum along the greater curvature of the stomach [12].

Through-the-scope (TTS) balloon inflation is usually performed under direct endoscope visualization, using a balloon dilator that is lowered through the endoscope channel. The center of the balloon should be centered at the narrowest point in the stricture with a dilation pressure ranging between 30 and 45 psi, varying in relation to the size of the balloon. When compared to the Savary-Gilliard, the TTS balloon dilator does not provide longitudinal compressive force because it is positioned in a static position between strictures during dilation. In addition, it is important to know the full anatomy (e.g., length and angulation) of the esophagus before balloon dilation is performed. The balloon must completely cross the stricture to avoid asymmetrical pressure across the stricture area, which can increase the risk of perforation [12]. Dilation using an endoscopic balloon is recommended in certain conditions where longitudinal pressure may be harmful, for example, in epidermolysis bullosa. In conditions where there is a tear of the esophageal mucosa (mucosal tear), it is important to carefully choose the size of the dilator, the target of the dilator and the time of dilation. It is said that dilation with an endoscopic balloon may be more advisable than using a rigid dilator in conditions with impaired continuity of the esophageal mucosa [12]. However, to date, there is no clear difference regarding the effectiveness and safety of the Savary-Gilliard bougie when compared to the endoscopic balloon (TTS) for the treatment of benign esophageal strictures [2,12]. However, the dilation of esophageal stricture due to corrosive injury using the Savary-Gilliard bougie rarely needs fluoroscopy, has shorter duration and is more economical than balloon endoscopy [13]. Ideally, the best interval between initial dilation sessions is between 2 and 4 weeks. After the goal of estimating the optimal diameter is achieved, the interval can be increased based on the patient's expectations of the dysphagia complaints they are experiencing [12]. In the case study presented, erosion and bleeding were seen in the dilated area during the second EGD, so the dilation method was changed from the Savary-Gilliard bougie to the CRE balloon to prevent further trauma to the esophageal mucosa. Esophageal dilation in this case was performed within 1 week between the first and second dilations, followed by an interval every 2 weeks for the next episodes of dilation.

Esophageal stricture develops over time, and the prognosis depends on the timing of evaluation and treatment, and the underlying cause of the stricture. Although esophageal dilation is the first line of management in cases of benign esophageal stricture, there is a 10–40% chance of restenosis [1,14]. A stricture is considered recurrent if there is an inability to maintain a satisfactory luminal diameter for 4 weeks after achieving the target diameter of 14 mm. Whereas, a stricture is said to be refractory if the dysphagia score remains to be two (can only eat soft foods) or more as a result of the inability to achieve a diameter of 14 mm in five dilation sessions, which are carried out at intervals of every 2 weeks [1]. In the presented case, the patient was only able to eat soft foods (e.g., porridge) until the end of the fourth dilation session, so it is very likely that the patient had a refractory esophageal stricture even though she had not met the number of sessions (i.e., at least five sessions of dilation) criteria.

Stricture recurrence is a serious problem that has the potential to increase the risk and cost of treatment. The prevalence of recurrent esophageal stricture is 11.1 per 100 person-years [3]. Predictors for stricture recurrence include the presence of complex stricture, persistent epigastric pain symptoms, presence of non-peptic stricture and undiagnosed eosinophilic esophagitis. Patients with long, narrow strictures are most likely to require repeat dilation. There is no clear limit on the number of dilation sessions needed by a patient [14]. However, one study found that "bougination" or bougie dilation of esophageal stricture due to corrosive injury has a low clinical success (i.e., being able to eat a normal diet 2 months after dilation without any special procedure) rate (approximately 22.5%), when compared with other causes of strictures. The clinical success rate was significantly higher in patients with a stricture length of less than 2 cm (47.2%), those with pre-procedure dysphagia on a semi-solid or soft diet (51.3%) and those with a dilation of 13 mm or more (46.1%) [15]. In the presented case, based on the results of the MSCT scan, it was found that the narrowing of the esophagus was 4.5 cm long and dilation with serial bougie and ballooning up to the fourth session was not able to dilate the esophagus for at least 12 mm. In addition, in the pre-procedure (i.e., the first EGD), the patient could not even drink water, and the cause of the stricture was gasoline which contains corrosive substances, so it is very likely that the clinical success of repeated dilation in this patient is very small and will require repetitive dilation and other adjuvant treatments.

In general, peptic strictures have an excellent prognosis when treated promptly with endoscopic dilation and long-term PPI therapy. To improve the prognosis in terms of reducing stricture recurrence, intramural steroid injection therapy or oral steroid therapy has been used and has shown promising clinical results [1,14]. An analysis of 13 studies involving 361 subjects with corrosive esophageal injuries found that steroid therapy was not beneficial in mild corrosive injuries but could be useful in preventing strictures in moderate and severe corrosive injuries [16]. Although the mechanism of action of steroids on strictures is not completely understood, it is supposed that steroids can affect collagen deposition and increase its breakdown, thereby reducing the formation of fibrous tissue [14]. Stents are primarily used in cases of benign strictures where repeated dilation is inadequate and where symptom control is poor. In cases of malignant strictures, the prognosis depends on the type of cancer, tumor invasion, and stage of disease. Surgical resection shows a better prognosis for cancer that has not invaded the lymph nodes and surrounding tissues. In malignant strictures, stent placement can be used as palliative therapy in cases of advanced cancer or as temporary therapy in cases of ongoing neoadjuvant treatment [1].

5. Summary

Here, we reported the case study of a patient with complex (refractory) esophageal stricture due to chronic gasoline ingestion. The patient initially complained of difficulty swallowing which was marked by vomiting a few seconds after eating and drinking. The patient then underwent two sessions of EGD and esophageal dilation during hospitalization and was scheduled to undergo another round of EGD/dilation within 2 weeks of the last esophageal dilation session. During discharge, the patient was able to eat soft food (e.g., porridge) and drink without vomiting. During the next EGD procedure, an esophageal stricture together with esophageal polyps, masses (i.e., granulation tissue) on the cardia and ulcers on the gastric antrum were observed. Then the patient underwent another esophageal dilation, this time with a CRE balloon, and a histopathological examination of gastric tissue was performed. To date, the patient has undergone at least four EGD sessions with repeated esophageal dilation. Vomiting when eating/drinking and the swallowing issue have significantly been reduced, even though endoscopically the lumen of the esophagus is still narrow (the scope was unable to be traversed by a 12 mm scope).

Author Contributions: Conceptualization; formal analysis; investigation; resources; data curation, H.S. and A.V.; writing—original draft preparation, H.S.; writing—review and editing, H.S. and A.V.; visualization, H.S.; supervision, A.V. All authors have read and agreed to the published version of the manuscript.

Funding: This research received no external funding.

Institutional Review Board Statement: Not applicable.

Informed Consent Statement: Written informed consent has been obtained from the patient to publish this paper.

Data Availability Statement: Data is unavailable due to privacy of the patient.

Conflicts of Interest: The authors declare no conflict of interest.

References

1. Desai, J.P.; Moustarah, F. Esophageal Stricture. In *StatPearls*; StatPearls Publishing: Treasure Island, FL, USA, 2023.
2. Siersema, P.D. Treatment options for esophageal strictures. *Nat. Rev. Gastroenterol. Hepatol.* 2008, *5*, 142–152. [CrossRef] [PubMed]
3. Ruigómez, A.; Rodríguez, L.A.G.; Wallander, M.-A.; Johansson, S.; Eklund, S. Esophageal Stricture: Incidence, Treatment Patterns, and Recurrence Rate. *Am. J. Gastroenterol.* 2006, *101*, 2685–2692. [CrossRef] [PubMed]
4. Mowry, J.B.; Spyker, D.A.; Cantilena, L.R.; McMillan, N.; Ford, M. 2013 Annual Report of the American Association of Poison Control Centers' National Poison Data System (NPDS): 31st Annual Report. *Clin. Toxicol.* 2014, *52*, 1032–1283. [CrossRef] [PubMed]
5. Hall, A.H.; Jacquemin, D.; Henny, D.; Mathieu, L.; Josset, P.; Meyer, B. Corrosive substances ingestion: A review. *Crit. Rev. Toxicol.* 2019, *49*, 637–669. [CrossRef] [PubMed]
6. Vulimiri, S.V.; Pratt, M.M.; Kulkarni, S.; Beedanagari, S.; Mahadevan, B. Reproductive and Developmental Toxicity of Solvents and Gases. In *Reproductive and Developmental Toxicology*, 2nd ed.; Gupta, R.C., Ed.; Academic Press: Cambridge, MA, USA, 2017; p. iii, ISBN 978-0-12-804239-7.
7. Pace, F.; Greco, S.; Pallotta, S.; Bossi, D.; Trabucchi, E.; Porro, G.B. An uncommon cause of corrosive esophageal injury. *World J. Gastroenterol.* 2008, *14*, 636–637. [CrossRef] [PubMed]
8. Matějovský, L.; Macák, J.; Pospíšil, M.; Baroš, P.; Staš, M.; Krausová, A. Study of Corrosion of Metallic Materials in Ethanol–Gasoline Blends: Application of Electrochemical Methods. *Energy Fuels* 2017, *31*, 10880–10889. [CrossRef]
9. Sarma, M.S.; Tripathi, P.R.; Arora, S. Corrosive upper gastrointestinal strictures in children: Difficulties and dilemmas. *World J. Clin. Pediatr.* 2021, *10*, 124–136. [CrossRef] [PubMed]
10. Hernandez, L.J.; Jacobson, J.W.; Harris, M. Comparison among the perforation rates of Maloney, balloon, and Savary dilation of esophageal strictures. *Gastrointest. Endosc.* 2000, *51*, 460–462. [CrossRef] [PubMed]
11. Soytürk, M.; Isik, A.; Firat, D.; Peker, K.; Sayar, I.; Idiz, O. A case report of esophageal perforation: Complication of nasogastric tube placement. *Am. J. Case Rep.* 2014, *15*, 168–171. [CrossRef] [PubMed]
12. Parekh, P.J.; Johnson, D.A. Esophageal Dilation: An Overview. In *Practical Gastroenterology and Hepatology Board Review Toolkit*; Wallace, M.B., Aqel, B.A., Lindor, K.D., Talley, N.J., Devault, K.R., Eds.; John Wiley & Sons, Ltd.: Oxford, UK, 2016; pp. 1–7, ISBN 978-1-119-12743-7.
13. Fakıoglu, E.; Güney, L.H.; Ötgün, İ. Esophageal Dilation via Bouginage or Balloon Catheters in Children, as the Treatment of Benign Esophageal Strictures: Results, Considering the Etiology and the Methods. *Turk. J. Trauma Emerg. Surg.* 2023, *29*, 574–581. [CrossRef]
14. Ferguson, D.D. Evaluation and management of benign esophageal strictures. *Dis. Esophagus* 2005, *18*, 359–364. [CrossRef] [PubMed]
15. Park, J.Y.; Park, J.M.; Shin, G.-Y.; Kim, J.S.; Cho, Y.K.; Kim, T.H.; Kim, B.-W.; Choi, M.-G. Efficacy of bougie dilation for normal diet in benign esophageal stricture. *Scand. J. Gastroenterol.* 2023, *58*, 199–207. [CrossRef] [PubMed]
16. Howell, J.M.; Dalsey, W.C.; Hartsell, F.; Butzin, C.A. Steroids for the treatment of corrosive esophageal injury: A statistical analysis of past studies. *Am. J. Emerg. Med.* 1992, *10*, 421–425. [CrossRef] [PubMed]

Disclaimer/Publisher's Note: The statements, opinions and data contained in all publications are solely those of the individual author(s) and contributor(s) and not of MDPI and/or the editor(s). MDPI and/or the editor(s) disclaim responsibility for any injury to people or property resulting from any ideas, methods, instructions or products referred to in the content.

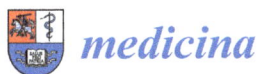

Systematic Review

Diagnosis of Liver Fibrosis Using Artificial Intelligence: A Systematic Review

Stefan Lucian Popa [1], Abdulrahman Ismaiel [1,*], Ludovico Abenavoli [2], Alexandru Marius Padureanu [3], Miruna Oana Dita [3], Roxana Bolchis [3], Mihai Alexandru Munteanu [4], Vlad Dumitru Brata [3], Cristina Pop [5], Andrei Bosneag [3], Dinu Iuliu Dumitrascu [6], Maria Barsan [7] and Liliana David [1]

1. 2nd Medical Department, "Iuliu Hatieganu" University of Medicine and Pharmacy, 400000 Cluj-Napoca, Romania; popa.stefan@umfcluj.ro (S.L.P.)
2. Department of Health Sciences, University "Magna Graecia", 88100 Catanzaro, Italy; l.abenavoli@unicz.it
3. Faculty of Medicine, "Iuliu Hatieganu" University of Medicine and Pharmacy, 400000 Cluj-Napoca, Romania; alexandru.padureanu@outlook.com (A.M.P.); miruna.dita@outlook.com (M.O.D.); bolchis.roxana@yahoo.com (R.B.)
4. Department of Medical Disciplines, Faculty of Medicine and Pharmacy, University of Oradea, 410087 Oradea, Romania
5. Department of Pharmacology, Physiology, and Pathophysiology, Faculty of Pharmacy, Iuliu Hatieganu University of Medicine and Pharmacy, 400347 Cluj-Napoca, Romania
6. Department of Anatomy, UMF "Iuliu Hatieganu" Cluj-Napoca, 400000 Cluj-Napoca, Romania
7. Department of Occupational Health, "Iuliu Hatieganu" University of Medicine and Pharmacy, 400000 Cluj-Napoca, Romania
* Correspondence: abdulrahman.ismaiel@yahoo.com

Abstract: *Background and Objectives*: The development of liver fibrosis as a consequence of continuous inflammation represents a turning point in the evolution of chronic liver diseases. The recent developments of artificial intelligence (AI) applications show a high potential for improving the accuracy of diagnosis, involving large sets of clinical data. For this reason, the aim of this systematic review is to provide a comprehensive overview of current AI applications and analyze the accuracy of these systems to perform an automated diagnosis of liver fibrosis. *Materials and Methods*: We searched PubMed, Cochrane Library, EMBASE, and WILEY databases using predefined keywords. Articles were screened for relevant publications about AI applications capable of diagnosing liver fibrosis. Exclusion criteria were animal studies, case reports, abstracts, letters to the editor, conference presentations, pediatric studies, studies written in languages other than English, and editorials. *Results*: Our search identified a total of 24 articles analyzing the automated imagistic diagnosis of liver fibrosis, out of which six studies analyze liver ultrasound images, seven studies analyze computer tomography images, five studies analyze magnetic resonance images, and six studies analyze liver biopsies. The studies included in our systematic review showed that AI-assisted non-invasive techniques performed as accurately as human experts in detecting and staging liver fibrosis. Nevertheless, the findings of these studies need to be confirmed through clinical trials to be implemented into clinical practice. *Conclusions*: The current systematic review provides a comprehensive analysis of the performance of AI systems in diagnosing liver fibrosis. Automatic diagnosis, staging, and risk stratification for liver fibrosis is currently possible considering the accuracy of the AI systems, which can overcome the limitations of non-invasive diagnosis methods.

Keywords: liver fibrosis; hepatic fibrosis; percutaneous liver biopsy; artificial intelligence; machine learning; computer scan; ultrasonography; digital pathology

Citation: Popa, S.L.; Ismaiel, A.; Abenavoli, L.; Padureanu, A.M.; Dita, M.O.; Bolchis, R.; Munteanu, M.A.; Brata, V.D.; Pop, C.; Bosneag, A.; et al. Diagnosis of Liver Fibrosis Using Artificial Intelligence: A Systematic Review. *Medicina* 2023, 59, 992. https://doi.org/10.3390/medicina59050992

Academic Editor: Sorin Tiberiu Alexandrescu

Received: 24 March 2023
Revised: 4 May 2023
Accepted: 19 May 2023
Published: 21 May 2023

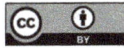

Copyright: © 2023 by the authors. Licensee MDPI, Basel, Switzerland. This article is an open access article distributed under the terms and conditions of the Creative Commons Attribution (CC BY) license (https://creativecommons.org/licenses/by/4.0/).

1. Introduction

Chronic liver diseases (CLD) represent an important public health issue, accounting for significant morbidity and mortality globally and resulting in approximately 2 million deaths annually [1].

The precise etiology, geographic region, and presumably additional factors (sex, race, and socioeconomic status) have a significant impact on the incidence and prevalence of CLD [2].

Underlying etiology in CLD comprise alcohol-related liver disease, nonalcoholic fatty liver disease (NAFLD), chronic viral hepatitis B and C, autoimmune liver diseases (such as primary biliary cirrhosis, primary sclerosing cholangitis, and autoimmune hepatitis), hereditary diseases (Wilson's disease, haemochromatosis, and alpha1-anti-trypsin deficiency) [3]. Regardless of the etiology, the course of CLD is characterized by a lengthy process of chronic parenchymal injury, prolonged inflammatory response, sustained activation of hepatic fibrogenesis, and continued activation of the wound healing response [4].

The development of hepatic fibrosis is a turning point in CLD, its presence and severity across the etiology being correlated with prognosis [3]. Liver fibrosis and fibrogenesis are key factors of the progression of any form of CLD towards liver cirrhosis and hepatic failure [4]. Liver fibrosis is characterized by hepatocellular damage (release of signals such as reactive oxygen species), the recruitment and activation of inflammatory cells (macrophages and lymphocytes generate multiple types of cytokines, including transforming growth factor-β and platelet-derived growth factor), and the excessive deposition of extracellular matrix proteins (differentiation of hepatic stellate cells towards myofibroblasts, dysregulated by cytokines) [5,6].

When fibrosis progresses, there is a worsening of the hepatic architecture, leading to bridging fibrosis and, eventually, cirrhosis (diffuse nodules of regenerating hepatocytes outlined by dense fibrotic tissue), causing hepatocellular dysfunction and distorted hepatic vasculature, which will result in hepatic insufficiency and portal hypertension [5].

Liver biopsy is the gold standard for fibrosis assessment because it allows detailed evaluation and localization and captures a larger amount of fibrosis [5]. However, its well-known drawbacks have made this procedure unappealing to doctors and patients (technical considerations, invasiveness, and potential severe complications) [7].

Considering this, efforts have been made in the last years for developing non-invasive strategies for assessing liver fibrosis. The several broad categories include serological markers (direct and indirect), imaging studies consisting of computed tomography (CT), magnetic resonance imaging (MRI), positron emission tomography–computed tomography (PET–CT), and methods assessing physical properties of the liver tissue (liver stiffness, attenuation, and viscosity) [2]. Methodologies that accurately and reproducibly evaluate liver anatomy and function without invasive procedures are urgently needed.

A new era of precision medicine in hepatology will begin once artificial intelligence's (AI) ability to analyze data from digital imaging and pathology will be validated [8]. This will gradually revolutionize clinical practice, both from the perspective of understanding disease mechanisms and drug development. AI algorithms offer innovative prospects to forecast the likelihood of progression from early-stage CLDs toward cirrhosis-related consequences, with the goal of precision medicine [9]. For instance, certain AI programs have already been developed and have shown promising results regarding the screening of cirrhosis complications, such as esophageal varices and hepatocellular carcinoma [10–12]. Moreover, often requiring a thorough differential diagnosis and various imaging methods, focal liver lesions also represent a field in which AI could provide much needed assistance, with research suggesting an overall accuracy comparable with human experts [13]. State-of-the-art AI technologies are also being used in predicting the overall outcome of patients with liver tumors, as well as the overall response to therapy, by assessing the microvascular invasion before and after therapy [14,15]. Continuing initiatives must push past the tendency to oppose change and encourage the acceptance and use of these developing technologies.

In the last decade, AI applications used for automatic diagnosis have revolutionized radiology. AI algorithms can analyze images, such as X-rays, CT scans, and MRIs, to diagnose and classify abnormalities with a better precision than human experts. Furthermore, AI algorithms can recognize patterns and features that are not visible to human experts, making automatic diagnosis faster and more accurate. Because this technology can improve patient outcomes and reduce healthcare costs, the aim of this systematic review is to provide a comprehensive overview of current AI applications and analyze the accuracy of these systems in order to perform an automated diagnosis of liver fibrosis.

2. Materials and Methods

This systematic review was conducted in accordance with the preferred reporting items for systematic reviews (PRISMA) guidelines [16]. PubMed, EMBASE, Cochrane Library, and WILEY databases were searched for relevant publications about AI applications used for an autonomous diagnosis in liver fibrosis. The search terms included: (liver fibrosis OR hepatic fibrosis) AND (artificial intelligence OR machine learning OR neural networks OR deep learning OR automated diagnosis OR computer-aided diagnosis OR digital pathology OR automated ultrasound OR automated computer tomography OR automated magnetic imaging). We included articles indexed by the queried databases and returned by our search strategies, for which the full text was available, only in English, or if an English version was available. We considered all original research studies as eligible. Exclusion criteria were animal studies, case reports, abstracts, letters to the editor, conference presentations, pediatric studies, studies written in languages other than English, and editorials.

Two independent authors (S.L.P and A.I.) reviewed, for eligibility, titles, abstracts, and the full text of eligible articles. Data extraction was also conducted independently by both reviewers, with data on the authors' names, year of publication, country or study population, sample size, study design, gender ratio, number and percentage of liver fibrosis patients, the method used to diagnose liver fibrosis, and artificial intelligence application being analyzed. Figure 1 shows the search strategy using the PRISMA flow diagram.

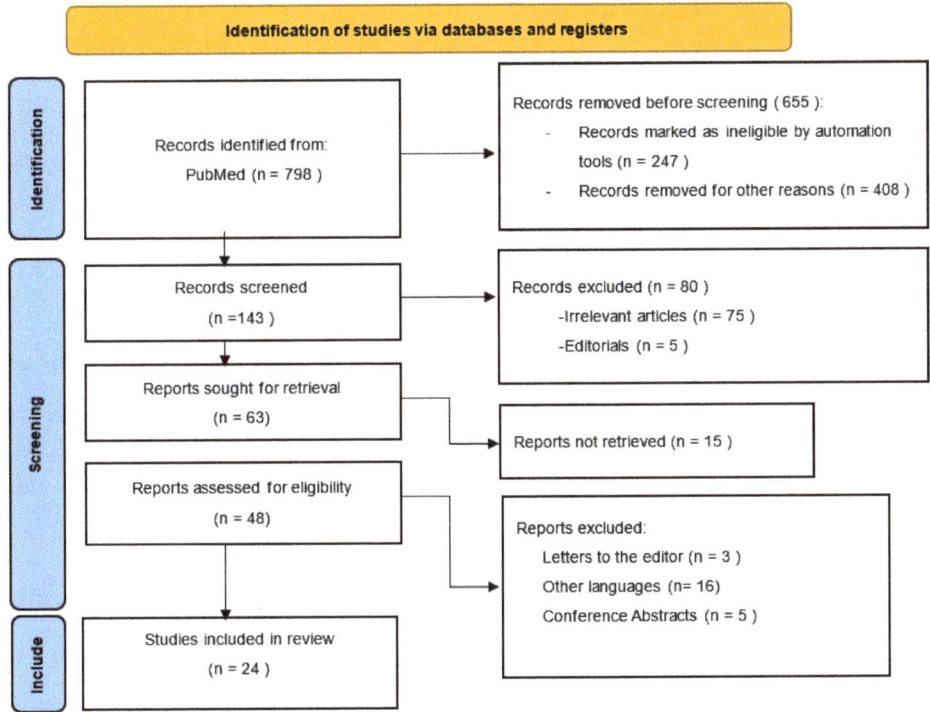

Figure 1. PRISMA flow diagram for study selection.

The initial search retrieved a total of 798 studies. We screened a total of 143 studies, and we excluded 119 articles as follows: irrelevant original studies to this review topic (n = 75), other languages (n = 16), conference abstracts (n = 5), articles not retrieved (15), and editorials or letters to the editor (n = 8). Finally, a total of 24 studies fulfilled our inclusion and exclusion criteria and were included in the systematic review as demonstrated in Figure 1.

3. Results

Histopathological analysis of liver tissue obtained via percutaneous biopsy is the current gold standard for identifying and staging hepatic fibrosis. However, there are some disadvantages accompanying biopsy, including peri-procedural pain, severe bleeding, and the potential of sampling bias due to the examination of only a limited area of liver parenchyma [17]. To overcome these drawbacks, non-invasive imaging-based approaches have been investigated as substitutes for biopsy: conventional MRI, magnetic resonance elastography (MRE), perfusion CT, and other experimental methods such as perfusion MRI, MR spectroscopy, and fibro CT [18].

Deep learning (DL) methods prove useful by aiding the clinician in making decisions. By combining the clinical point of view together with multiple paraclinical findings, such as laboratory and imaging findings, the diagnostic value rises. DL methods should be able to provide early identification of liver fibrosis, considering that early identification and accurate staging of liver fibrosis are critical for preventing or delaying clinical decompensation and the necessity for liver transplantation.

Clinically, it appears logical that in the case of severe liver fibrosis, the DL model focuses on both the liver and the spleen, because both organs undergo morphological changes when cirrhosis advances, as well as complications such as ascites, collateral circulation, and esophageal varices [19]. Therefore, these models should not only focus on the liver when describing liver fibrosis but also on the complications caused by advanced liver disease. These complications can be systemic, and for future perspectives, DL algorithms can be combined with blood parameters to help stage liver disease.

3.1. Artificial Intelligence Techniques and CT Imaging

The main studies analyzing the efficiency of AI algorithms in assessing liver fibrosis on CT images are illustrated in Table 1.

Table 1. Studies assessing AI techniques and CT imaging for the diagnosis of liver fibrosis.

First Author	Year	Total Number of Images	Diagnosis	Main Findings
Yasaka et al. [20]	2018	496	Liver fibrosis	Magnified CT images were analyzed by deep learning to diagnose and stage liver fibrosis, revealing a moderate correlation with histopathological staging.
Li et al. [21]	2020	1041	Liver fibrosis	The residual neural network (ResNet) is an efficient non-invasive diagnostic method for diagnosing liver fibrosis using plain CT images.
Choi et al. [22]	2018	7461	Liver fibrosis	The deep learning system was able to diagnose and stage live fibrosis with high accuracy (79.4%).
Yin et al. [23]	2021	252	Liver fibrosis	By using contrast-enhanced CT images and deep learning algorithms, liver fibrosis can be successfully diagnosed and staged.
Yin et al. [24]	2022	252	Liver fibrosis	Splenic radiomic features are an important and useful addition to hepatic radiomic features when staging liver fibrosis.
Budai et al. [25]	2020	354	Liver fibrosis	In order to differentiate between low- and high-grade fibrosis, CT texture analysis can be used for prognosis calculations of chronic liver disease.
Wu et al. [26]	2022	112	Liver cirrhosis and liver fibrosis	AI segmentation algorithms can be used to diagnose liver fibrosis in a clinical context.

CT: computed tomography.

Yasaka et al. investigated if liver fibrosis could be effectively staged through deep learning techniques. They used a deep convolutional neural network (DCNN) trained and tested on 496 liver CT scans for the evaluation of the fibrosis stage in comparison to histopathological results. The study revealed that liver fibrosis could be staged with moderate performance based on dynamic contrast-enhanced portal phase CT images. For this particular AI model, the AUCs for diagnosing significant fibrosis, advanced fibrosis, and cirrhosis were 0.74, 0.76, and 0.73, respectively. Further improvements to the model are necessary in order for it to be used in clinical settings [20].

Li et al. conducted a study aimed at evaluating the performance of a residual neural network (ResNet) for staging liver fibrosis through plain CT images. The study involved liver CT scans from 347 patients with diagnosed CLD. Three different CT sections from adjacent levels were obtained for each patient, pre-processed through manual outlining of the interest area performed by two radiologists, and merged into a single sample for each patient. All the values obtained by the ResNet were the result of a cross-validation that was repeated five times between the CT image sample and the pathology report obtained from the assessment of liver biopsies. The accuracy of the ResNet model was higher than 0.82 for each category of fibrosis assessed through the METAVIR score, thus making the ResNet effective in evaluating fibrosis staging on plain CT images [21].

Using portal venous phase CT scans, Choi et al. created a deep learning system (DLS) to stage liver fibrosis. The DLS consists of two separate algorithms based on a convolutional neural network (CNN) in order to perform liver segmentation and fibrosis staging. In 707 of 891 individuals, the DLS correctly predicted the fibrosis stage, yielding a staging accuracy of 79.4%. The DLS created in this investigation was resilient across a variety of clinical settings and imaging situations with findings suggesting that the DLS's accuracy in staging fibrosis was not reliant on CT scan methodology, patient demographic variables, or the presence of a liver focal mass. The diagnosis of intermediate stage fibrosis with the DLS was less accurate than the diagnosis of cirrhosis; the pathologic fibrosis stage was the only significant independent factor that significantly influenced the performance of the DLS [22].

Yin et al. used a new technique to better understand the interpretation of DL models when they staged liver fibrosis. The liver fibrosis staging network (LFS network) was created using contrast-enhanced CT scans taken during the portal venous phase of 252 individuals with histologically established liver fibrosis. Gradient-weighted Class Activation Mapping (Grad-cam) was used to locate where the LFS network focuses when predicting liver fibrosis stages. The corresponding location map revealed that the network strongly focused on the liver surface rather than the liver parenchyma when it came to a healthy liver, whereas in the case of cirrhosis (F4 liver fibrosis), the network focused more on the spleen and the central parts of the liver parenchyma [23]. The same group further used a combination of liver and splenic CT-based radiomics analysis to quantify liver fibrosis. Radiomics analysis, as opposed to DL, employs manually created features taken from CT scans. The model can show which types of symptoms on images are more essential to the model, and the results paralleled previous research. This means that the current radiomic analysis results might supplement the Grad-cam location maps by demonstrating the emphasis of DLS for predicting liver fibrosis stages [24].

Other directions for radiomics related studies include CT-texture analysis (CTTA) methods for the prediction of liver fibrosis and even differentiating between fibrosis grades. CTTA can quantify the heterogeneity and distribution of pixel or voxel grey levels on CT images. CTTA is based on extensive quantitative imaging characteristics that are undetectable to the naked eye and are created through numerous mathematical descriptors of the original picture. In their work, Budai et al. used CTTA software for processing liver CT images and predicting the fibrosis grade of each liver segment. A set of 354 CT images from 32 patients was used to extract quantitative parameters before texture analysis was performed. Results showed that CTTA-based models can not only detect fibrosis, but they also can differentiate between low- or high-grade fibrosis [25].

Wu et al. investigated the use of multi-slice spiral computed tomography (MSCT), which is centered on an AI segmentation algorithm, to diagnose liver cirrhosis and liver fibrosis. There were 112 patients included in the study and there were three indexes evaluated: hepatic arterial fraction (HAF), blood flow (BF), blood volume (BV), and mean transit time (MTT). Both patients with moderate liver fibrosis and those with substantial hepatic fibrosis had significantly higher HAF levels than those in the control group. Other indexes also achieved significant performance with authors concluding that larger sample sizes are needed to improve this method [26].

3.2. Artificial Intelligence Techniques and MRI Imaging

We found five studies assessing the accuracy of AI algorithms in diagnosing liver fibrosis on MRI images, as depicted in Table 2.

Table 2. Studies assessing AI techniques and MRI imaging for the diagnosis of liver fibrosis.

First Author	Year	Total Number of Images	Diagnosis	Main Findings
Nowak et al. [27]	2021	713	Liver cirrhosis	Two pre-trained convolutional neural networks were successfully used to detect liver cirrhosis on standard T2-weighted MRIs.
Kato et al. [28]	2007	52	Liver fibrosis	The computer algorithm revealed a potential usefulness for the diagnosis of hepatic fibrosis.
Hectors et al. [29]	2021	355	Liver fibrosis	Deep learning algorithm, based on gadoxetic acid-enhanced MRI data, was comparable to MR elastography analysis.
Strotzer et al. [30]	2022	112	Liver cirrhosis and liver fibrosis	A multiphase Gd-EOB-DTPA-enhanced liver MRI was used to diagnose fibrosis stage or cirrhosis.
Soufi et al. [31]	2019	51	Liver fibrosis	PLSR-based SSM could help to better understand the variations associated with liver fibrosis staging and diagnosis.

MRI: Magnetic resonance imagine; MR: magnetic resonance; Gd-EOB-DTPA: Gadolinium ethoxybenzyl-diethylenetriaminepentaacetic acid; PLSR: partial least squares regression; SSM: statistical shape models.

Nowak et al. conducted a study analyzing how a deep transfer learning (DTL) method can identify liver cirrhosis in standard transverse T2-weighted MRI images with accuracy compared to the assessments made by two radiologists. The study used two CNNs which were trained on a large natural data set of images obtained from the ImageNet archive. Then the transfer learning method was applied: the pre-trained CNN was adapted to identify liver cirrhosis in T2-weighted MRI scans. The AI was tested on 713 MRI scans from patients, 553 with confirmed liver cirrhosis and 160 with no history of liver disease. The DTL analysis utilized a single-slice MRI image, taken at the level of the caudate lobe for each entry. Two separate processing pipelines were used to analyze the images. The first one consisted of images priorly processed through a segmentation network and the second one utilized unsegmented images. The accuracy with which the DTL analysis correctly identified the presence of liver cirrhosis on the testing images was 0.97 for the pre-segmented set and 0.95 for the unsegmented set [27].

In the study conducted by Kato et al., the goal was to assess if the finite difference method paired with an artificial neural network (ANN) could be useful in identifying fibrosis in various acquisitions of MRI images. The study included 52 patients who underwent partial hepatectomy surgery for various liver tumors. The results obtained by the algorithm were compared to assessments made by two radiologists, and the fibrotic stage was also determined by a pathologist through semi-quantitative methods. On the samples, 10 areas of interest were marked by a radiologist prior to analysis. The ANN calculated seven texture parameters for each of the pre-determined areas on the samples and then compiled a probability for the presence of fibrosis in the whole liver. The AI model proved to be superior to the radiologists' assessment, although no strong correlation between the radiologists' grading and the ANN's output could be established [28].

Hectors et al. created a DL algorithm based on gadoxetic acid-enhanced hepatobiliary phase (HBP) MRI in order to stage liver fibrosis. A secondary objective was to compare the diagnostic performance of DL vs. MRE. To reduce bias generated by the manual extraction of features and region of interest (ROI) placement as well as interobserver variability, it would be desired that DL models work fully automated. DL adopting CNNs can collect texture information in the initial convolutional layers, allowing picture texture analysis without the requirement for hand-crafted feature extraction. The group discovered that the algorithm performed well for predicting fibrosis severity with AUCs ranging from 0.77–0.91 for various fibrosis stages. Upon validation in different sets, the DL method may serve for noninvasive assessment of liver fibrosis without any need for extra MRI equipment, mainly because it had a similar performance compared to MRE [29].

Another MRI–DL technique combination which was recently introduced showed promising results in grading liver fibrosis after automatic segmentation of the liver. The method also uses a type of CNN for processing MRI Gadolinium ethoxybenzyl-diethylenetriaminepentaacetic acid (Gd-EOB-DTPA)-enhanced liver images from 121 livers pathologically confirmed as fibrotic or even cirrhotic (Ishak scores 0–6). It has been shown that CNNs with a U-shaped architecture are efficient at both segmenting organs and classifying them based on those segments. Because the model assigns an Ishak fibrosis score to each individual voxel, it is possible to make location-specific predictions about the amount of fibrosis. The approach functioned effectively, especially in situations where there was no fibrosis (Ishak 0) or cirrhosis (Ishak 6). Moderate fibrosis stages had a lower prediction rate, for which the authors suggest that the model's capacity could be improved by integrating alternative sequences, such as T2 or diffusion-weighted imaging (DWI) [30].

Soufi et al. implemented a statistical shape modeling (SSM) technique based on partial least squares regression (PLSR), which directly uses the fibrosis stage as data to comprehend the liver shape and calculate a PSLR score. This was further used on the test data set to predict the fibrosis stage associated with this score in contrast-enhanced MR images. The SSM based on PLSR showed locally detailed variations in addition to generally recognized differences associated with liver fibrosis, such as shrinking of the entire right lobe or growth of the enlarged left lobe. The anterior section of the right lobe shrinks, while the caudate lobe and posterior part of the right lobe increase. As future perspectives, this method can be deeper explored by integrating the PLSR scores with other image features reflecting liver parenchyma properties, for example DL models combining CNNs as well as physiological information, such as serum or blood parameters, to increase fibrosis classification accuracy [31].

3.3. Artificial Intelligence Techniques and Ultrasonography

The main studies analyzing the accuracy of AI algorithms in detecting liver fibrosis on ultrasonography images are illustrated in Table 3.

The study conducted by Brattain et al. focused on developing an automated framework aimed to assess fibrosis grades in Sheer Wave Elastography (SWE) samples. The algorithm was meant to assess the quality of the SWE image, to automatically select an area of interest, and to decide whether that area presents a lesser or greater stage of fibrosis than stage F2. The study utilized several AI methods, and the best results were obtained by using the CNN model, with a performance assessed through the area under the curve of 0.89 [32].

Other imaging studies are also combined with machine learning (ML), as in, for example, the study conducted by Li et al. in which multiparametric ultrasound features served as input data for multiple ML algorithms. The types of parameters that were measured consisted of ultrasound images, radiofrequency data, and contrast-enhanced micro-flow images focused on a 2 cm ROI from the sixth liver segment. All these acquisitions, together with the ML models, are described as ultrasomics—a clinical decision support system based on large amounts of data which can predict liver fibrosis staging, necroinflammatory activity, and steatosis degree. The models combining morphological and hemodynamic characteristics performed better. This discovery indicates that using multiparametric ultrasomics from various pathophysiological procedures might improve the effectiveness of the clinical decision support system. The authors conclude that multicentric, whole-liver studies should be considered to increase the robustness of the multiparameter ultrasomics analysis [33].

Table 3. Studies assessing artificial intelligence techniques and ultrasonography for the diagnosis of liver fibrosis.

First Author	Year	Total Number of Images	Diagnosis	Main Findings
Brattain et al. [32]	2018	3392	Liver fibrosis	A new method of diagnosis for liver fibrosis that is based on a single image per decision compared to previous methods which used 10 images per decision.
Li et al. [33]	2019	144	Chronic hepatitis B	Machine-learning-based analysis of ultrasonography images can help stage liver fibrosis.
Xie et al. [34]	2022	640	Chronic hepatitis B and cirrhosis	The GoogLeNet model shows promising results in terms of recognition of lesions and diagnosis.
Zhang et al. [35]	2012	239	Liver fibrosis or cirrhosis	The ANN model presented high sensitivity and specificity for the non-invasive diagnosis of liver fibrosis.
Lee et al. [36]	2020	13,608	Liver fibrosis	Deep convolutional neural network accurately classified the ultrasonography images for cirrhosis diagnosis.
Gatos et al. [37]	2017	126	chronic liver disease	Color information quantification, from SWE images, by machine-learning can dissociate between chronic liver disease and healthy patients.

ANN: artificial neural network.

Xie et al. used four network model structure schemes—AlexNet, VGG-16, VGG-19, and GoogLeNet—to find the most appropriate CNN model for ultrasound images of liver fibrosis analysis. Therefore, 640 samples in total from 780 individuals with cirrhosis and chronic hepatitis B were chosen for analysis. The GoogLeNet model was chosen as the best network model, because it performs recognition more accurately than other models. With a batch size of 32, a learning rate of 0.0005 as the parameter of the model, and a total of 10 iterations, the GoogLeNet model has the best classification and recognition effect in the analysis of ultrasound images of liver fibrosis and may eliminate the subjectivity of manual classification and increase the precision of assessing the severity of liver fibrosis, allowing for complete liver fibrosis prevention and therapy [34].

Zhang et al. looked to demonstrate, in their study, how an ANN may provide a duplex US-based non-invasive grading evaluation for hepatic fibrosis using data from 239 patients with different stages of liver fibrosis, with respect to cirrhosis. Five ultrasonographic measurements—the liver parenchymal, spleen thickness, hepatic vein waveform, hepatic artery pulsatile index (HAPI), and hepatic vein damping index (HVDI)—were chosen as the input neurons, because statistical analysis revealed a difference between the fibrosis group and the cirrhosis group in these five variables. This model can accurately identify liver cirrhosis when utilizing ultrasonography, according to certain predictive indices, including sensitivity, specificity, misdiagnosis rate (MR), and ROC curves for the ANN [35].

Using a total of 13,608 ultrasound scans from 3446 patients who had surgical resection, biopsy, or transient elastography, Lee et al. aimed to develop a CNN for METAVIR score prediction using B-mode ultrasound images. The AUC of the CNN was 0.866 for the classification of significant fibrosis (F2 or greater) in the test set, and for the classification of liver cirrhosis (F4), the algorithm achieved an AUC of 0.857. Most importantly, when utilizing US pictures to identify cirrhosis (F4), the CNN surpassed five radiologists. In the simulated US examination utilizing the test set, the CNN system had an AUC of 0.857, which was higher than that of each radiologist (AUC range, 0.656–0.816) [36].

Gatos et al., with the clinical data of 126 patients, used an algorithm based on ML and a stiffness value clustering to classify CLD using ultrasonic SWE imaging. Two radiologists' clinical evaluations produced accuracy results of 75.3% and 76.6%, as well as sensitivity/specificity results of 72.2/80.1 and 73.8/81.3, respectively, proving that, in identifying healthy people from CLD patients, the proposed system performed better than all clinical and automated investigations and expert radiologists [37].

3.4. Artificial Intelligence Techniques and Liver Biopsy

Table 4 illustrates the main findings of studies analyzing the efficiency of AI algorithms in detecting liver fibrosis on liver biopsies.

Table 4. Studies assessing artificial intelligence techniques and liver biopsy studies for the diagnosis of liver fibrosis.

First Author	Year	Total Number of Images	Diagnosis	Main Findings
Astbury et al. [38]	2021	20	Liver cirrhosis	Standardization between staining methods is still very important, as computational tools cannot yet normalize samples when performing analysis.
Sarvestany et al. [39]	2022	1703	Liver fibrosis	MLAs are able to help differentiate between patients with different prognoses concerning chronic liver disease.
Matalka et al. [40]	2006	260	Liver fibrosis	The automated quantification system differentiated between normal biopsies and samples with liver fibrosis, with an accuracy of 98.46%, and classified each sample with fibrosis according to the Ishak scoring system, with a precision of 94.69%.
Qiu et al. [41]	2020	369	Liver fibrosis	Radiomics analysis of liver images can accurately diagnose liver disease, resulting in a superior diagnosis tool compared to liver biopsy.
Wei et al. [42]	2019	141	Liver fibrosis	The multi-variable model developed can be useful for the evaluation of the clinical evolution of patients with chronic HBV-induced liver fibrosis.
Wang et al. [43]	2018	1990	Chronic hepatitis B	Deep learning Radiomics of elastography (DLRE) is useful for the non-invasive staging of liver fibrosis in patients infected with HBV.

MLAs: Machine learning algorithms; HBV: Hepatitis B virus.

Astbury et al. examined the effectiveness of a DL model with simple color space thresholding and human assessment in determining scar percentage in picrosirius red (PSR)-stained liver sections obtained from 20 cirrhotic explant livers. A quantitative evaluation of collagen or elastin throughout the entire region can be carried out using a color space threshold based on hue, saturation, and brightness (HSB). As opposed to HSB thresholding, computational approaches, particularly those based on AI, should allow the collection of data from liver biopsies while also minimizing the subjectivity inherent in the scoring process. Despite the issue seemingly favoring computational methods, there was significant residual inconsistency in the calculated scar percentage by the DL algorithm, and human observers consistently outperformed these methods. Because intra- and interlaboratory staining variation significantly reduces consistent PSR quantitative measurements using computer-aided methods and the section age may contribute to intra-laboratory variation if a standard timeframe between sectioning and staining is not respected, these findings suggest that quality control measures such as staining standardization and color adjustment will be necessary if AI-assisted scoring of stains is to be widely used [38].

Sarvestany et al. conducted a retrospective cohort study aimed to identify patients with liver fibrosis of any cause by using ML algorithms (MLAs). The study used 1703 liver biopsy specimens and associated demographic data and laboratory parameters provided by the Toronto Liver Clinic and McGill University Health Centre for testing the MLAs. The five validation sets comprised biopsies and data originating from the same health care facilities. Five standard MLAs as well as a combination of standard MLAs were used to differentiate between F0, F1, and F2 fibrosis stages regarded as one category and stages F3 and F4 considered as the other category. The ensemble of five MLAs proved superior to the other MLAs studied and also to other fibrosis detection methods that are not based on imaging techniques, such as APRI, FIB-4, or ENS, in identifying stages F3 and F4. The study claims that such MLAs could be used in the future for the screening of cirrhosis and advanced stage fibrosis [39].

The study conducted by Matalka et al. used an automated quantification system (AQS) to evaluate the degree of fibrosis in specimens of liver biopsy. The aim of the AQS was to identify the architecture of the fibrosis in tested samples through the recognition of textures and shapes that were representative of the fibrous expansion in the parenchyma. All images were pre-processed for clarity and brightness and segmented for better analysis of structural differences differentiating fibrosis stages. The AQS performed two different tasks: the first one being to differentiate between samples without fibrosis and fibrous samples of any stage and the second one to classify each fibrous sample to one of the six categories of the Ishak scoring system. The study included 260 samples, 50 without fibrosis and 210 with various Ishak stages of fibrosis, divided into a training and a testing set. The AQS differentiated non-fibrous samples from samples with varying degrees of fibrosis with an accuracy of 98.46%. Regarding the second stage of the AQS process, the accuracy for the testing lot was 94.69%. To further test the model, nine more samples were introduced in the algorithm, and the results obtained from the AQS were compared to those of two pathologists. The correlation between the AQS and the pathologists' results were 0.9648 and 0.9125, respectively, after correcting the overlapping of the 5th and 6th Ishak stages in the ASQ analysis [40].

Qiu et al. developed a radiomics model in order to accurately stage liver fibrosis and detect early-stage cirrhosis, using a feature extraction technique from the DWI-MRI images of 369 patients from a single hospital. A biopsy with histopathology interpretation was used as the standard reference, with 108 patients presenting with liver fibrosis and early-stage cirrhosis and 146 with a healthy liver. Two radiologists performed volume of interest (VOI) extraction from these MRI images [35]. For maximal accuracy, the research team compared two analysis plans, of which the most proficient one achieved an AUC of 0.973 (95% CI 0.946–1.000) for the training dataset and an AUC of 0.948 (95% CI 0.903–0.993) for the independent testing dataset used for validation. At the time, the ML-assisted DWI-MRI diagnostic tool demonstrated utility in assessing liver fibrosis staging, with the goal of eventually replacing invasive biopsy for this purpose [41].

Wei et al. conducted a prospective study in which an ANN was constructed in order to isolate and predict biomarkers for fibrosis reversal in 141 treatment-naïve HBV patients with fibrosis S2/S3 staging between two treatment groups [42]. One consisted of 2 years of Entecavir therapy, and the other was Entecavir alternating with Entecavir combined with pegylated interferon (Peg-IFN). Patients included in the study were assessed using serum biomarkers every 6 months and liver biopsies at baseline and after 1.5 years post-treatment. The dataset was randomly divided into a training (80% patients) and testing set (20% of patients) and detected AST (aspartate aminotransferase), PLT (platelet count), WBC (white blood cell), CHE (cholinesterase), LSM (liver stiffness measurement), ALT (alanine aminotransferase), and gender as statistically significant parameters for liver fibrosis reverse prediction, using cross-sectional validation for the ANN's performance. As a result, with a sensitivity and specificity of 83.1% and 85.2%, respectively, and an AUC of 0.809 in accurately classifying fibrosis with liver biopsy as the gold standard, these markers could constitute an accurate tool for predicting fibrosis reverse after antiviral therapy [42].

Wang et al. proposed a radiomics-based DL-algorithm for assessing liver fibrosis staging that was trained and validated with 1990 images from 398 patients of shear wave elastography and achieved an AUC of 0.97 for F4, 0.98 for $\geq$F3, and 0.85 for F2 [43]. Its performance was compared to that of conventional 2D-SWE and serum biomarkers (APRI model, using ASL, ALT, and FIB-4), using liver biopsy as a reference standard. The DL classifier performed better than 2D-SWE and biomarkers for all fibrosis types when more than one elastography image per patient was used as input, with the exception of F2 fibrosis, where the fibrosis heterogeneity is greater. There was no statistically significant difference between DLRE and 2D-SWE. The images were randomly, without overlap, divided into training (1330 images from 266 patients) and testing (660 images from 132 patients). The 2D-SWEs were manually cropped into an ROI, and that was used as the input layer of the DL. The DLRE's accuracy, as expected, increased with the number of ROI input images in the training set, up to three images, with no significant improvement in the AUC between three and five images [43].

This DL classifier represented a diagnostic efficacy of fibrosis staging similar to the histopathological interpretation and performed significantly better than conventional 2D elastography and biomarkers. Another valuable feature was the DLRE's diagnostic consistency when given data from various hospitals, suggesting the classifier's robustness. However, testing other ethnic groups could bring different results [43].

4. Discussion

Most studies assessing computer-aided diagnostic tools for fibrosis detection and staging need a reference standard to compare their accuracy with, namely, biopsy with histopathological interpretation. Different types of ML-algorithms have been used for maximal diagnostic accuracy, such as DL (CNN-based classifiers), support vector machines (SVM), automated quantification systems, and random forest classifiers. In most cases, model overfitting of feature selection was avoided by using independent validation sets [20,39,40,42], and/or other methods, such as the RELIEFF algorithm, bootstrapping, and k-fold cross-validation [21,42]. However, some studies with low AUCs and an appropriate population size for ML-algorithm performance should consider these methods for validation.

The AI's diagnostic performance was compared to radiologists' interpretation performance and other non-invasive tests that represent current fibrosis staging guidelines, such as aspartate aminotransferase-to-platelet ratio index (APRI), Fibrosis-4 score (FIB-4), and alpha-fetoprotein (AFP) [39,43], as well as imaging techniques, such as 2D elastography [44] and MRE [30], demonstrating the AI's diagnostic superiority. These comparisons are significant because, while AI-assisted tools may not be accurate enough to replace the gold standard, they may outperform other non-invasive alternatives.

Additionally, an inappropriate population study size could raise the error probability in the statistical analysis. Studies presenting such an issue would need a global database expansion [28,38,44] or merely regarding subgroups, such as additional data on cirrhotic patients [32]. Furthermore, while some studies used controls, other classifiers have been trained on unbalanced data with no control patients or in regard to cirrhosis and fibrosis patient distribution.

Different AI-assisted non-invasive techniques have achieved different diagnostic performances. While some studies showed high AUCs of 0.948 (95% CI 0.903–0.993) when using DWI-MRI images' features when extracting features from SWE for maximal classification accuracy [41], others had a low AUC only ranging from 0.72 to 0.77 for the classification of fibrosis stages F0 vs. F1-4 and moderate performance and stages F0-1 vs. F2-4, F0-2 vs. F3-4, and F0-3 vs. 4. This shows the level of influence on diagnosis accuracy that different types of image techniques have, with elastography being shown to be more prone to disease heterogeneity errors [45]. However, elastography diagnostic accuracy can be raised with the use of SVM [46,47] and DL.

On the same note, a systematic review concluded that AI-assisted ultrasonography of NAFLD showed the highest diagnostic performance of all AI-assisted tools for NAFLD or NASH diagnosis or fibrosis detection [48]. It yielded a sensitivity and specificity of 0.97 (95% CI: 0.91–0.99) and 0.98 (95% CI: 0.89–1.00), respectively, an AUC of 0.98, and low heterogeneity. The next highest in terms of diagnostic performance was the AI-supported clinical diagnosis of NAFLD, with a sensitivity and specificity of 0.75 (95% CI: 0.66–0.82) and 0.82 (95% CI: 0.74–0.88), respectively, and an AUC of 0.85 with a slightly higher degree of heterogeneity. AI-supported clinical data sets performed comparably to conventional TE and slightly lower than MRI. Consequently, the information gathered on patient admission could be used as a screening method for at-risk patients for NAFLD. On the other hand, AI-assisted diagnostic tools for NASH diagnosis and fibrosis staging achieved a sensitivity of 80% (95% CI: 0.75–0.85) and a specificity of 0.69 (95% CI: 0.53–0.82).

This integration of clinical features (e.g., BMI, laboratory markers, gender, and comorbidities) along with the non-invasive procedures as input to the AI classifier with great diagnostic results has been successfully achieved in other studies [33,39]. Radiomics feature selection in combination with ML algorithms has been used, with ROI or VOI selection from 2D-SWE and DWI-MRI images made by experienced radiologists [24,41,43].

AI-based systems can help overcome the limitations of non-invasive methods by providing a more accurate and reliable diagnosis and staging of liver fibrosis. By combining the technology used in NAFLD and liver cirrhosis automatic diagnosis, researchers can develop AI-based systems that can accurately diagnose and stage liver fibrosis. Moreover, with the increasing availability of electronic health records, AI-based systems can be used to identify patients at high risk of developing liver fibrosis and provide timely interventions to prevent disease progression [49].

A timely and accurate diagnosis of liver fibrosis is essential for avoiding poor prognosis. However, liver biopsy, the current gold standard for diagnosis, is invasive and costly, with limited accuracy due to sampling error and intra- and interobserver agreement. Hence, the ability to assess fibrosis staging, steatosis, and inflammation with non-invasive techniques is crucial. Several studies have shown that ML algorithms can accurately diagnose fibrosis staging, with DL (CNN-based classifiers), SVM, and random forest classifiers achieving high accuracy. Although these AI-assisted tools may not replace liver biopsy, they can outperform other non-invasive alternatives, such as biomarkers and imaging techniques. AI-assisted non-invasive techniques have immense potential in accurately diagnosing liver fibrosis, allowing for timely risk factor modification and appropriate treatment. Researchers must expand the global database and validate the models using independent validation sets, additional data on controls, and increase the population study size to reduce the error probability in statistical analysis.

Due to the high prevalence of CLD, together with the lack of an adequate non-invasive diagnosis tests that would try to replace the liver biopsy, the subject of implementing AI algorithms into the diagnosis and management of liver fibrosis is of great importance. In this systematic review, the main imaging and diagnosis methods of liver fibrosis have been included, namely liver ultrasound, CT, MRI, and liver biopsy.

Nevertheless, the findings of the previously mentioned studies need to be confirmed through clinical trials. However, many studies had discrepancies regarding methodology, design, and outcomes. For this reason, international collaboration on AI systems can improve outcomes and provide a useful tool to human radiologists.

5. Conclusions

The current systematic review provides a comprehensive analysis of the performance of AI systems in diagnosing liver fibrosis. Automatic diagnosis, staging, and risk stratification for liver fibrosis is currently possible considering the accuracy, sensibility, and specificity of AI systems, which is comparable to human experts.

Author Contributions: Conceptualization, S.L.P., A.I. and L.D.; methodology, S.L.P., A.I. and A.M.P.; writing—original draft preparation, S.L.P., M.O.D., R.B., M.A.M., V.D.B., M.B. and L.D.; writing—review and editing, C.P., A.B., D.I.D. and L.A.; supervision, S.L.P., L.A. and L.D. All authors have read and agreed to the published version of the manuscript.

Funding: This research received no external funding.

Data Availability Statement: Not applicable.

Conflicts of Interest: The authors declare no conflict of interest.

References

1. Asrani, S.K.; Devarbhavi, H.; Eaton, J.; Kamath, P.S. Burden of liver diseases in the world. *J. Hepatol.* **2019**, *70*, 151–171. [CrossRef] [PubMed]
2. Marcellin, P.; Kutala, B.K. Liver diseases: A major, neglected global public problem requiring urgent actions and large-scale screening. *Liver Int.* **2018**, *38*, 2–6. [CrossRef] [PubMed]
3. European Association for the Study of the Liver. EASL Clinical Practice Guidelines on non-invasive tests for evaluation of liver disease severity and prognosis—2021 update. *J. Hepatol.* **2021**, *75*, 659–689. [CrossRef] [PubMed]
4. Parola, M.; Pinzani, M. Liver fibrosis: Pathophysiology, pathogenetic targets and clinical issues. *Mol. Asp. Med.* **2019**, *65*, 37–55. [CrossRef]
5. Lambrecht, J.; van Grunsven, L.A.; Tacke, F. Current and emerging pharmacotherapeutic interventions for the treatment of liver fibrosis. *Expert Opin. Pharm.* **2020**, *21*, 1637–1650. [CrossRef]
6. Wang, F.D.; Zhou, J.; Chen, E.Q. Molecular Mechanisms and Potential New Therapeutic Drugs for Liver Fibrosis. *Front. Pharm.* **2022**, *13*, 787748. [CrossRef]
7. Lai, M.; Afdhal, N.H. Liver fibrosis determination. *Gastroenterol. Clin. N. Am.* **2019**, *48*, 281–289. [CrossRef]
8. Friedman, S.L.; Pinzani, M. Hepatic Fibrosis 2022: Unmet Needs and a Blueprint for the Future. *Pathology* **2022**, *75*, 473–488. [CrossRef]
9. Dana, J.; Venkatasami, A.; Saviano, A.; Lupberger, J.; Hoshida, Y.; Vilgrain, V.; Nahon, P.; Reinhold, C.; Gallix, B.; Baumert, T.F. Conventional and artificial intelligence-based imaging for biomarker discovery in chronic liver disease. *Hepatol. Int.* **2022**, *16*, 509–522. [CrossRef]
10. Marozas, M.; Zykus, R.; Sakalauskas, A.; Kupčinskas, L.; Lukoševičius, A. Noninvasive Evaluation of Portal Hypertension Using a Supervised Learning Technique. *J. Healthc. Eng.* **2017**, *2017*, 6183714. [CrossRef]
11. Bayani, A.; Hosseini, A.; Asadi, F.; Hatami, B.; Kavousi, K.; Aria, M.; Zali, M.R. Identifying predictors of varices grading in patients with cirrhosis using ensemble learning. *Clin. Chem. Lab. Med.* **2022**, *60*, 1938–1945. [CrossRef] [PubMed]
12. Kim, H.Y.; Lampertico, P.; Nam, J.Y.; Lee, H.C.; Kim, S.U.; Sinn, D.H.; Seo, Y.S.; Lee, H.A.; Park, S.Y.; Lim, Y.S.; et al. An artificial intelligence model to predict hepatocellular carcinoma risk in Korean and Caucasian patients with chronic hepatitis B. *J. Hepatol.* **2022**, *76*, 311–318. [CrossRef] [PubMed]
13. Popa, S.L.; Grad, S.; Chiarioni, G.; Masier, A.; Peserico, G.; Brata, V.D.; Dumitrascu, D.I.; Fantin, A. Applications of Artificial Intelligence in the Automatic Diagnosis of Focal Liver Lesions: A Systematic Review. *J. Gastrointest. Liver Dis.* **2023**, *32*, 77–85. [CrossRef] [PubMed]
14. Xu, X.; Zhang, H.-L.; Liu, Q.-P.; Sun, S.-W.; Zhang, J.; Zhu, F.-P.; Yang, G.; Yan, X.; Zhang, Y.-D.; Liu, X.-S. Radiomic analysis of contrast-enhanced CT predicts microvascular invasion and outcome in hepatocellular carcinoma. *J. Hepatol.* **2019**, *70*, 1133–1144. [CrossRef]
15. Abajian, A.; Murali, N.; Savic, L.J.; Laage-Gaupp, F.M.; Nezami, N.; Duncan, J.S.; Schlachter, T.; Lin, M.; Geschwind, J.-F.; Chapiro, J. Predicting treatment response to intra-arterial therapies for hepatocellular carcinoma with the use of supervised machine learning-an artificial intelligence concept. *J. Vasc. Interv. Radiol.* **2018**, *29*, 850–857.e1. [CrossRef] [PubMed]
16. Page, M.J.; McKenzie, J.E.; Bossuyt, P.M.; Boutron, I.; Hoffmann, T.C.; Mulrow, C.D.; Shamseer, L.; Tetzlaff, J.M.; Akl, E.A.; Brennan, S.E.; et al. The PRISMA 2020 statement: An updated guideline for reporting systematic reviews. *BMJ* **2021**, *372*, n71. [CrossRef]
17. Lurie, Y.; Webb, M.; Cytter-Kuint, R.; Shteingart, S.; Lederkremer, G.Z. Non-invasive diagnosis of liver fibrosis and cirrhosis. *World J. Gastroenterol.* **2015**, *21*, 11567–11583. [CrossRef]
18. Tsochatzis, E.A.; Bosch, J.; Burroughs, A.K. Liver cirrhosis. *Lancet* **2014**, *383*, 1749–1761. [CrossRef]
19. Li, L.; Duan, M.; Chen, W.; Jiang, A.; Li, X.; Yang, J.; Li, Z. The spleen in liver cirrhosis: Revisiting an old enemy with novel targets. *J. Transl. Med.* **2017**, *15*, 111. [CrossRef]
20. Yasaka, K.; Akai, H.; Kunimatsu, A.; Abe, O.; Kiryu, S. Deep learning for staging liver fibrosis on CT: A pilot study. *Eur. Radiol.* **2018**, *28*, 4578–4585. [CrossRef]
21. Li, Q.; Yu, B.; Tian, X.; Cui, X.; Zhang, R.; Guo, Q. Deep residual nets model for staging liver fibrosis on plain CT images. *Int. J. CARS* **2020**, *5*, 1399–1406. [CrossRef] [PubMed]
22. Choi, K.J.; Jang, J.K.; Lee, S.S.; Sung, Y.S.; Shim, W.H.; Kim, H.S.; Yun, J.; Choi, J.-Y.; Lee, Y.; Kang, B.-K.; et al. Development and Validation of a Deep Learning System for Staging Liver Fibrosis by Using Contrast Agent-enhanced CT Images in the Liver. *Radiology* **2018**, *289*, 688–697. [CrossRef] [PubMed]
23. Yin, Y.; Yakar, D.; Dierckx, R.A.J.O.; Mouridsen, K.B.; Kwee, T.C.; de Haas, R.J. Liver fibrosis staging by deep learning: A visual-based explanation of diagnostic decisions of the model. *Eur. Radiol.* **2021**, *31*, 9620–9627. [CrossRef] [PubMed]
24. Yin, Y.; Yakar, D.; Dierckx, R.A.J.O.; Mouridsen, K.B.; Kwee, T.C.; de Haas, R.J. Combining Hepatic and Splenic CT Radiomic Features Improves Radiomic Analysis Performance for Liver Fibrosis Staging. *Diagnostics* **2022**, *12*, 550. [CrossRef]
25. Budai, B.K.; Tóth, A.; Borsos, P.; Frank, V.G.; Shariati, S.; Fejér, B.; Folhoffer, A.; Szalay, F.; Bérczi, V.; Kaposi, P.N. Three-dimensional CT texture analysis of anatomic liver segments can differentiate between low-grade and high-grade fibrosis. *BMC Med. Imaging* **2020**, *20*, 108. [CrossRef]

26. Wu, L.; Ning, B.; Yang, J.; Chen, Y.; Zhang, C.; Yan, Y. Diagnosis of Liver Cirrhosis and Liver Fibrosis by Artificial Intelligence Algorithm-Based Multislice Spiral Computed Tomography. *Comput. Math. Methods Med.* **2022**, *2022*, 1217003. [CrossRef]
27. Nowak, S.; Mesropyan, N.; Faron, A.; Block, W.; Reuter, M.; Attenberger, U.I.; Luetkens, J.A.; Sprinkart, A.M. Detection of liver cirrhosis in standard T2-weighted MRI using deep transfer learning. *Eur. Radiol.* **2021**, *31*, 8807–8815. [CrossRef]
28. Kato, H.; Kanematsu, M.; Zhang, X.; Saio, M.; Kondo, H.; Goshima, S.; Fujita, H. Computer-Aided Diagnosis of Hepatic Fibrosis: Preliminary Evaluation of MRI Texture Analysis Using the Finite Difference Method and an Artificial Neural Network. *Am. J. Roentgenol.* **2007**, *189*, 117–122. [CrossRef]
29. Hectors, S.J.; Kennedy, P.; Huang, K.H.; Stocker, D.; Carbonell, G.; Greenspan, H.; Friedman, S.; Taouli, B. Fully automated prediction of liver fibrosis using deep learning analysis of gadoxetic acid–enhanced MRI. *Eur. Radiol.* **2021**, *31*, 3805–3814. [CrossRef]
30. Strotzer, Q.D.; Winther, H.; Utpatel, K.; Scheiter, A.; Fellner, C.; Doppler, M.C.; Ringe, K.I.; Raab, F.; Haimerl, M.; Uller, W.; et al. Application of A U-Net for Map-like Segmentation and Classification of Discontinuous Fibrosis Distribution in Gd-EOB-DTPA-Enhanced Liver MRI. *Diagnostics* **2022**, *12*, 1938. [CrossRef]
31. Soufi, M.; Otake, Y.; Hori, M.; Moriguchi, K.; Imai, Y.; Sawai, Y.; Ota, T.; Tomiyama, N.; Sato, Y. Liver shape analysis using partial least squares regression-based statistical shape model: Application for understanding and staging of liver fibrosis. *Int. J. CARS* **2019**, *14*, 2083–2093. [CrossRef] [PubMed]
32. Brattain, L.J.; Telfer, B.A.; Dhyani, M.; Grajo, J.R.; Samir, A.E. Objective liver fibrosis estimation from shear wave elastography. *Annu. Int. Conf. IEEE Eng. Med. Biol. Soc.* **2018**, *2018*, 1–5. [CrossRef] [PubMed]
33. Li, W.; Huang, Y.; Zhuang, B.W.; Liu, G.J.; Hu, H.T.; Li, X.; Liang, J.-Y.; Wang, Z.; Huang, X.-W.; Zhang, C.-Q.; et al. Multiparametric ultrasomics of significant liver fibrosis: A machine learning-based analysis. *Eur. Radiol.* **2019**, *29*, 1496–1506. [CrossRef]
34. Xie, Y.; Chen, S.; Jia, D.; Li, B.; Zheng, Y.; Yu, X. Artificial Intelligence-Based Feature Analysis of Ultrasound Images of Liver Fibrosis. *Comput. Intell. Neurosci.* **2022**, *2022*, 2859987. [CrossRef] [PubMed]
35. Zhang, L.; Li, Q.Y.; Duan, Y.Y.; Yan, G.Z.; Yang, Y.L.; Yang, R.J. Artificial neural network aided non-invasive grading evaluation of hepatic fibrosis by duplex ultrasonography. *BMC Med. Inform. Decis. Mak.* **2012**, *12*, 55. [CrossRef]
36. Lee, J.H.; Joo, I.; Kang, T.W.; Paik, Y.H.; Sinn, D.H.; Ha, S.Y.; Kim, K.; Choi, C.; Lee, G.; Yi, J.; et al. Deep learning with ultrasonography: Automated classification of liver fibrosis using a deep convolutional neural network. *Eur. Radiol.* **2020**, *30*, 1264–1273. [CrossRef]
37. Gatos, I.; Tsantis, S.; Spiliopoulos, S.; Karnabatidis, D.; Theotokas, I.; Zoumpoulis, P.; Loupas, T.; Hazle, J.D.; Kagadis, G.C. A Machine-Learning Algorithm Toward Color Analysis for Chronic Liver Disease Classification, Employing Ultrasound Shear Wave Elastography. *Ultrasound Med. Biol.* **2017**, *43*, 1797–1810. [CrossRef]
38. Astbury, S.; Grove, J.I.; Dorward, D.A.; Guha, I.N.; Fallowfield, J.A.; Kendall, T.J. Reliable computational quantification of liver fibrosis is compromised by inherent staining variation. *J. Pathol. Clin. Res.* **2021**, *7*, 471–481. [CrossRef]
39. Sarvestany, S.S.; Kwong, J.C.; Azhie, A.; Dong, V.; Cerocchi, O.; Ali, A.F.; Karnam, R.S.; Kuriry, H.; Shengir, M.; Candido, E.; et al. Development and validation of an ensemble machine learning framework for detection of all-cause advanced hepatic fibrosis: A retrospective cohort study. *Lancet Digit. Health* **2022**, *4*, e188–e199. [CrossRef]
40. Matalka, I.I.; Al-Jarrah, O.M.; Manasrah, T.M. Quantitative assessment of liver fibrosis: A novel automated image analysis method. *Liver Int.* **2006**, *26*, 1054–1064. [CrossRef]
41. Qiu, Q.T.; Zhang, J.; Duan, J.H.; Wu, S.Z.; Ding, J.L.; Yin, Y. Development and validation of radiomics model built by incorporating machine learning for identifying liver fibrosis and early-stage cirrhosis. *Chin. Med. J.* **2020**, *133*, 2653–2659. [CrossRef] [PubMed]
42. Wei, W.; Wu, X.; Zhou, J.; Sun, Y.; Kong, Y.; Yang, X. Noninvasive Evaluation of Liver Fibrosis Reverse Using Artificial Neural Network Model for Chronic Hepatitis B Patients. *Comput. Math. Methods Med.* **2019**, *2019*, 7239780. [CrossRef] [PubMed]
43. Wang, K.; Lu, X.; Zhou, H.; Gao, Y.; Zheng, J.; Tong, M.; Wu, C.; Liu, C.; Huang, L.; Jiang, T.; et al. Deep learning Radiomics of shear wave elastography significantly improved diagnostic performance for assessing liver fibrosis in chronic hepatitis B: A prospective multicentre study. *Gut* **2019**, *68*, 729–741. [CrossRef]
44. Eslam, M.; Newsome, P.N.; Sarin, S.K.; Anstee, Q.M.; Targher, G.; Romero-Gomez, M.; Zelber-Sagi, S.; Wong, V.W.-S.; Dufour, J.-F.; Schattenberg, J.M.; et al. A new definition for metabolic dysfunction-associated fatty liver disease: An international expert consensus statement. *J. Hepatol.* **2020**, *73*, 202–209. [CrossRef] [PubMed]
45. Lefebvre, T.; Wartelle-Bladou, C.; Wong, P.; Sebastiani, G.; Giard, J.M.; Castel, H.; Murphy-Lavallée, J.; Olivié, D.; Ilinca, A.; Sylvestre, M.-P.; et al. Prospective comparison of transient, point shear wave, and magnetic resonance elastography for staging liver fibrosis. *Eur. Radiol.* **2019**, *29*, 6477–6488. [CrossRef]
46. Durot, I.; Akhbardeh, A.; Sagreiya, H.; Loening, A.M.; Rubin, D.L. A New Multimodel Machine Learning Framework to Improve Hepatic Fibrosis Grading Using Ultrasound Elastography Systems from Different Vendors. *Ultrasound Med. Biol.* **2020**, *46*, 26–33. [CrossRef] [PubMed]
47. Kagadis, G.C.; Drazinos, P.; Gatos, I.; Tsantis, S.; Papadimitroulas, P.; Spiliopoulos, S.; Karnabatidis, D.; Theotokas, I.; Zoumpoulis, P.; Hazle, J.D. Deep learning networks on chronic liver disease assessment with fine-tuning of shear wave elastography image sequences. *Phys. Med. Biol.* **2020**, *65*, 215027. [CrossRef] [PubMed]

48. Decharatanachart, P.; Chaiteerakij, R.; Tiyarattanachai, T.; Treeprasertsuk, S. Application of artificial intelligence in non-alcoholic fatty liver disease and liver fibrosis: A systematic review and meta-analysis. *Therap. Adv. Gastroenterol.* **2021**, *14*, 17562848211062807. [CrossRef]
49. Popa, S.L.; Ismaiel, A.; Cristina, P.; Cristina, M.; Chiarioni, G.; David, L.; Dumitrascu, D.L. Non-Alcoholic Fatty Liver Disease: Implementing Complete Automated Diagnosis and Staging. A Systematic Review. *Diagnostics* **2021**, *11*, 1078. [CrossRef]

Disclaimer/Publisher's Note: The statements, opinions and data contained in all publications are solely those of the individual author(s) and contributor(s) and not of MDPI and/or the editor(s). MDPI and/or the editor(s) disclaim responsibility for any injury to people or property resulting from any ideas, methods, instructions or products referred to in the content.

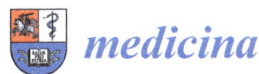

Case Report

Orthotopic Liver Transplantation of a SARS-CoV-2 Negative Recipient from a Positive Donor: The Border between Uncertainty and Necessity in a Pandemic Era- Case Report and Overview of the Literature

Gabriela Droc [1,2,†], Cristina Martac [1,†], Cristina Georgiana Buzatu [1], Miruna Jipa [1], Maria Daniela Punga [1] and Sebastian Isac [1,3,*]

1. Department of Anesthesiology and Intensive Care I, 'Fundeni' Clinical Institute, 022328 Bucharest, Romania; gabriela.droc@umfcd.ro (G.D.); christtina_martac@yahoo.com (C.M.); cristina.buzatu944@gmail.com (C.G.B.); mirunaa.jipa@gmail.com (M.J.); pungadaniela@yahoo.com (M.D.P.)
2. Department of Anesthesiology and Intensive Care I, Carol Davila University of Medicine and Pharmacy, 020021 Bucharest, Romania
3. Department of Physiology, Faculty of Medicine, Carol Davila University of Medicine and Pharmacy, 020021 Bucharest, Romania
* Correspondence: sebastian.isac@umfcd.ro
† These authors contributed equally to this work.

Abstract: (1) *Introduction*: Liver transplantation represents the gold-standard therapy in eligible patients with acute liver failure or end-stage liver disease. The COVID-19 pandemic dramatically affected the transplantation landscape by reducing patients' addressability to specialized healthcare facilities. Since evidence-based acceptance guidelines for non-lung solid organ transplantation from SARS-CoV-2 positive donors are lacking, and the risk of bloodstream-related transmission of the disease is debatable, liver transplantation from SARS-CoV-2 positive donors could be lifesaving, even if long-term interactions are unpredictable. The aim of this case report is to highlight the relevance of performing liver transplantation from SARS-CoV-2 positive donors to negative recipients by emphasizing the perioperative care and short-term outcome. (2) *Case presentation*: A 20-year-old female patient underwent orthotropic liver transplantation for Child-Pugh C liver cirrhosis secondary to overlap syndrome, from a SARS-CoV-2 positive brain death donor. The patient was not infected nor vaccinated against SARS-CoV-2, and the titer of neutralizing antibodies against the spike protein was negative. The liver transplantation was performed with no significant complications. As immunosuppression therapy, the patient received 20 mg basiliximab (Novartis Farmacéutica S.A., Barcelona, Spain) and 500 mg methylprednisolone (Pfizer Manufacturing Belgium N.V, Puurs, Belgium) intraoperatively. Considering the risk of non-aerogene-related SARS-CoV-2 reactivation syndrome, the patient received remdesivir 200 mg (Gilead Sciences Ireland UC, Carrigtohill County Cork, Ireland) in the neo-hepatic stage, which was continued with 100 mg/day for 5 days. The postoperative immunosuppression therapy consisted of tacrolimus (Astellas Ireland Co., Ltd., Killorglin, County Kerry, Ireland) and mycophenolate mofetil (Roche România S.R.L, Bucharest, Romania) according to the local protocol. Despite the persistent negative PCR results for SARS-CoV-2 in the upper airway tract, the blood titer of neutralizing antibodies turned out positive on postoperative day 7. The patient had a favorable outcome, and she was discharged from the ICU facility seven days later. (3) *Conclusions*: We illustrated a case of liver transplantation of a SARS-CoV-2 negative recipient, whose donor was SARS-CoV-2 positive, performed in a tertiary, university-affiliated national center of liver surgery, with a good outcome, in order to raise the medical community awareness on the acceptance limits in the case of COVID-19 incompatibility for non-lung solid organs transplantation procedures.

Keywords: liver transplantation; SARS-CoV-2 positive donor; liver surgery; immunosuppression therapy

Citation: Droc, G.; Martac, C.; Buzatu, C.G.; Jipa, M.; Punga, M.D.; Isac, S. Orthotopic Liver Transplantation of a SARS-CoV-2 Negative Recipient from a Positive Donor: The Border between Uncertainty and Necessity in a Pandemic Era- Case Report and Overview of the Literature. *Medicina* **2023**, *59*, 836. https://doi.org/10.3390/medicina59050836

Academic Editor: Jai Young Cho

Received: 14 March 2023
Revised: 19 April 2023
Accepted: 24 April 2023
Published: 26 April 2023

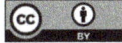

Copyright: © 2023 by the authors. Licensee MDPI, Basel, Switzerland. This article is an open access article distributed under the terms and conditions of the Creative Commons Attribution (CC BY) license (https:// creativecommons.org/licenses/by/ 4.0/).

1. Introduction

Liver transplantation represents, nowadays, the standard of care for patients with end-stage liver disease or acute liver failure. The main causes for developing liver cirrhosis are alcohol abuse, chronic viral hepatitis, autoimmune hepatitis, primary biliary cholangitis, cryptogenic hepatitis, overlap syndrome, or Wilson disease [1]. The leading cause of liver cirrhosis depends on country-related socio-economic factors; in developing countries, the main cause is chronic hepatitis, while alcohol abuse represents the main cause in industrialized countries [1].

Due to the COVID-19 pandemic, the addressability of patients with chronic conditions, including various liver pathologies, to healthcare providers decreased while their conditions worsened [2]. The severe acute respiratory syndrome coronavirus type 2 (SARS-CoV-2) has caused millions of victims worldwide since its outbreak in 2020 not only from the virus itself but also from the lack of appropriate treatment for their chronic diseases [3,4]. Thus, in the context of a preexisting worldwide donor crisis, and despite various national strategies, the pandemic affected, even more, the organ donation process, in the absence of acceptance patterns [5].

As the COVID-19 pandemic continued, major abdominal surgeries, including liver transplantation suffered a delay due to the need to find appropriate SARS-CoV-2 negative donors [6]. Data from the literature points out that cirrhotic patients or patients with advanced liver disease are prone to complications and death in this pandemic context [7]. Moreover, COVID-19 acts as a systemic disease, as it affects the lungs, kidneys, heart, brain, and liver [8,9]. The gastrointestinal tract and liver represent also important features of the disease [8]. Due to its prolonged shedding from the gastrointestinal tract, as stool samples from symptomatic and even asymptomatic patients have shown, the virus could reach through portal circulation in the liver [10,11]. Hepatic cell injury could result from either a direct viral infection, the antiviral drugs cytotoxicity, or the inflammatory response of the liver immune system [12].

Consequently, liver transplant recipients could have an even higher morbidity risk because of their fragile immune state and particular liver-specific tropism of the virus. The data from the literature revealed, however, conflicting results [13,14]. We have also previously shown that patients infected with SARS-CoV-2 following the liver transplantation surgery had good outcomes, and the survival rate was the same as for those without COVID-19 [15].

The immunosuppression therapy, following liver transplantation, involves a combination of drugs like corticosteroids, calcineurin inhibitors (CNI) (cyclosporine or tacrolimus), and antiproliferative agents (mycophenolate mofetil—MMF) according to local guidelines [16]. Tacrolimus could offer protection and lower mortality in SARS-CoV-2-positive liver recipients [17,18].

Even if the lungs represent the main transmission gateway of the SARS-CoV-2 virus, the uncertainty of infection through non-lung solid organ transplantation procedures remains [19]. The persistence of viral particles in the blood and endothelium could influence the decision to exclude SARS-CoV-2-positive donors from the non-lung solid organ transplantation [20].

Since evidence-based acceptance guidelines for non-lung solid organ transplantation from SARS-CoV-2-positive donors are lacking, and the risk of bloodstream-related transmission of the disease is debatable, some specialized surgery centers perform transplantation surgery using solid organs from SARS-CoV-2-positive donors [21–24].

This case report aims to highlight the relevance of performing liver transplantation from a SARS-CoV-2-positive donor to a negative recipient by presenting the perioperative care and outcome. Furthermore, this case should raise the clinician's awareness in extending the pool of eligible liver donors in order to include those with present COVID-19 disease who check all the other mandatory requests.

2. Case Presentation

A 20-year-old female patient, 65 kg, 171 cm, underwent orthotopic liver transplantation for Child-Pugh C liver cirrhosis secondary to overlap syndrome from a SARS-CoV-2-positive donor.

The donor was a 16-year-old female patient, a victim of a car accident that, due to severe traumatic brain damage, was declared brain dead 48 h after admission. No other chronic condition was observed in her medical records. The vaccination status against SARS-CoV-2 was unknown. Furthermore, the donor did not show any pulmonary complications during the ICU stay, despite the positive PCR test for SARS-CoV-2 from the upper airway tract at admission. Since all criteria for organ harvesting were met, the medical team proceeded without any additional blood sampling in accordance with the national guidelines for solid organ transplantation.

The recipient's preoperative model for end-stage liver disease (MELD) score was 17 points. The anamnesis revealed that the patient was not vaccinated for SARS-CoV-2, nor did she get the disease. The titer of SARS-CoV-2 neutralizing antibodies against the spike protein was undetectable before transplantation, as was the PCR test from the upper airway tract. Her medical records revealed an episode of upper digestive hemorrhage due to variceal rupture one year before surgery.

The preoperative blood sample analysis revealed cirrhosis-related pancytopenia (mild leucopenia, moderate normochromic and normocytic anemia, moderate thrombocytopenia), cirrhosis-specific coagulopathy (International Normalized Ratio of 1.95, an activated partial thromboplastin time of 62.7 s, normal range 23–36 s, prothrombin time of 25 s, normal range 10.4–14.3 s, and fibrinogen levels of 154 mg/de, normal range 200–400 mg/dL). Biochemical results revealed elevated aspartate aminotransferase (160 U/L, normal range 0–34 U/L) and cholestasis (total bilirubin of 2 mg/dL, normal range 0.1–1.2 mg/dL, alkaline phosphatase of 323 U/L, normal range 43–132 U/L and gamma-glutamic transferase of 81 U/L, normal range 0–38 U/L). The preoperative chest X-ray revealed no structural changes (Figure 1).

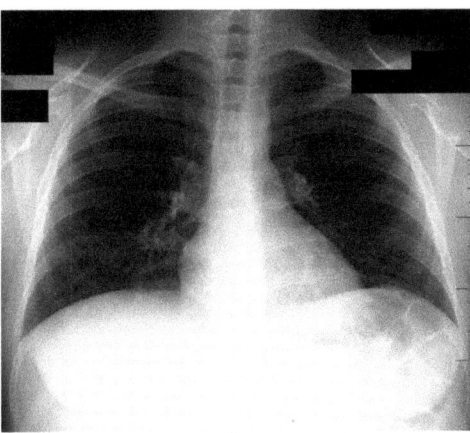

Figure 1. Chest X-ray before surgery (anteroposterior view).

Since the donor did not manifest any gastrointestinal symptoms related to a possible SARS-CoV-2 infection, no targeted liver biopsy was performed.

The patient underwent standard intravenous induction using fentanyl (Chiesi Pharmaceuticals GmbH, Wien, Austria), propofol (Fresenius Kabi GmbH, Graz, Austria), and succinylcholine (Takeda Austria GmbH) in accordance with the local guidelines. General anesthesia was maintained with sevoflurane (Abbvie Deutschland GmbH & Co., Ludwigshafen, Germany), fentanyl, and rocuronium (N.V. Organon, Oss, Holland). The respiratory and hemodynamically parameters were monitored continuously during the procedure [25]. The urine output was recorded hourly while the hemostasis and metabolic changes were monitored and corrected intermittently, at the discretion of the clinician, using thromboelastometry and blood–gas analysis.

Overall, the total fluid output consisted of 8000 mL ascites, 6000 mL blood loss, and 3100 mL urine, which was balanced with crystalloid infusion and albumin solution. The anhepatic phase lasted for 20 min. As primary prophylaxis against acute organ rejection syndrome, the patient received 20 mg basiliximab (Novartis Farmacéutica S.A., Barcelona, Spain) and 500 mg methylprednisolone (Pfizer Manufacturing Belgium N.V, Puurs, Belgium) intraoperatively. Considering the risk of lung-independent SARS-CoV-2 reactivation, the patient received antiviral therapy with remdesivir 200 mg/day (Gilead Sciences Ireland UC, Carrigtohill County Cork, Ireland) immediately after graft reperfusion (in the neo-hepatic stage).

Further, in the ICU, immunosuppression was maintained with tacrolimus (Astellas Ireland Co., Ltd. Killorglin, County Kerry, Ireland) and mycophenolate mofetil (Roche România S.R.L, Bucharest, Romania) at doses guided by daily tacrolinemia and blood sample analysis. A second dose of basiliximab (Novartis Farmacéutica S.A., Barcelona, Spain) was administered on the fourth postoperative day, in accordance with the local protocol. Further, the antiviral therapy with remdesivir 100 mg daily was maintained for 5 days.

On the first postoperative day, the patient was weaned from the ventilator and repeated SARS-CoV-2 PCR test from the upper airway tract turned out negative. Additionally, on postoperative day 7, the titer of neutralizing antibodies against the spike protein was 1442 U/mL. The chest X-ray showed no structural changes (Figure 2).

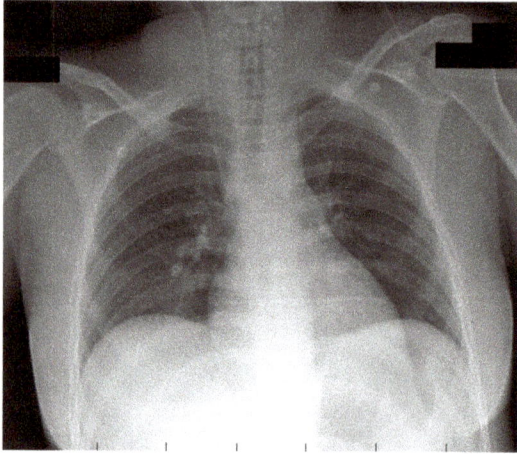

Figure 2. Chest X-ray seven days after surgery (anteroposterior view).

As a differential diagnosis of the presence of postoperative neutralizing antibodies against the spike protein, we considered the passive immunity, once the new vascular liver anastomosis was made, or a non-lung-related SARS-CoV-2 reactivation. Since no other symptoms occurred, additional SARS-CoV-2-specific immunologic testing or liver biopsy were not needed.

The patient had a favorable postoperative outcome, without any clinical or biological signs of SARS-CoV-2 infection. She was discharged from the ICU facility seven days later.

3. Discussion

The decision to recover organs from donors with active COVID-19 should evaluate the risk of virus transmission, severe COVID-19 in an immunosuppressed patient, the recipient's mortality risk, and long-term allograft outcome. These risks must be balanced against the life-saving benefit of a liver transplant in patients with end-stage liver disease since no other evidence-based recommendations state against their use. Our patient was a young patient with no other severe associated comorbidity, which had a good outcome after surgery and no short-term COVID-19-related complications.

Moreover, the patient was not vaccinated against SARS-CoV-2 prior to surgery, which raises an ethical issue regarding the importance of preoperative immunization against SARS-CoV-2 in this pandemic milieu. Sufficient data highlights the need for preoperative immunization since postoperative immunosuppression could exacerbate any infectious disease, including COVID-19 [26]. Kates et al. analyzed ethically two perspectives of SARS-CoV-2 vaccination for transplant candidates: the mandatory vaccination for recipients in the light of a potential increase in the number of SARS-CoV-2-positive donors and the optional vaccination [26]. Mandatory vaccination could constrain patients' autonomy, while the optional vaccination programs should be enforced with valid strategies to increase the patient's acceptance for vaccination, time-dependent on the organ availability. Since no further isolation strategies are used in most countries worldwide, immunization approaches should be prioritized and regulated.

The predominant mechanism of transmission is contact with droplets of respiratory secretions from an infectious individual- aerosol transmission. Angiotensin-converting enzyme 2 (ACE2-R) is the receptor for SARS-CoV-2, which is expressed not only in the lung but also in the liver [12]. Since the virus can be detected in specimens from other sites, other transmission mechanisms must be considered. According to Jayalakshmi Vallamkondu et al., the entry of SARS-CoV-2 into host cells is mediated by the interaction between the spike proteins and Angiotensin-Converting Enzyme-2 (ACE-2) receptors causing endocytic entry of the virus [27]. ACE 2 receptor is strongly expressed in the liver (liver cells, bile duct cells, liver endothelial cells), but its presence alone does not predict organ infection.

According to H. Y. Lei et al., SARS-CoV-2 particles could be detected in liver tissue, using the RT-PCR technique [12]. Additionally, in vitro, experiments have shown the ability of SARS-CoV-2 to infect and replicate in liver tissue [28]. In addition, studies that used human liver ductal organoids have demonstrated that SARS-CoV-2 can also damage the liver tissue [29]. Furthermore, the endothelium is also a target cell for SARS-CoV-2 [20]. The virus can cause endothelial cell dysfunction, leading to increased permeability, and adherence to the blood vessel wall, thrombosis, and multiorgan injury. Our patient had no anti-spike antibodies before surgery, but tested positive 7 days after, with no other symptoms. Therefore, two options could explain a possible recipient infection: through either endothelial cells and blood preserved in the donor's liver or directly through hepatocytes and cholangiocytes. Furthermore, passive immunity could also explain the immunological results.

The risk of blood-related transmission of SARS-CoV-2 is supported by the reports of the detection of viral RNA in the blood of some infected individuals [30]. In addition, no transfusion-acquired SARS-CoV-2 has been reported, even when the transfusion was made from infected donors [31]. Moreover, studies have shown that a minimum RNA load is required to establish the correlation between the presence of viral RNA in a biological sample and infectivity, which is rarely detected in the blood [30]. Therefore, very low levels of infectious SARS-CoV-2 particles affect other organs through blood. These studies conclude that the risk of transmission of SARS-CoV-2 through blood remains theoretical [31,32].

The outcome of SARS-CoV-2-infected patients after liver transplantation could depend also on the infection time point, considering that immunosuppression intensity is also time-dependent and related to the drugs used [15,33].

Immunosuppression represents usually a risk factor for severe COVID-19 in liver-transplanted patients. The antiproliferative agents (mycophenolate mofetil) decrease the clonal expansion of alloreactive T cells resulting in high viral load and increased mortality in experimental settings [34]. These data are, however, not confirmed in clinical settings [33,35].

Conversely, some drugs used for immunosuppression could be helpful in reducing COVID-19 severity. Tacrolimus seems to improve the survival rate for liver-transplanted patients with COVID-19 [36]. Consequently, its dose is kept the same after a liver transplant regardless of COVID-19 infection in patients under 70 years old [17]. Studies have shown that tacrolimus has an inhibitory effect on the viral replication of other coronaviruses [37]. The mechanism of action of calcineurin inhibitors could be the protein–protein interactions between SARS-CoV-2 and the human host proteins [38]. This could explain the reduced number of SARS-CoV-2-positive patients among liver transplant recipients and the less severe COVID-19 disease progression in solid organ transplant recipients compared to the immunocompetent population [18]. Even if mycophenolate mofetil should be resumed in cases of severe infections, our patient received intraoperatively a combination of corticosteroids and basiliximab, and for long-term immunosuppression, mycophenolate mofetil, and tacrolimus, in the absence of any other COVID-19-related symptoms and in accordance with our national guidelines for immunosuppression after liver transplantation.

Finally, SARS-CoV-2 infection could cause liver graft dysfunction. Immune-mediated cholangitis could be a common finding in long-COVID syndrome as well as in chronic graft failure after liver transplantation [39,40]. Those cases are difficult to distinguish, while the treatment is basically different: intensive immunosuppression and corticotherapy and liver transplantation, respectively. Our patient presented, however, a good short-term outcome, with no further immune-mediated complications, even if the anti-spike antibodies turned out positive postoperatively in the absence of any positive PCR COVID-19 test from the upper airway.

4. Conclusions

We revealed a case of a SARS-CoV-2 negative liver recipient, whose donor was SARS-CoV-2 positive, and whose surgery was performed in a tertiary, university-affiliated national center of liver transplantation and surgery, with a good outcome, in order to raise the medical community awareness on the border between uncertainty and necessity of COVID-19 incompatibility transplantation procedures. Moreover, vaccination strategies and screening for SARS-CoV-2 in liver transplant candidates should be further prioritized since the isolation of infected persons is no longer practiced in many countries. Finally, proactive graft recovery from SARS-CoV-2 positive donors could represent a valid option for select cases that could be beneficial for the recipient with proven immunity against it.

Author Contributions: Conceptualization, S.I.; methodology, G.D. and C.M.; software, C.G.B.; validation, M.J.; formal analysis S.I. and M.D.P.; investigation, G.D.; resources, C.M., C.G.B. and M.D.P.; data curation, S.I.; writing—original draft preparation, G.D., C.G.B., M.J. and S.I.; writing—review and editing, S.I. and G.D.; visualization, G.D. and C.M.; supervision, S.I.; project administration, G.D. All authors have read and agreed to the published version of the manuscript.

Funding: This research received no external funding.

Institutional Review Board Statement: The study was conducted in accordance with the Declaration of Helsinki and approved by the Institutional Review Board of the Fundeni Clinical Institute (13409/13.03.2023).

Informed Consent Statement: Informed consent was obtained from the patient involved in the study. Written informed consent has been obtained from the patient to publish this paper.

Data Availability Statement: Not applicable.

Conflicts of Interest: The authors declare no conflict of interest.

References

1. Wang, X.; Lin, S.X.; Tao, J.; Wei, X.Q.; Liu, Y.T.; Chen, Y.M.; Wu, B. Study of liver cirrhosis over ten consecutive years in Southern China. *World J. Gastroenterol. WJG* **2014**, *20*, 13546. [CrossRef] [PubMed]
2. Andrei, S.; Isac, S.; Jelea, D.; Martac, C.; Stefan, M.G.; Cotorogea-Simion, M.; Buzatu, C.G.S.; Ingustu, D.; Abdulkareem, I.; Vasilescu, C.; et al. COVID-19 Pandemic Was Associated with Lower Activity but Not Higher Perioperative Mortality in a Large Eastern European Center. *Med. Sci. Monit. Int. Med. J. Exp. Clin. Res.* **2022**, *28*, e935809-1. [CrossRef] [PubMed]
3. Fekadu, G.; Bekele, F.; Tolossa, T.; Fetensa, G.; Turi, E.; Getachew, M.; Abdisa, E.; Assefa, L.; Afeta, M.; Demisew, W.; et al. Impact of COVID-19 pandemic on chronic diseases care follow-up and current perspectives in low resource settings: A narrative review. *Int. J. Physiol. Pathophysiol. Pharmacol.* **2021**, *13*, 86. [PubMed]
4. Horton, R. Offline: COVID-19 and the NHS—"A national scandal". *Lancet* **2020**, *395*, 1022. [CrossRef]
5. Ahmed, O.; Brockmeier, D.; Lee, K.; Chapman, W.C.; Doyle, M.B.M. Organ donation during the COVID-19 pandemic. *Am. J. Transplant.* **2020**, *20*, 3081. [CrossRef]
6. Søreide, K.; Hallet, J.; Matthews, J.B.; Schnitzbauer, A.A.; Line, P.D.; Lai, P.B.S.; Otero, J.; Callegaro, D.; Warner, S.G.; Baxter, N.N.; et al. Immediate and long-term impact of the COVID-19 pandemic on delivery of surgical services. *Br. J. Surg.* **2020**, *107*, 1250. [CrossRef]
7. Singh, S.; Khan, A. Clinical Characteristics and Outcomes of Coronavirus Disease 2019 among Patients with Preexisting Liver Disease in the United States: A Multicenter Research Network Study. *Gastroenterology* **2020**, *159*, 768. [CrossRef]
8. Barnes, E. Infection of liver hepatocytes with SARS-CoV-2. *Nat. Metab.* **2022**, *4*, 301–302. [CrossRef]
9. Pavel, B.; Moroti, R.; Spataru, A.; Popescu, M.R.; Panaitescu, A.M.; Zagrean, A.-M. Neurological Manifestations of SARS-CoV2 Infection: A Narrative Review. *Brain Sci.* **2022**, *12*, 1531. [CrossRef]
10. Cerrada-Romero, C.; Berastegui-Cabrera, J.; Camacho-Martínez, P.; Goikoetxea-Aguirre, J.; Pérez-Palacios, P.; Santibáñez, S.; Blanco-Vidal, M.J.; Valiente, A.; Alba, J.; Rodríguez-Álvarez, R.; et al. Excretion and viability of SARS-CoV-2 in feces and its association with the clinical outcome of COVID-19. *Sci. Rep.* **2022**, *12*, 7397. [CrossRef]
11. Xiao, F.; Tang, M.; Zheng, X.; Liu, Y.; Li, X.; Shan, H. Evidence for Gastrointestinal Infection of SARS-CoV-2. *Gastroenterology* **2020**, *158*, 1831–1833.e3. [CrossRef] [PubMed]
12. Lei, H.Y.; Ding, Y.H.; Nie, K.; Dong, Y.M.; Xu, J.H.; Yang, M.L.; Liu, M.Q.; Wei, L.; Nasser, M.I.; Xu, L.Y.; et al. Potential effects of SARS-CoV-2 on the gastrointestinal tract and liver. *Biomed. Pharmacother.* **2021**, *133*, 111064. [CrossRef] [PubMed]
13. Guarino, M.; Cossiga, V.; Loperto, I.; Esposito, I.; Ortolani, R.; Fiorentino, A.; Pontillo, G.; De Coppi, L.; Cozza, V.; Lanza, A.G.; et al. COVID-19 in liver transplant recipients: Incidence, hospitalization and outcome in an Italian prospective double-centre study. *Sci. Rep.* **2022**, *12*, 4831. [CrossRef] [PubMed]
14. Kulkarni, A.V.; Tevethia, H.V.; Premkumar, M.; Arab, J.P.; Candia, R.; Kumar, K.; Kumar, P.; Sharma, M.; Rao, P.N.; Reddy, D.N. Impact of COVID-19 on liver transplant recipients-A systematic review and meta-analysis. *EClinicalMedicine* **2021**, *38*, 101025. [CrossRef]
15. Punga, D.; Isac, S.; Paraipan, C.; Cotorogea, M.; Stefan, A.; Cobilinschi, C.; Vacaroiu, I.A.; Tulin, R.; Ionescu, D.; Droc, G. Impact of COVID-19 Infection on Liver Transplant Recipients: Does It Make Any Difference? *Cureus J. Med. Sci.* **2022**, *14*, 22687. [CrossRef] [PubMed]
16. Millson, C.; Considine, A.; Cramp, M.E.; Holt, A.; Hubscher, S.; Hutchinson, J.; Jones, K.; Leithead, J.; Masson, S.; Menon, K.; et al. Adult liver transplantation: UK clinical guideline—Part 2: Surgery and post-operation. *Frontline Gastroenterol.* **2020**, *11*, 385–396. [CrossRef]
17. Belli, L.S.; Fondevila, C.; Cortesi, P.A.; Conti, S.; Karam, V.; Adam, R.; Coilly, A.; Ericzon, B.G.; Loinaz, C.; Cuervas-Mons, V.; et al. Protective Role of Tacrolimus, Deleterious Role of Age and Comorbidities in Liver Transplant Recipients with COVID-19: Results from the ELITA/ELTR Multi-center European Study. *Gastroenterology* **2021**, *160*, 1151. [CrossRef]
18. Cheng, G.S.; Evans, S.E. The paradox of immunosuppressants and COVID-19. *Eur. Respir. J.* **2021**, *59*, 2102828. [CrossRef]
19. Peghin, M.; Grossi, P.A. COVID-19 positive donor for solid organ transplantation. *J. Hepatol.* **2022**, *77*, 1198–1204. [CrossRef]
20. Xu, S.; Ilyas, I.; Weng, J. Endothelial dysfunction in COVID-19: An overview of evidence, biomarkers, mechanisms and potential therapies. *Acta Pharmacol. Sin.* **2022**, *44*, 695–709. [CrossRef]
21. Schold, J.D.; Koval, C.E.; Wee, A.; Eltemamy, M.; Poggio, E.D. Utilization and outcomes of deceased donor SARS-CoV-2-positive organs for solid organ transplantation in the United States. *Am. J. Transplant. Off. J. Am. Soc. Transplant. Am. Soc. Transpl. Surg.* **2022**, *22*, 2217–2227. [CrossRef] [PubMed]
22. Eichenberger, E.M.; Coniglio, A.C.; Milano, C.; Schroder, J.; Bryner, B.S.; Spencer, P.J.; Haney, J.C.; Klapper, J.; Glass, C.; Pavlisko, E.; et al. Transplanting thoracic COVID-19 positive donors: An institutional protocol and report of the first 14 cases. *J. Heart Lung Transplant.* **2022**, *41*, 1376. [CrossRef] [PubMed]
23. Samuel, T.K.; Amit, I.; Alan, H.; Weingarten, N.; Helmers, R.M.; Pavan, A. Abstract 12504: Outcomes of COVID-19 Positive Donor Heart Transplantation in the United States. *Circulation* **2022**, *146*, A12504.
24. Perlin, D.V.; Dymkov, I.N.; Terentiev, A.V.; Perlina, A.V. Is Kidney Transplantation from a COVID-19-Positive Deceased Donor Safe for the Recipient? *Transplant. Proc.* **2021**, *53*, 1138–1142. [CrossRef] [PubMed]
25. Liton, E.; Morgan, M. The PiCCO monitor: A review. *Anaesth. Intensive Care* **2012**, *40*, 393–409. [CrossRef] [PubMed]

26. Kates, O.S.; Stock, P.G.; Ison, M.G.; Allen, R.D.M.; Burra, P.; Jeong, J.C.; Kute, V.; Muller, E.; Nino-Murcia, A.; Wang, H.; et al. Ethical review of COVID-19 vaccination requirements for transplant center staff and patients. *Am. J. Transplant.* **2022**, *22*, 371–380. [CrossRef]
27. Vallamkondu, J.; John, A.; Wani, W.Y.; Ramadevi, S.P.; Jella, K.K.; Reddy, P.H.; Kandimalla, R. SARS-CoV-2 pathophysiology and assessment of coronaviruses in CNS diseases with a focus on therapeutic targets. *Biochim. Biophys. Acta (BBA) Mol. Basis Dis.* **2020**, *1866*, 165889. [CrossRef]
28. Chu, H.; Chan, J.F.-W.; Yuen, T.T.-T.; Shuai, H.; Yuan, S.; Wang, Y.; Hu, B.; Yip, C.C.; Tsang, J.O.; Huang, X.; et al. Comparative tropism, replication kinetics, and cell damage profiling of SARS-CoV-2 and SARS-CoV with implications for clinical manifestations, transmissibility, and laboratory studies of COVID-19: An observational study. *Lancet Microbe* **2020**, *1*, 14–23. [CrossRef]
29. Zhao, B.; Ni, C.; Gao, R.; Wang, Y.; Yang, L.; Wei, J.; Lv, T.; Liang, J.; Zhang, Q.; Xu, W.; et al. Recapitulation of SARS-CoV-2 infection and cholangiocyte damage with human liver ductal organoids. *Protein Cell* **2020**, *11*, 771–775. [CrossRef]
30. Chang, L.; Yan, Y.; Wang, L. Coronavirus Disease 2019: Coronaviruses and Blood Safety. *Transfus. Med. Rev.* **2020**, *34*, 75. [CrossRef]
31. Chiem, C.; Alghamdi, K.; Nguyen, T.; Han, J.H.; Huo, H.; Jackson, D. The Impact of COVID-19 on Blood Transfusion Services: A Systematic Review and Meta-Analysis. *Transfus. Med. Hemother.* **2022**, *49*, 107. [CrossRef] [PubMed]
32. Matthews, P.C.; Andersson, M.I.; Arancibia-Carcamo, C.V.; Auckland, K.; Baillie, J.K.; Barnes, E.; Beneke, T.; Bibi, S.; Brooks, T.; Carroll, M. SARS-CoV-2 RNA detected in blood products from patients with COVID-19 is not associated with infectious virus. *Wellcome Open Res.* **2020**, *5*, 181.
33. Schoot, T.S.; Kerckhoffs, A.P.M.; Hilbrands, L.B.; Van Marum, R.J. Immunosuppressive Drugs and COVID-19: A Review. *Front. Pharmacol.* **2020**, *11*, 1333. [CrossRef] [PubMed]
34. Lui, S.L.; Ramassar, V.; Urmson, J.; Halloran, P.F. Mycophenolate mofetil reduces production of interferon-dependent major histocompatibility complex induction during allograft rejection, probably by limiting clonal expansion. *Transpl. Immunol.* **1998**, *6*, 23–32. [CrossRef]
35. Sajgure, A.; Kulkarni, A.; Joshi, A.; Sajgure, V.; Pathak, V.; Melinkeri, R.; Pathak, S.; Agrawal, S.; Naik, M.; Rajurkar, M.; et al. Safety and efficacy of mycophenolate in COVID-19: A nonrandomised prospective study in western India. *Lancet Reg. Health Southeast Asia* **2023**, *11*, 100154. [CrossRef]
36. Yin, S.; Wang, X.; Song, T. Tacrolimus Use and COVID-19 Infection in Patients After Solid Organ Transplantation. *Gastroenterology* **2021**, *161*, 728. [CrossRef]
37. Hage, R.; Schuurmans, M.M. Calcineurin Inhibitors and COVID-19. *Reumatol. Clin.* **2022**, *18*, 314. [CrossRef]
38. Bremer, S.; Vethe, N.T.; Bergan, S. Monitoring Calcineurin Inhibitors Response Based on NFAT-Regulated Gene Expression. Personalized Immunosuppression in Transplantation: Role of Biomarker Monitoring and Therapeutic Drug Monitoring. *Br. J. Clin. Pharmacol.* **2016**, *11*, 259–290.
39. Yanny, B.; Alkhero, M.; Alani, M.; Stenberg, D.; Saharan, A.; Saab, S. Post-COVID-19 Cholangiopathy: A Systematic Review. *J. Clin. Exp. Hepatol.* **2022**. [CrossRef]
40. Bernal, R.B.; Medina-Morales, E.; Goyes, D.; Patwardhan, V.; Bonder, A.; Lai, Q. Management of Autoimmune Liver Diseases after Liver Transplantation. *Transplantology* **2021**, *2*, 162–182. [CrossRef]

Disclaimer/Publisher's Note: The statements, opinions and data contained in all publications are solely those of the individual author(s) and contributor(s) and not of MDPI and/or the editor(s). MDPI and/or the editor(s) disclaim responsibility for any injury to people or property resulting from any ideas, methods, instructions or products referred to in the content.

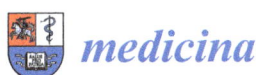

Case Report

Enterolith Treated with a Combination of Double-Balloon Endoscopy and Cola Dissolution Therapy

Kei Nomura, Tomoyoshi Shibuya *, Masashi Omori, Rina Odakura, Kentaro Ito, Takafumi Maruyama, Mayuko Haraikawa, Keiichi Haga, Osamu Nomura, Hirofumi Fukushima, Takashi Murakami, Dai Ishikawa, Mariko Hojo and Akihito Nagahara

Department of Gastroenterology, Juntendo University School of Medicine, 2-1-1 Hongo, Bunkyo-ku, Tokyo 113-0033, Japan
* Correspondence: tomoyosi@juntendo.ac.jp; Tel.: +81-3-3813-3111

Abstract: A 71-year-old woman with rheumatoid arthritis who had been taking NSAIDs for many years consulted our hospital for abdominal pain. She was diagnosed with a small bowel obstruction due to an enterolith according to an abdominal CT scan that showed dilation from the enterolith in the small intestine on the oral side. It was considered that the intestinal stone was formed due to stagnation of intestinal contents and had gradually increased in size, resulting in an intestinal obstruction. We performed antegrade double-balloon endoscopy (DBE) to observe and remove the enterolith. We used forceps and a snare to fracture the enterolith. During this attempt, we found a seed in the center of the enterolith. Since the intestinal stone was very hard, cola dissolution therapy was administered from an ileus tube for 1 week. The following week, DBE was performed again, and it was found that the stone had further softened, making attempts at fracture easier. Finally, the enterolith was almost completely fractured. Intestinal stenosis, probably due to ulcers caused by NSAIDs, was found. Small bowel obstruction with an enterolith is rare. In this case, it was considered that the seed could not pass through the stenotic region of the small intestine and the intestinal contents had gradually built up around it. It has been suggested that DBE may be a therapeutic option in cases of an enterolith. Further, cola dissolution therapy has been shown to be useful in treating an enterolith, with the possible explanation that cola undergoes an acid–base reaction with the enterolith. In summary, we report, for the first time, treatment of an enterolith with a combination of DBE and cola dissolution therapy, thereby avoiding surgery and its risks.

Keywords: enterolith; double-balloon endoscopy; cola dissolution therapy

Citation: Nomura, K.; Shibuya, T.; Omori, M.; Odakura, R.; Ito, K.; Maruyama, T.; Haraikawa, M.; Haga, K.; Nomura, O.; Fukushima, H.; et al. Enterolith Treated with a Combination of Double-Balloon Endoscopy and Cola Dissolution Therapy. *Medicina* 2023, 59, 573. https://doi.org/10.3390/medicina59030573

Academic Editors: Jan Bilski, Marcello Candelli and Ludovico Abenavoli

Received: 31 January 2023
Revised: 2 March 2023
Accepted: 13 March 2023
Published: 15 March 2023

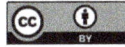

Copyright: © 2023 by the authors. Licensee MDPI, Basel, Switzerland. This article is an open access article distributed under the terms and conditions of the Creative Commons Attribution (CC BY) license (https://creativecommons.org/licenses/by/4.0/).

1. Introduction

Enteroliths are an uncommon medical condition [1], with prevalence ranging from 0.3% to 10% in selected populations. Various sized enteroliths are more common than anticipated because they typically remain underreported in the absence of clinical symptoms or due to their diminutive size that permits intermittent passage and may not always be visualized on radiologic images. The majority of enteroliths are discovered in symptomatic patients, who have abdominal pain or small bowel obstruction. Therefore, the prevalence of asymptomatic enteroliths is still largely unknown. Enteroliths are classified into primary and secondary types. Furthermore, primary enteroliths are divided into false and true enteroliths, with most classified as false. Primary false enteroliths have been shown to result from orally ingested substances, such as trichobezoar, phytobezoar, varnish stone, and fecalith. On the other hand, primary true enteroliths are originally created within the intestine by substances present, such as calcium and choleric acid. Conversely, secondary enteroliths occur from outside the intestine due to the migration of gall stones through a fistula. A detailed history and physical examination are required to diagnose enteroliths. Sudden or recurrent abdominal pain with vomiting in a patient who is in a population at risk for enteroliths should raise suspicion of the possibility of an enterolith. Important risk factors include intraluminal stricture or stenosis seen in Crohn's disease, tuberculous and radiation enteritis; surgical anastomoses; intestinal malignancy; extraluminal kinking or angulation found in the setting of intra-abdominal adhesions, external compressions, or incarcerated hernias [1–12]. Radiological imaging has been useful for early diagnosis of enteroliths. Plain abdominal roentgenograms can detect stones in up to one-third of cases [13]. Computed tomography (CT) may also be useful in identifying the number of enteroliths and their exact location.

Optimal treatment of enteroliths should focus on enterolith removal and correction of the underlying pathology to prevent future formation of additional enteroliths. Enteroliths are asymptomatic in most cases. However, when symptoms appear, such as abdominal distension and/or abdominal pain, critical clinical conditions that require surgical treatment may arise because of ileus and intestinal perforation due to intestinal obstruction. Recently, it was suggested that double-balloon endoscopy (DBE) may be a therapeutic option in selected cases as it can approach the whole small intestine [14–16]. The benefit of using DBE for the treatment of enteroliths is that the risk of treatment complications is relatively lower than with surgery. Further, cola has been used to treat enteroliths [17,18]. Cola dissolution therapy has been useful for softening enteroliths and is simpler than surgery. Although each of these treatments is useful for treatment of enteroliths, the combination of DBE and cola dissolution therapy has not been reported. We, herein, present the first report of treatment of an enterolith using a combination of DBE and cola dissolution therapy.

2. Case Report

A 71-year-old woman with rheumatoid arthritis had been taking NSAIDs for many years. Seven years ago, she consulted our hospital for anemia. Gastroscopy and colonoscopy were normal and showed no evidence of bleeding. DBE was performed to detect small intestinal bleeding, and multiple small intestinal ulcers and membranous stenosis were found. Biopsy and stool cultures were negative; infections, vasculitis, and Crohn's disease were ruled out. Moreover, since these findings had almost disappeared after not taking NSAIDs, she was diagnosed as having an NSAID ulcer in the small intestine. At the follow-up two years ago, a patency capsule was retained, and small bowel stenosis was found again by DBE. Aspirin, which had been started for coronary arteriosclerosis, was stopped, and balloon dilation was planned after the ulcer had healed. However, she did not return to our hospital for two years. Then, after two years, she consulted our hospital for abdominal pain from several days ago and was admitted. Blood testing revealed a leukocyte count of 5.3×10^9/L and C-reactive protein level of 24.2 mg/L at admission. Abdominal X-ray revealed intestinal gas. As she had a history of an NSAID ulcer and stenosis in the small intestine, CT was performed to examine the intestine. She was diagnosed as having a small bowel obstruction by an enterolith according to an abdominal CT that showed dilation from the enterolith in the small intestine on the oral side (Figure 1a). It was considered that the intestinal stone was formed due to stagnation of intestinal contents and had gradually increased in size, resulting in intestinal obstruction. Upon the diagnosis of the small bowel obstruction, an ileus tube was placed and conservative treatment was administered. We recommended that she undergo surgery to remove the enterolith, but she refused surgery. Therefore, after intestinal decompression via the ileus tube and improvement in abdominal pain, we performed antegrade DBE (EN-580T®, Fujifilm, Tokyo, Japan) to observe and remove the enterolith (Figure 1b).

We used forceps (EndoJaw®, Olympus, Tokyo, Japan) and a snare (Snaremaster®, Olympus, Tokyo, Japan) to fracture the enterolith (Figure 2a,b). While attempting to fracture the enterolith, we found a seed at its center (Figure 2c). Since the intestinal stone was very hard, 500 mL/day of cola (Coca-Cola®) was injected from an ileus tube for 1 week to dissolve the stone. The following week, DBE was performed again, and the stone had further softened and was more easily fractured. Finally, the enterolith was almost completely fractured. Intestinal stenosis, probably due to ulcers caused by NSAIDs, was found (Figure 2d and Supplementary Material Video S1). After 1 week, we confirmed that there were no stones, and balloon dilation was performed. The patient began to eat and continued to be well upon discharge. Our follow-up of the patient has remained uneventful for three years.

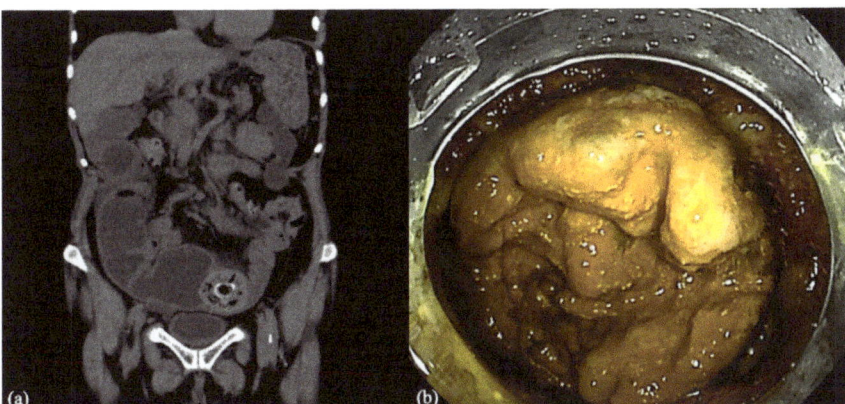

Figure 1. (a) Dilation of the small intestine and findings of an enterolith on CT. (b) Endoscopic view of the enterolith in the small intestine.

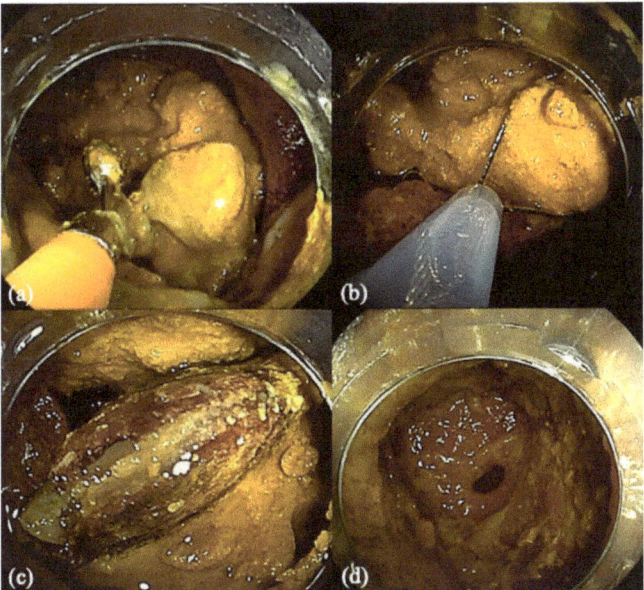

Figure 2. (a) We used forceps and (b) a snare in attempting to fracture the enterolith. (c) Seed in the center of the enterolith. (d) Small intestinal stenosis found after fracturing the enterolith.

3. Discussion

Small bowel obstruction by an enterolith is rare [1,19]. It is assumed that the formation of primary enteroliths is related to intestinal stenosis due to Crohn's disease and/or intestinal tuberculosis. In addition, primary enteroliths may occur in the area of stasis due to the existence of intestinal diverticulum, afferent loops after surgery, incarcerated hernias, small intestinal tumors, and intestinal kinking from intra-abdominal adhesions [1–12]. In the present case, it was considered that the seed could not pass through the stenotic region of the small intestine due to the NSAID ulcer and the intestinal contents gradually built up around it. In most cases, surgical management is the main treatment for enteroliths because they are not discovered until the occurrence of clinical conditions, such as ileus or intestinal perforation. A comparatively large number of cases are diagnosed by laparotomy or autopsy [1]. Although it is difficult to diagnose asymptomatic enteroliths, once enteroliths are diagnosed, enteroscopy may become an effective but invasive treatment option. Several reports have suggested that DBE may be a therapeutic option in cases of an enterolith [15,16]. Moreover, DBE is useful in searching for an underlying pathology for enteroliths. In cases of intestinal stricture, stenosis, or an anastomotic defect, an attempt at endoscopic segment dilatation and stone retrieval, may be considered first [2,20]. Endoscopic snaring, electrohydraulic lithotripsy, and mechanical lithotripsy have been previously described [21–24]. It is generally believed that stones with a diameter > 25 mm may cause intestinal obstruction in the absence of luminal stricture or stenosis [25]. On the other hand, stones < 20 mm in diameter can pass through without symptoms. Thus, even if an enterolith cannot be removed completely, just fragmentizing it using a device through an enteroscope may be an effective treatment. However, it is possible that remnants may become a nidus for future stones. Importantly, enterolith formation may be the first clue to the existence of a compromised intestinal anatomy and every effort should be made to decrease future stone formation by recognizing and treating underlying medical conditions. Medical, endoscopic, or surgical correction of inflammatory, infectious, or structural pathology may provide chronic symptom relief and benefit the long-term outcome in many cases [26]. In the present case, balloon dilation was performed after fracturing the enterolith. Our follow-up of the patient has remained uneventful for a long time. The benefit of using DBE for the treatment of enteroliths is that the risk of treatment complications is relatively lower than surgery.

Further, cola dissolution therapy was reported as useful for an enterolith [17,18]. A possible explanation among its properties for dissolution is that cola undergoes an acid–base reaction with an enterolith. Ladas et al. reported that fine bubbles of carbon dioxide permeate the fine irregularities on the gastrolith surface and soften the fibrous bonds [27]. Cola dissolution therapy is a simpler treatment than surgery and is considered to be feasible in many facilities. However, the risks associated with injecting cola include mucosal damage due to carbonic acid and increased intestinal pressure due to carbon dioxide production. In particular, increased intestinal pressure during the acute phase of colitis may cause colonic perforation and bacterial translocation, leading to aggravation of sepsis. If intestinal necrosis occurs, prompt surgery is the principal treatment, and indications for surgery should be carefully considered.

In this case, it was difficult to fracture the enterolith using DBE because the intestinal stone was very hard. Generally, surgery is often selected for enteroliths in the small intestine if endoscopic treatment is not able to remove an enterolith. However, we ultimately administered cola to our patient via an ileus tube because she refused invasive treatment such as surgery. Cola dissolution therapy further softened the stone, making it easier to fracture, which may have served as an adjunct to endoscopic treatment and avoided surgery and its attendant risks. It is considered worth trying cola dissolution therapy before endoscopic treatment if enteroliths are hard and large.

4. Conclusions

In summary, we report, for the first time, treatment of an enterolith using a combination of DBE and cola dissolution therapy, thereby avoiding surgery and its attendant risks. This combination therapy may be a non-invasive treatment option for enteroliths.

Supplementary Materials: The following supporting information can be downloaded at: https://www.mdpi.com/article/10.3390/medicina59030573/s1, Video S1: Enterolith fractured by forceps and a snare using a double-balloon endoscopy.

Author Contributions: Conceptualization, K.N. and T.S.; methodology, T.S.; validation, T.S., M.O., R.O., K.I., T.M. (Takafumi Maruyama), M.H. (Mayuko Haraikawa), K.H., O.N., H.F., T.M. (Takashi Murakami), D.I. and M.H. (Mariko Hojo); investigation, K.N.; data curation, K.N.; writing—original draft preparation, K.N.; writing—review and editing, T.S.; supervision, A.N. All authors have read and agreed to the published version of the manuscript.

Funding: This research received no external funding.

Institutional Review Board Statement: Not applicable.

Informed Consent Statement: The patient signed informed consent for video endoscopy and the possible publication of images guaranteeing anonymity.

Data Availability Statement: The data presented in this study are available on request from the corresponding author. The data are not publicly available due to patient's privacy.

Conflicts of Interest: The authors declare no conflict of interest.

References

1. Gurvits, G.E.; Lan, G. Enterolithiasis. *World J. Gastroenterol.* **2014**, *20*, 17819–17829. [CrossRef] [PubMed]
2. Muthukumarasamy, G.; Nairn, E.R.; McMillan, I. Enterolith and small bowel perforation in Crohn's disease. *Inflamm. Bowel Dis.* **2011**, *17*, E126–E127. [CrossRef] [PubMed]
3. Tewari, A.; Weiden, J.; Johnson, J.O. Small-bowel obstruction associated with Crohn's enterolith. *Emerg. Radiol.* **2013**, *20*, 341–344. [CrossRef]
4. Hirakawa, Y.; Shigyo, H.; Katagiri, Y.; Hashimoto, K.; Katsumoto, M.; Tomoeda, H.; Nakano, M. Nontraumatic perforation of the small intestine caused by true primary enteroliths associated with radiation enteritis: A case report. *Surg. Case Rep.* **2021**, *7*, 102. [CrossRef]
5. Tan, W.S.; Chung, A.Y.; Low, A.S.; Cheah, F.K.; Ong, S.C. Enterolith formation in the roux limb hepaticojejunostomy. *Dig. Dis. Sci.* **2007**, *52*, 3214–3216. [CrossRef]
6. Gupta, N.M.; Pinjla, R.K.; Talwar, B.L. Calcific enterolithiasis. *Indian J. Gastroenterol.* **1986**, *5*, 29–30. [PubMed]
7. Wilson, I.; Parampalli, U.; Butler, C.; Ahmed, I.; Mowat, A. Multiple large enteroliths associated with an incisional hearnia: A rare case. *Ann. R. Coll. Surg. Engl.* **2012**, *94*, e227–e229. [CrossRef]
8. Gin, F.M.; Maglinte, D.D.; Chua, G.T. General case of the day. Enterolith in a blind pouch (blind pouch syndrome secondary to side-to-side enteroanastomosis). *Radiographics* **1993**, *13*, 965–967. [CrossRef]
9. Kia, D.; Dragstedt, L.R. Enterolithiasis associated with side-to-side intestinal anastomosis. *Arch. Surg.* **1967**, *95*, 898–901. [CrossRef]
10. Paige, M.L.; Ghahremani, G.G.; Brosnan, J.J. Laminated radiopaque enteroliths: Diagnostic clues to intestinal pathology. *Am. J. Gastroenterol.* **1987**, *82*, 432–437. [PubMed]
11. Khan, A.; Schreiber, S.; Hopkins, W.; Berkelhammer, C. Enterolith-induced perforation in small bowel carcinoid tumor. *Am. J. Gastroenterol.* **2001**, *96*, 261. [CrossRef]
12. Lorimer, J.W.; Allen, M.W.; Tao, H.; Burns, B. Small-bowel carcinoid presenting in association with a phytobezoar. *Can. J. Surg.* **1991**, *34*, 331–333. [PubMed]
13. Athey, G.N. Unusual demonstration of a Meckel's diverticulum containing enteroliths. *Br. J. Radiol.* **1980**, *53*, 365–368. [CrossRef] [PubMed]
14. Kim, H.J.; Moon, J.H.; Choi, H.J.; Koo, H.C.; Park, S.J.; Cheon, Y.K.; Cho, Y.D.; Lee, M.S.; Shin, C.S. Endoscopic removal of an enterolith causing afferent loop syndrome using electrolithotripsy. *Dig. Endosc.* **2010**, *22*, 220–222. [CrossRef]
15. Ishioka, M.; Jin, M.; Matsuhashi, T.; Arata, S.; Suzuki, Y.; Watanabe, N.; Sawaguchi, M.; Kanazawa, N.; Onochi, K.; Hatakeyama, N.; et al. True primary enterolith treated by balloon-assisted enteroscopy. *Intern. Med.* **2015**, *54*, 2439–2442. [CrossRef]
16. Kikuchi, T.; Yamasaki, Y.; Fujimoto, T.; Tanaka, S. Strategy for removing an impacted enterolith using double-balloon enteroscopy in crohn's disease. *Eur. J. Case Rep. Intern. Med.* **2021**, *8*, 002266. [PubMed]
17. Komaki, Y.; Kanmura, S.; Tanaka, A.; Nakashima, M.; Komaki, F.; Iwaya, H.; Arima, S.; Sasaki, F.; Nasu, Y.; Tanoue, S.; et al. Cola dissolution therapy via ileus tube was effective for ileus secondary to small bowel obstruction induced by an enterolith. *Intern. Med.* **2019**, *58*, 2473–2478. [CrossRef] [PubMed]
18. Oshiro, K.; Okai, K.; Yoshii, H.; Ohara, K.; Yamada, A.; Tadauchi, A. A case of obstructive colitis treated with Cola dissolution therapy administered via a transanal ileus tube. *JJAAM* **2021**, *32*, 517–522.
19. Muacevic, A.; Adler, R.J. Jejunal enterolith: A rare case of small bowel obstruction. *Cureus* **2020**, *12*, e8427.
20. Van Gossum, A.; Gay, F.; Cremer, M. Enteroliths and Crohn's disease stricture treated by transendoscopic balloon dilation. *Gastrointest. Endosc.* **1995**, *42*, 597. [CrossRef]
21. Agaoglu, N. Meckel's diverticulum enterolith: A rare cause of acute abdomen. *Acta Chir. Belg.* **2009**, *109*, 513–515. [CrossRef] [PubMed]

22. Moriai, T.; Hasegawa, T.; Fuzita, M.; Kimura, A.; Tani, T.; Makino, I. Successful removal of massive intragastric gallstones by endoscopic electrohydraulic lithotripsy and mechanical lithotripsy. *Am. J. Gastroenterol.* **1991**, *86*, 627–629. [PubMed]
23. Alves, A.R.; Almeida, N.; Ferreira, A.M.; Tome, L. Endoscopic management of afferent loop syndrome caused by enteroliths and anastomotic stricture. A case report. *Rev. Esp. Enferm. Dig.* **2017**, *109*, 457–458. [PubMed]
24. Tang, L.; Huang, L.Y.; Cui, J.; Wu, C.R. Effect of double-balloon enteroscopy on diagnosis and treatment of small-bowel disease. *Chin. Med. J.* **2018**, *131*, 1321–1326. [CrossRef] [PubMed]
25. Nakao, A.; Okamoto, Y.; Sunami, M.; Fujita, T.; Tsuhi, T. The oldest patient with gall stone ileus: Report of a case and review of 176 cases in Japan. *Kurume Med. J.* **2008**, *55*, 29–33. [CrossRef]
26. Yu, Z.; Shibata, R.; Nishida, Y.; Nomura, Y.; Tada, H.; Maeda, T. A case report of incarcerated enteroliths treated successfully by double balloon dilation using a two-channel endoscope. *Gastroenterol. Endosc.* **2020**, *62*, 59–64.
27. Ladas, S.D.; Triantafyllou, K.; Tzathas, C.; Tassios, P.; Rokkas, T.; Raptis, S.A. Gastric phytobezoars may be treated by nasogastric Coca-Cola lavage. *Eur. J. Gastroenterol. Hepatol.* **2002**, *14*, 801–803. [CrossRef]

Disclaimer/Publisher's Note: The statements, opinions and data contained in all publications are solely those of the individual author(s) and contributor(s) and not of MDPI and/or the editor(s). MDPI and/or the editor(s) disclaim responsibility for any injury to people or property resulting from any ideas, methods, instructions or products referred to in the content.

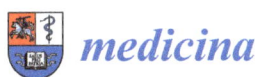

Case Report

Persistence of Abdominal Pain: Did You Check for Mesenteric Vessels?

Jessica Piroddu [1], Maria Pina Dore [1,2,*], Giovanni Mario Pes [1], Pier Paolo Meloni [3] and Giuseppe Manzoni [1]

1. Dipartimento di Medicina, Chirurgia e Farmacia, University of Sassari, Viale San Pietro, No. 43, 07100 Sassari, Italy
2. Baylor College of Medicine, One Baylor Plaza, Houston, TX 77023, USA
3. General Practitioner, Azienda Sanitaria Locale No. 1, 07100 Sassari, Italy
* Correspondence: mpdore@uniss.it; Tel.: +39-079-229886

Abstract: The incidence of abnormalities regarding the celiac-mesenteric trunk (CMT) has been reported to be between 1% and 2.7%, whereas for visceral aneurysms the incidence is between 0.1% and 0.2% of the general population. Anatomical variations in the CMT may be the result of abnormal embryogenesis of the primitive segmental splanchnic arteries that supply the bowel and several abdominal organs. The clinical presentation may range from vague abdominal symptoms to aneurysm rupture with a significant mortality risk. In this case, we describe the clinical history of a 37-year-old man with postprandial abdominal pain likely related to the celiac-mesenteric trunk enlargement, associated with high resistance flow in the proximal site. Postprandial symptoms improved by avoiding large meals and surveillance for the CMT anomalies was recommended by cross-imaging including the echo-color-Doppler to assess blood flow modification.

Keywords: vessel abnormalities; celiac-mesenteric trunk; aneurysms

Citation: Piroddu, J.; Dore, M.P.; Pes, G.M.; Meloni, P.P.; Manzoni, G. Persistence of Abdominal Pain: Did You Check for Mesenteric Vessels? . *Medicina* 2023, 59, 442. https://doi.org/10.3390/medicina59030442

Academic Editor: Ludovico Abenavoli

Received: 18 January 2023
Revised: 21 February 2023
Accepted: 21 February 2023
Published: 23 February 2023

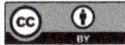

Copyright: © 2023 by the authors. Licensee MDPI, Basel, Switzerland. This article is an open access article distributed under the terms and conditions of the Creative Commons Attribution (CC BY) license (https://creativecommons.org/licenses/by/4.0/).

1. Introduction

Albrecht Von Haller, a Swiss anatomist and physiologist, was the first to describe the anatomy of the celiac-mesenteric trunk (CMT) [1]. The celiac tripod, also known as the celiac trunk or celiac artery, is the first branch of the abdominal aorta arising anteriorly at the level of the vertebral bodies T12–L1. Approximately 1.5–2 cm from the aortic origin the celiac trunk continues by dividing into three major branches: (i) the common hepatic artery; (ii) the gastric artery; and (iii) the splenic artery, being the primary arterial supply of the liver, stomach, abdominal esophagus, spleen, the upper portion of the duodenum and pancreas [1].

The arrangement of the anatomical structures, and the relationship between organs, the blood, and the lymphatic vessel network are the result of the growth process, rotation, and migration during embryogenesis and fetal development [2].

Progenitor cell movement and aggregation during organogenesis are responsible for the final organs' morphology and can be the cause of variations in arterial and venous vessels. More specifically, during embryogenesis, the main visceral arteries develop from four vascular roots derived from the primitive dorsal abdominal aorta. These four roots are joined by ventral longitudinal anastomosis. In the course of normal maturation, the gastric, hepatic, and splenic roots join to form the main celiac axis, while the fourth root develops separately into the superior mesenteric artery. An interruption of the ventral anastomosis process may lead to a wide variety of vascular anomalies [3]. Several anatomical and radiological descriptions of CMT abnormalities have been reported in the literature, including common trunks and anastomoses between the celiac trunk and the superior mesenteric artery, the inter-mesenteric arch between the superior and the inferior mesenteric arteries, or a common arterial trunk between the celiac trunk and the superior and inferior mesenteric arteries [4–6]. In some individuals, the celiac trunk is completely absent [4].

Therefore, anatomical variants of the celiac trunk branches may be the result of anomalous embryogenesis of the primitive segmental splanchnic arteries [7].

CMT anatomic variations are rare; they have been reported to range between 1% and 2.7% of cases [8], whereas the incidence of visceral aneurysms ranges between 0.1% and 0.2% in the general population [9]. CMT aneurysm is even rarer and occurs in only 0.25% of all visceral artery anomalies. For example, in the last 52 years, only 26 cases have been reported in the literature [10–24]. Depending on the location and size of the aneurysm, the mortality rate is 10–90% after rupture. The majority of visceral aneurysms occur in the splenic artery, accounting for nearly 60% of the total, while the superior mesenteric and celiac artery aneurysms account for 5% and 4%, respectively [25].

In the absence of aneurysm rupture, symptoms may be insidious and progressive with malaise, postprandial epigastric/abdominal pain or discomfort, sometimes associated with back pain, early satiety, nausea, and/or vomiting often attributed to another etiology or functional disorder, leading to delay in diagnosis [3,5,26,27].

A physical examination is usually not helpful for diagnosis. In cases where the aneurysm has expanded to a large size, it may present as a palpable mass in thin individuals [28], albeit this is uncommon. Laboratory studies are generally non-specific. Differential diagnosis may be difficult, requiring an extensive workup. The single most important step in diagnosing CMT anomalies is to suspect the disorder from the patient's initial presentation.

Ultrasonography and cross-sectional abdominal vascular imaging, including computed tomography (CT) and magnetic resonance (MR), provide an accurate diagnosis of CMT anomalies. Echo-color-Doppler is particularly helpful for measuring blood flow inside the abnormal trunk. Moreover, imaging can simultaneously exclude additional conditions.

The suggested approach to a visceral aneurysm is early intervention. However, observation with surveillance could be an option for some small aneurysms and accordingly for trunk enlargement [29].

2. Case Presentation

A 37-year-old white Caucasian man came to our attention during a gastroenterological visit. Anthropometric features were: height 185 cm, weight 100 kg (body mass index 29.2 kg/m^2). He was a former cigarette smoker and did not practice physical exercise. At the visit time, he was unemployed and consumed a balanced diet. The patient complained of gastroesophageal reflux disease (GERD) symptoms, motility-like dyspepsia, and abdominal pain localized in the epigastric region and right hypochondrium occurring nearly 30 min after meals, lasting approximately 30–60 min and exacerbated by sitting, usually improving within two hours. Additionally, the patient complained of constipation and a weight loss of 5 kg in the last two years. He had no significant comorbidities, except for appendectomy and two inguinal hernia repairs on both sides in his youth. The family history was negative for major disorders.

Physical examination did not show specific signs, although a deep palpation of the periumbilical area was able to evoke mild pain. There was no chronic therapy ongoing.

For the above-mentioned abdominal pain, the patient had undergone extensive workup over the past 2 years, including invasive and non-invasive tests suggested by different specialists, mostly surgeons. All records were carefully checked during the gastroenterological visit.

Routine and specific blood and stool tests (according to the diseases' epidemiology in our region, Sardinia, Italy) for hepatic, pancreatic, intestinal, infectious, celiac, autoimmune, and hematological diseases showed normal results. The upper endoscopy and colonoscopy were negative for significant findings. Interestingly, in the ultrasound scan of the abdomen cavity, we noticed agenesis of the left hepatic lobe, splenomegaly, and enlargement (1.89 cm at the ostium and 1.53 cm downstream) of the CMT (normally ranging between 0.7 to 1 cm) (Figure 1).

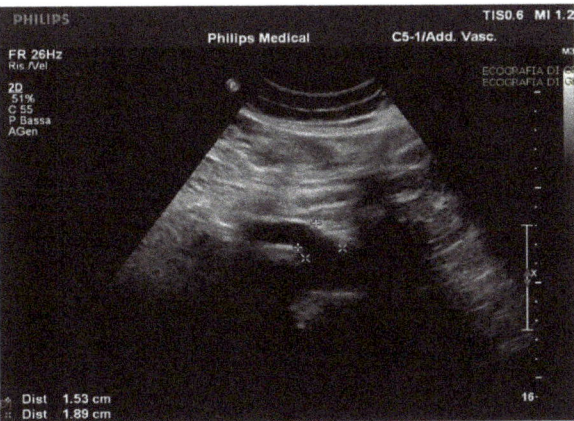

Figure 1. The celiac-mesenteric trunk observed by an ultrasound scan of the abdomen, indicating the size of the proximal and distal site.

Abnormalities were also present in the CT scan with and without contrast medium (Figures 2 and 3).

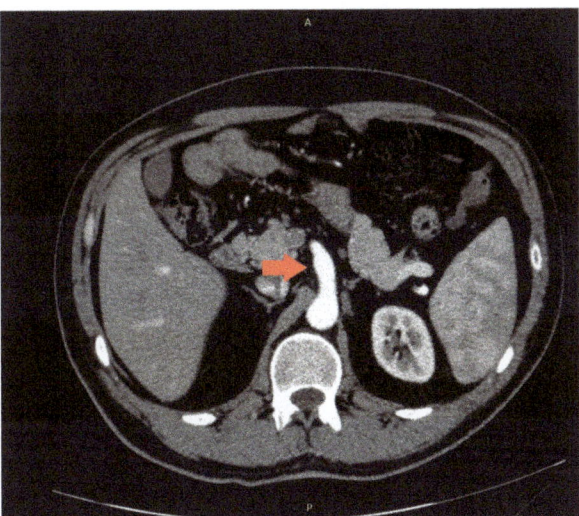

Figure 2. The computer tomography scan confirmed the agenesis of the left hepatic lobe, splenomegaly, and an enlarged celiac-mesenteric trunk (red arrow).

The echo-color-Doppler revealed a high resistance flow in the proximal site of the CMT (Figure 4).

By comparing previous and current imaging tests, an increase of 5 mm in CMT diameter in 5 years was observed.

The consulted team of vascular surgeons recommended surveillance over intervention for the CMT anomalies by cross-imaging, according to the guidelines of the European Society of Vascular Surgery [30].

High doses of second-generation proton pump inhibitors twice daily, in addition to prokinetics, were prescribed, and lifestyle with dietary modification was proposed. In the follow-up visit (three weeks later), the patient reported an improvement in GERD and motility-like dyspepsia symptoms, despite the persistence of the post-prandial pain exacerbated by large meals. Because of this, the patient was asked to avoid large meals with high fat content. More specifically, the patient was advised to reduce the main meal portion sizes (lunch and dinner) and, in case of hunger, to add snacks between meals. At the third follow-up visit (2 months later), the patient reported an improvement in abdominal symptoms and quality of life through the adoption of a different eating pattern. Moreover, he maintained a steady weight.

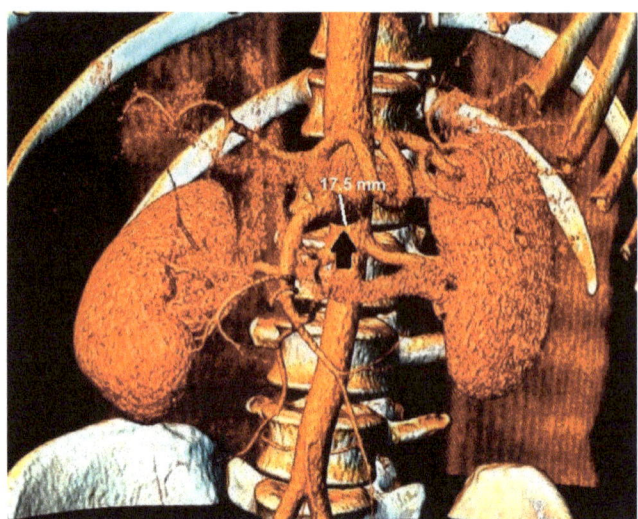

Figure 3. In the 3D reconstruction of CT scan images, the enlarged celiac-mesenteric trunk can be observed indicated by a black arrow.

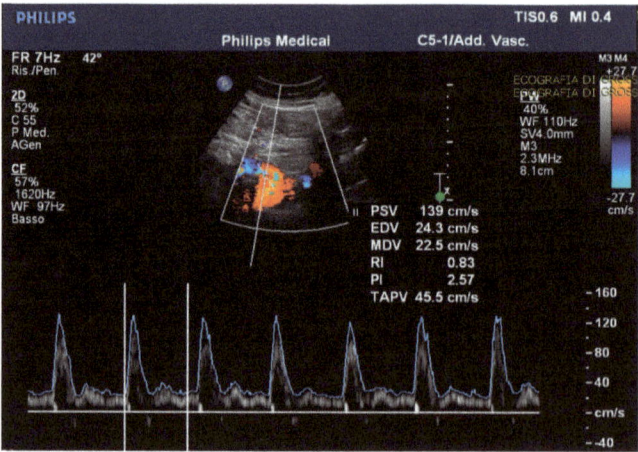

Figure 4. The echo-color-Doppler detected a high resistance flow in the proximal site of the celiac-mesenteric trunk, usually ranging from systolic velocity peaks between 90–100 cm/s (PSV); 30–65 cm/s end diastolic velocity peaks (EDV); and a pulsatility index (PI) of 1.5 ± 0.02.

3. Discussion

Causes of chronic abdominal pain and weight loss in adults are several and frequently prompt an extensive workup. More specifically, our patient complained of upper abdominal pain located in the right upper quadrant and epigastric region, characteristic locations for biliary and/or liver etiologies. However, laboratory studies were normal over time, excluding hepatobiliary disorders. Due to their rarity, visceral artery anomalies and associated modifications in blood flow are often unsuspected in patients reporting abdominal complaints. The majority of visceral abnormalities and/or aneurysms are asymptomatic and detected during autopsy. In our case, the CMT anomaly was labeled by the radiologist as an enlargement. Although there are no specific symptoms reported in the literature for CMT anomalies, in the case of a hepatic aneurysm, symptoms are represented by nausea and pain in the right hypochondrium or mesoepigastrium radiating to the back. Patients with splenic artery aneurysms complain of nausea and vague abdominal discomfort in the mesoepigastric quadrant or left hypochondrium, associated sometimes with left shoulder discomfort due to diaphragm irritation. Almost half of patients with splenic artery aneurysms present with moderate splenomegaly [26]. Most celiac artery aneurysms are asymptomatic and rarely associated with mesoepigastrium pain radiating to the back, mimicking the symptoms of pancreatitis [27]. Symptoms related to an aneurysm of the superior mesenteric artery are generally nonspecific, but if there is an aneurysm-related thrombus, ischemic symptoms may occur, resulting in pain after meals [5]. Similarly, to angina abdominis, our patient also complained of abdominal pain after meals that almost completely resolved after changing eating pattern, although a different cause of the pain could not be ruled out.

4. Conclusions

This case of unexplained abdominal pain includes a difficult-to-diagnose condition that is not frequently encountered by most clinicians but is nonetheless important to accurately recognize. The clinical presentation of CTM anomalies may range from vague abdominal symptoms to aneurysm rupture with a significant mortality risk especially when complicated by a high blood flow resistance. Postprandial symptoms improved by avoiding large meals and surveillance was recommended by cross-imaging, including echo-color-Doppler, to assess the magnitude of blood flow modification.

Author Contributions: J.P., M.P.D., P.P.M. and G.M. collected all patient data. J.P., M.P.D. and G.M.P. drafted and edited the manuscript. J.P., M.P.D. and P.P.M. participated in the care of the patient. All authors have read and agreed to the published version of the manuscript.

Funding: This research received no external funding.

Institutional Review Board Statement: Not applicable.

Informed Consent Statement: Informed consent of the patient was obtained.

Data Availability Statement: Data and material are available on reasonable request.

Conflicts of Interest: The authors declare no conflict of interest.

References

1. Haller, V.A. *Icones Anatomicae quibus Praecipuae Aliquae Partes Corporis Humani Delineatae Proponuntur et Arteriarum Potissimum Historia Continetur*; Vandenhoeck, Abraham: Gottingen, Germany, 1756.
2. Sadler, T.W. *Langman's Medical Embryology*, 11th ed.; Lippincott Williams & Wilkins: New Dehli, India, 2009.
3. Abbas, M.A.; Fowl, R.J.; Stone, W.M.; Panneton, J.M.; Oldenburg, W.A.; Bower, T.C.; Cherry, K.J.; Gloviczki, P. Hepatic artery aneurysm: Factors that predict complications. *J. Vasc. Surg.* **2003**, *38*, 41–45. [CrossRef]
4. Sumalatha, S.; Hosapatna, M.; Bhat, K.R.; D'Souza, A.S.; Kiruba, L.; Kotian, S.R. Multiple variations in the branches of the coeliac trunk. *Anat. Cell Biol.* **2015**, *48*, 147–150. [CrossRef]
5. Pilleul, F.; Beuf, O. Diagnosis of splanchnic artery aneurysms and pseudoaneurysms, with special reference to contrast enhanced 3D magnetic resonance angiography: A review. *Acta Radiol.* **2004**, *45*, 702–708. [CrossRef]
6. Saeed, M.; Murshid, K.R.; Rufai, A.A.; Elsayed, S.E.; Sadiq, M.S. Coexistence of multiple anomalies in the celiac-mesenteric arterial system. *Clin. Anat.* **2003**, *16*, 30–36. [CrossRef]
7. Karamanidi, M.; Chrysikos, D.; Samolis, A.; Protogerou, V.; Fourla, N.; Michalis, I.; Papaioannou, G.; Troupis, T. Agenesis of the coeliac trunk: A case report and review of the literature. *Folia Morphol.* **2021**, *80*, 718–721. [CrossRef]
8. Cavdar, S.; Sehirli, U.; Pekin, B. Celiacomesenteric trunk. *Clin. Anat.* **1997**, *10*, 231–234. [CrossRef]

9. VonDerHaar, R.J.; Shah, A.; Nissen, N.N.; Gewertz, B.L. Primary intra-aneurysmal surgical repair of a celiomesenteric trunk aneurysm. *J. Vasc. Surg. Cases* **2015**, *1*, 50–52. [CrossRef]
10. Alam, W.; Kamareddine, M.H.; Geahchan, A.; Ghosn, Y.; Feghaly, M.; Chamseddine, A.; Bou Khalil, R.; Farhat, S. Celiacomesenteric trunk associated with superior mesenteric artery aneurysm: A case report and review of literature. *SAGE Open Med. Case Rep.* **2020**, *8*, 1–5. [CrossRef]
11. Bailey, R.W.; Riles, T.S.; Rosen, R.J.; Sullivan, L.P. Celiomesenteric anomaly and aneurysm: Clinical and etiologic features. *J. Vasc. Surg.* **1991**, *14*, 229–234. [CrossRef]
12. Detroux, M.; Anidjar, S.; Nottin, R. Aneurysm of a common celiomesenteric trunk. *Ann. Vasc. Surg.* **1998**, *12*, 78–82. [CrossRef]
13. Guntani, A.; Yamaoka, T.; Kyuragi, R.; Honma, K.; Iwasa, K.; Matsumoto, T.; Nishizaki, T.; Maehara, Y. Successful treatment of a visceral artery aneurysm with a celiacomesenteric trunk: Report of a case. *Surg. Today* **2011**, *41*, 115–119. [CrossRef]
14. Higashiyama, H.; Yamagami, K.; Fujimoto, K.; Koshiba, T.; Kumada, K.; Yamamoto, M. Open surgical repair using a reimplantation technique for a large celiac artery aneurysm anomalously arising from the celiomesenteric trunk. *J. Vasc. Surg.* **2011**, *54*, 1805–1807. [CrossRef]
15. Iida, Y.; Obitsu, Y.; Sugimoto, T.; Yamamoto, K.; Yoshii, S.; Shigematsu, H. A case of abdominal aortic aneurysm associated with L-shaped crossed-fused renal ectopia. *Ann. Vasc. Surg.* **2010**, *24*, 1137.e1–1137.e5. [CrossRef] [PubMed]
16. Kalra, M.; Panneton, J.M.; Hofer, J.M.; Andrews, J.C. Aneurysm and stenosis of the celiomesenteric trunk: A rare anomaly. *J. Vasc. Surg.* **2003**, *37*, 679–682. [CrossRef] [PubMed]
17. Lipari, G.; Cappellari, T.F.; Giovannini, F.; Pancheri, O.; Piovesan, R.; Baggio, E. Treatment of an aneurysm of the celiac artery arising from a celiomesenteric trunk. Report of a case. *Int. J. Surg. Case Rep.* **2015**, *8*, 45–48. [CrossRef] [PubMed]
18. Mammano, E.; Cosci, M.; Zanon, A.; Picchi, G.; Tessari, E.; Pilati, P.; Nitti, D. Celiomesenteric trunk aneurysm. *Ann. Vasc. Surg.* **2009**, *23*, 257.e7–257.e10. [CrossRef]
19. Matsuda, H.; Ogino, H.; Ito, A.; Sasaki, H.; Minatoya, K.; Higashi, M.; Yagihara, T.; Kitamura, S. Aneurysm of the celiac artery arising from a celiomesenteric trunk. *J. Vasc. Surg.* **2006**, *44*, 660. [CrossRef]
20. Matsumoto, K.; Tanaka, K.; Ohsumi, K.; Nakamaru, M.; Obara, H.; Hayashi, S.; Kitajima, M. Celiomesenteric anomaly with concurrent aneurysm. *J. Vasc. Surg.* **1999**, *29*, 711–714. [CrossRef] [PubMed]
21. Obara, H.; Matsumoto, K.; Fujimura, N.; Ono, S.; Hattori, T.; Kitagawa, Y. Reconstructive surgery for a fusiform common celiomesenteric trunk aneurysm and coexistent abdominal aortic aneurysm: Report of a case. *Surg. Today* **2009**, *39*, 55–58. [CrossRef]
22. Stanley, J.C.; Thompson, N.W.; Fry, W.J. Splanchnic artery aneurysms. *Arch. Surg.* **1970**, *101*, 689–697. [CrossRef]
23. Wang, C.; Cai, X.; Liang, F.; Chu, F.; Chen, G.; Duan, Z. Surgical treatment of celiomesenteric trunk aneurysm-7 case report. *Biomed. Mater. Eng.* **2014**, *24*, 3487–3492. [CrossRef]
24. Wang, Y.; Chen, P.; Shen, N.; Yang, J.T.; Chen, J.H.; Zhang, W.G. Celiomesenteric trunk with concurrent aneurysm: Report of a case. *Surg. Today* **2010**, *40*, 477–481. [CrossRef]
25. Maatman, T.K.; Heimberger, M.A.; Lewellen, K.A.; Roch, A.M.; Colgate, C.L.; House, M.G.; Nakeeb, A.; Ceppa, E.P.; Schmidt, C.M.; Zyromski, N.J. Visceral artery pseudoaneurysm in necrotizing pancreatitis: Incidence and outcomes. *Can. J. Surg.* **2020**, *63*, E272–E277. [CrossRef] [PubMed]
26. Lakin, R.O.; Kashyap, V.S. *Splanchnic Artey Aneurysms*; Cronenwett, J.L., Johnston, K.W., Eds.; Elsevier Saunders: Philadelphia, PA, USA, 2014.
27. Nishida, O.; Moriyasu, F.; Nakamura, T.; Ban, N.; Miura, K.; Sakai, M.; Uchino, H.; Miyake, T. Hemodynamics of splenic artery aneurysm. *Gastroenterology* **1986**, *90*, 1042–1046. [CrossRef] [PubMed]
28. Tijani, Y.; Belmir, H.; Zahdi, O.; Khalki, L.; El Khloufi, S.; Sefiani, Y.; Elmesnaoui, A.; Lekehal, B. Giant anevrisms of the splenic artery about six cases. *J. Med. Vasc.* **2020**, *45*, 248–253. [CrossRef] [PubMed]
29. Chaer, R.A.; Abularrage, C.J.; Coleman, D.M.; Eslami, M.H.; Kashyap, V.S.; Rockman, C.; Murad, M.H. The Society for Vascular Surgery clinical practice guidelines on the management of visceral aneurysms. *J. Vasc. Surg.* **2020**, *72*, 3S–39S. [CrossRef] [PubMed]
30. Bjorck, M.; Koelemay, M.; Acosta, S.; Bastos Goncalves, F.; Kolbel, T.; Kolkman, J.J.; Lees, T.; Lefevre, J.H.; Menyhei, G.; Oderich, G.; et al. Editor's Choice—Management of the Diseases of Mesenteric Arteries and Veins: Clinical Practice Guidelines of the European Society of Vascular Surgery (ESVS). *Eur. J. Vasc. Endovasc. Surg.* **2017**, *53*, 460–510. [CrossRef]

Disclaimer/Publisher's Note: The statements, opinions and data contained in all publications are solely those of the individual author(s) and contributor(s) and not of MDPI and/or the editor(s). MDPI and/or the editor(s) disclaim responsibility for any injury to people or property resulting from any ideas, methods, instructions or products referred to in the content.

MDPI
St. Alban-Anlage 66
4052 Basel
Switzerland
www.mdpi.com

Medicina Editorial Office
E-mail: medicina@mdpi.com
www.mdpi.com/journal/medicina

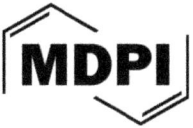

Disclaimer/Publisher's Note: The statements, opinions and data contained in all publications are solely those of the individual author(s) and contributor(s) and not of MDPI and/or the editor(s). MDPI and/or the editor(s) disclaim responsibility for any injury to people or property resulting from any ideas, methods, instructions or products referred to in the content.